MW01625765

Interventional Radiology in Women's Health

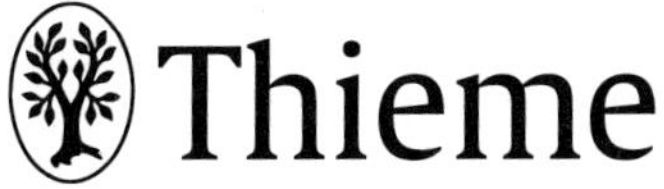

Interventional Radiology in Women's Health

Gary P. Siskin, MD
Professor and Chairman
Department of Radiology
Albany Medical Center
Albany, New York

Thieme
New York • Stuttgart

Thieme Medical Publishers, Inc.
333 Seventh Ave.
New York, NY 10001

Executive Editor: Timothy Hiscock
Vice President, Production and Electronic Publishing: Anne T. Vinnicombe
Production Editor: Heidi Grauel, Maryland Composition
Vice President, International Marketing and Sales: Cornelia Schulze
Chief Financial Officer: Peter Van Woerden
President: Brian D. Scanlan
Compositor: Manila Typesetting Company
Printer: Maple-Vail Book Manufacturing Group

Cover illustration by Markus Voll.
Library of Congress Cataloging-in-Publication Data

Interventional radiology in women's health / edited by Gary Siskin.
p. ; cm.
Includes bibliographical references and index.
ISBN 978-1-60406-046-1 — ISBN (invalid) 978-1-60406-153-6 1. Interventional radiology. 2. Women — Diseases — Radiotherapy.
3. Generative organs, Female — Diseases — Radiotherapy. I. Siskin, Gary.
[DNLM: 1. Radiography, Interventional — methods. 2. Women's Health. 3. Genital Diseases, Female — radiography. WN 200 I61225 2009]
RD33.55.I584 2009
617'.05--dc22

2008055905

Important note: Medical knowledge is ever-changing. As new research and clinical experience broaden our knowledge, changes in treatment and drug therapy may be required. The authors and editors of the material herein have consulted sources believed to be reliable in their efforts to provide information that is complete and in accord with the standards accepted at the time of publication. However, in view of the possibility of human error by the authors, editors, or publisher of the work herein or changes in medical knowledge, neither the authors, editors, nor publisher, nor any other party who has been involved in the preparation of this work, warrants that the information contained herein is in every respect accurate or complete, and they are not responsible for any errors or omissions or for the results obtained from use of such information. Readers are encouraged to confirm the information contained herein with other sources. For example, readers are advised to check the product information sheet included in the package of each drug they plan to administer to be certain that the information contained in this publication is accurate and that changes have not been made in the recommended dose or in the contraindications for administration. This recommendation is of particular importance in connection with new or infrequently used drugs.

Some of the product names, patents, and registered designs referred to in this book are in fact registered trademarks or proprietary names even though specific reference to this fact is not always made in the text. Therefore, the appearance of a name without designation as proprietary is not to be construed as a representation by the publisher that it is in the public domain.

Printed in the United States

5 4 3 2 1

ISBN 978-1-60406-046-1

I would like to dedicate this book to my wife Robin, who has been with me through it all and continues to provide me with unwavering love, support, and patience. Thank you also to my children Jordan, Matthew, Jake, and Ava because they serve as a constant reminder of everything that is good in life and inspire me to be the best person I can be. In addition, I want to thank my parents who have supported and encouraged me for my entire life.

I would also like to acknowledge the physicians and nurse practitioners I have had the privilege of working with through the years; the students, residents, and fellows I have had the opportunity to train and who have since moved on to make significant contributions to our field; and the hard work and dedication of my assistant Rachelle Stepnowski who is always appreciated because, without her, none of this would have happened.

Contents

Foreword

I am honored to be asked to contribute the Foreword to Dr. Gary Siskin's book, *Interventional Radiology in Women's Health*. It is timely that a book focused on women's health has been written. Advances in women's health and the fact that women are much more likely to investigate health alternatives for themselves and their families serve as an impetus for this text.

Dr. Siskin has recruited some of the leaders of interventional radiology and their counterparts in medicine and surgery to produce a text covering the spectrum of disorders primarily affecting women, including uterine fibroids, infertility, pelvic pain, osteoporosis, and varicose veins. Each section is introduced by a clinical review of the condition and ends with short chapters discussing the interventional and surgical or medical perspectives.

Image-guided therapies for uterine myomata, infertility, pelvic pain, osteoporosis, and varicose veins have been developed largely over the past 10 years, an amazing accomplishment that reflects the vibrancy and innovation within our specialty.

It is surprising that we have not seen more self-standing outpatient practices developed for women's health issues by interventional radiologists. Many of Dr. Siskin's contributors are quick to emphasize the importance of interventional radiologists developing their practices and offices. Hopefully, primary care physicians who read this book will realize they can directly refer to interventional radiologists. Practice development is an essential part of having a successful career as an interventional radiologist and "branding our specialty" is a priority of the leaders within our specialty. As the readers delve into each section, I believe they will be left with the same thought that I experienced after reading this text: why not develop more practices along these lines?

Congratulations to Dr. Siskin and his colleagues. It is quite a feat for Dr. Siskin to conceive of such a book and to contribute to 7 of 28 chapters. I am hopeful that primary care practitioners and internists will also find this book useful, as it contains much new information concerning women's health and the value of interventional radiology.

Robert I. White Jr., MD
Professor of Diagnostic Radiology
Yale University School of Medicine
Director of the Yale AVM Center
New Haven, Connecticut

Preface

One of the most interesting things about the field of interventional radiology is the ability to be involved in the care of so many different types of patients with a variety of medical conditions. The primary goal of this textbook is to focus on women's health and the role of interventional radiology within this area of medicine. Some of the conditions discussed are unique to women, while others are more common in women than they are in men. What ties them together is that these conditions, and the procedures performed to treat these conditions, often form the core of contemporary interventional radiology practice. The increased involvement of interventional radiology in the area of women's health has rejuvenated the entire field and has allowed many physicians to grow their practices at a time of increased competition. More importantly, the focus on women's health has changed interventional radiologists from providers of procedural care into providers of medical care.

It is my hope that interventional radiologists may find this text to be a single resource covering much of what they do on a daily basis in this particular area of their practice. The text itself has been designed as a clinical and procedural resource with comprehensive reviews of the major clinical entities treated within this patient population by interventional radiologists including uterine fibroids, pelvic pain, infertility, osteoporosis, and varicose veins, among others. These features, and the perspectives of physicians in several medical specialties regarding the role of interventional radiology in women's health, may also prove helpful for residents and fellows who are planning careers in interventional radiology. Finally, this text can serve as a resource for gynecologists, primary care physicians, and other providers who refer their patients to interventional radiologists for care and may wish to better understand these procedures.

There is enormous opportunity for interventional radiology in the area of women's health. This book and the procedures described within it represent only the beginning. As experience grows with local tumor therapy in the liver and lungs, it is easy to envision the role of interventional radiology increasing in the care of patients with primary breast cancer and metastatic disease to the liver and lungs from breast, ovarian, and other malignancies occurring uniquely or more commonly in women. Similarly, with a growing role in the treatment of varicose veins, it becomes easy to envision the role of interventional radiology increasing in the delivery of cosmetic procedures. Finally, many interventional radiologists remain quite active in the care of patients with vascular disease, and it is well known that there are significant gender-based differences in the manifestations of this disease and the response to treatment. With the continuing national and international focus on women's health, new advances and new opportunities are likely to come in the future. The topics described in this textbook are likely to provide the foundation for the involvement of interventional radiology in areas of which we are not yet aware.

As the editor of this project, I would like to thank those physicians within and outside the field of interventional radiology for their time and effort in making significant contributions to this book. I also appreciate the support of Timothy Hiscock and Dominik Pucek at Thieme, both of whom gave me the freedom to design a book that would uniquely address the physicians interested in the role of interventional radiology in women's health.

Contributors

R. Torrance Andrews, MD
Associate Professor and Chief
Section Chief, Vascular and Interventional Radiology
Director of Endovascular Therapy
University of Washington Medical Center
Seattle, Washington

Mark F. Brodie, MD
Interventional Radiologist
Department of Radiology
Naval Medical Center
San Diego, California

Kristof Chwalisz, MD, PhD
TAP Pharmaceutical Products, Inc.
Lake Forest, Illinois

Stephen Cohen, MD, FACOG
Associate Professor of Obstetrics and Gynecology
Albany Medical College
CNY Fertility Center
Albany and Syracuse, New York

Meridith Englander, MD
Assistant Professor of Radiology
Albany Medical Center
Albany, New York

Chieh-Min Fan, MD
Brigham and Women's Hospital
Angiography and Interventional Radiology
Boston, Massachusetts

Jay Goldberg, MD, MSCP
Clinical Associate Professor of Obstetrics and Gynecology
Director, Division of General Obstetrics and Gynecology
Director, Jefferson Fibroid Center
Department of Obstetrics and Gynecology
Jefferson Medical College
Philadelphia, Pennsylvania

Jafar Golzarian, MD
Professor
University of Iowa Hospitals and Clinics
Iowa City, Iowa

Michael F. Holick, PhD, MD
Department of Medicine, Section of Endocrinology, Nutrition, and Diabetes
Vitamin D, Skin and Bone Research Laboratory
Boston University Medical Center
Boston University School of Medicine
Boston, Massachusetts

Ann Honebrink, MD, FACOG
Associate Professor and Medical Director
Department of Obstetrics and Gynecology
Penn Health for Women
University of Pennsylvania School of Medicine
Radnor, Pennsylvania

David M. Hovsepian, MD
Interventional Radiology Section
Mallinckrodt Institute of Radiology
St. Louis, Missouri

Lowell S. Kabnick, MD, FACS, FACPh
New York University School of Medicine
New York University Langone Medical Center
Division of Vascular Surgery
Director, NYU Vein Center
Morristown Memorial Hospital–NJ
Clinical Assistant Professor, UMDNJ
New York, New York

David F. Kallmes, MD
Professor of Radiology
Mayo Clinic
Rochester, Minnesota

Colleen M. Kennedy, MD, MS
Assistant Professor of Obstetrics and Gynecology
Department of Gynecology
University of Iowa
Iowa City, Iowa

Todd L. Kooy, MD
Assistant Professor of Radiology
Fellowship Director, Vascular and Interventional Radiology
University of Washington
Seattle, Washington

Suzanne D. LeBlang, MD
Medical Director, MR Guided Focused Ultrasound
University MRI
Boca Raton, Florida

Hugh McSwain, MD
Neuro Interventional Radiology
University of California–San Francisco
San Francisco, California

Robert J. Min, MD, MBA
Chairman of Radiology
Weill Medical College of Cornell University
New York Presbyterian Hospital
New York, New York

Kieran Murphy, MD, BCH, FRCPC, FSIR
Professor, Vice Chair, and Director of Research
Department of Medical Imaging
University of Toronto
Deputy Chief of Medical Imaging
University Health Network
Toronto, Ontario, Canada

Anthony Andrew Nicholson, MSC, FRCR
Consultant Vascular Radiologist
Leeds University Teaching Hospitals
Department of Interventional Radiology
Leeds, United Kingdom

Gerald Niedzwiecki, FSIR
Advanced Intervention
Clearwater, Florida

Wayne J. Olan, MD
Clinical Professor Radiology and Neurosurgery
The George Washington University Medical Center
Director, Neuroradiology/MRI
Suburban Hospital
Bethesda, Maryland

C. Paul Perry, MD †
Director, C. Paul Perry Pelvic Pain Center
Chairman of the Board, International Pelvic Pain Society
Birmingham, Alabama

Joey Marie Robinson, MA
Consultant
Irvine, California

Mark Rosen, MD, PhD
Department of Radiology
University of Pennsylvania Medical Center
University of Pennsylvania School of Medicine
Hospital of the University of Pennsylvania
Philadelphia, Pennsylvania

† deceased

Richard Shlansky-Goldberg, MD
Associate Professor of Radiology
Division of Interventional Radiology
Hospital of the University of Pennsylvania
Philadelphia, Pennslyvania

Gary P. Siskin, MD
Professor and Chairman
Department of Radiology
Albany Medical Center
Albany, New York

James Spies, MD
Georgetown University Hospital
Department of Radiology
Washington, DC

Jeffrey M. Spivak, MD
Clinical Assistant Professor of Orthopaedic Surgery
Department of Orthopaedic Surgery
New York University for Joint Diseases
New York, New York

Brian F. Stainken, MD, FSIR
Adjunct Professor
Roger Williams Hospital
Providence, Rhode Island

Kenneth R. Tomkovich, MD
Director of Vascular and Interventional Radiology
CentraState Medical Center
Department of Radiology
Freehold, New Jersey

Jean-Claude Veille, MD
Perinatal Associates of Sacramento
Sacramento, California

Robert L. Worthington-Kirsch, MD
Department of Cardiovascular and Interventional Radiology
Pottstown Memorial Medical Center
Pottstown, Pennsylvania

Gerald Wyse, MD
Division of Interventional Neuroradiology
Johns Hopkins School of Medicine
Baltimore, Maryland

Burt Yaszay, MD
Clinical Instructor
Department of Orthopaedic Surgery
University of California–San Diego
San Diego, California

Fadi Youness, MD
Clinical Assistant Professor
Division of Interventional Radiology
Department of Radiology
University of Iowa
Iowa City, Iowa

I Women and Interventional Radiology

1 Clinical Patient Management

Brian F. Stainken and Gary P. Siskin

"For most of history, Anonymous was a woman."
Virginia Woolf

It is time for a textbook focused on women's health and interventional radiology (IR) for very many reasons. The most obvious, and possibly least significant, is that IR has matured as a subspecialty and we have begun to refine our body of knowledge as it concerns this field. We have learned, and now understand, that the anatomic and physiologic differences between women and men present unique challenges and merit considered approaches for the interventional radiologist. But there is a lot more below the surface. To a large degree, the success that IR has enjoyed in the transition from benchtop to clinic is because of women. This is because women have risen from the shadows to become the primary health care decision makers for themselves and for their families. It is because women were willing to join us and upset the status quo when we discovered a way to avoid uterine amputation for leiomyoma. Women saw us for what we are, what we could be, and how we could help address their unique health care needs. They were willing to come to our clinics and help us fight back those opposed to change. Women were willing to listen, to learn, to consider, and to believe.

■ Women's Health Care Needs

This text is offered as a beginning, an attempt to compile our work product, not by organ system but by patient gender. To the extent that the medical literature supports specific approaches or solutions, they are offered. Equally important is that this is a book about what we have yet to learn about these medical problems and the solutions that we hope to offer in the future.

The anatomic and physiologic differences between men and women and the resulting differences in their health care needs was recognized by the Federal Department of Health and Human Services in 1991 with the establishment of the Office on Women's Health. This office was established with the broad mandate of raising awareness of women's health issues and promoting activities that improve the health of women. In addition, its mission is to coordinate a comprehensive women's health agenda to address health care prevention and service delivery, research, public and health care professional education, and career advancement for women in the health professions.[1]

The attention paid to these issues has raised an awareness of several key concerns regarding the health care needs and utilization of women. These were highlighted by Brittle and Bird, in a report produced for the Office of Women's Health.[2] **Table 1.1**[3–11] outlines some specific examples from that report of how disease states may differ between the sexes.[2] Although these specific differences are important on a patient-to-patient basis, there are more general differences that demonstrate how gender impacts the relationship between female patients and the health care system. Brittle and Bird found that women utilize the health care system more often than men, primarily due to their higher use of preventive care services. This does not appear to carry over into better care of acute conditions in women. The cause of this discrepancy is likely multifactorial. In part, it may be because, though the differences outlined in **Table 1.1** are recognized, this recognition has not yet translated into tangible changes in how these disease processes are addressed in men and women.

Historically, women have not participated in clinical trials as often as men and therefore, it is not really known if many medical treatments are as appropriate for women as they are for men. The differences in the management of acute conditions in men and women may also be due to the fact that women typically have poorer access to health care than men. Despite the fact that slightly more women than men have health insurance coverage, women are more likely to be covered as dependents on a man's health insurance policy, which makes them vulnerable to disruptions in care and may limit access to care in times of acute need. Salganicoff et al[12] also found that for many women, counseling by physicians about health risks and health promoting behaviors is deficient. All of these findings have led to a growing movement toward a more gender-based system of care, which will also encourage research to support this model and demonstrate its effectiveness.

Fortuitously, IR has developed a focus in women's health during the past decade, at the same time that the above discussions have been going on at a national and global level. A quick glance at the Table of Contents of this textbook will show a list of solutions that are largely directed toward conditions prevalent in women, many of which, until recently, were not performed on a regular basis. In other words, the scope and nature of IR procedural care

Table 1.1 Examples of Gender-Related Differences in Health

Before menopause, women have lower blood pressure than men do. After menopause, systolic blood pressure in women is higher than in men.
Women with peripheral arterial disease are at greater risk for a compromise in daily function and quality of life than are men.
Women are more likely than are men to experience coronary vascular injury and bleeding complications after percutaneous coronary interventions.
Women have more advanced disease than men do when colon cancer is first diagnosed.
Women are at a significantly higher risk for autoimmune disease than are men.
Men experience more deaths due to cancer than women do (57% to 43%).
Thyroid cancers are more prevalent in women than they are men.
Women with Alzheimer disease are more likely to exhibit severe cognitive impairment than do men.
Women have a later age of onset of schizophrenia than do men.

Source: Data from Kim JK, Alley D, Seeman T, Karlamangla A, Crimmins E. Recent changes in cardiovascular risk factors among women and men. J Womens Health (Larchmt) 2006;15:734–746; Collins TC, Suarez-Almazor M, Bush RL, Petersen NJ. Gender and peripheral arterial disease. J Am Board Fam Med 2006;19:132–140; Argulian E, Patel AD, Abramson JL, et al. Gender differences in short-term cardiovascular outcomes after percutaneous coronary interventions. Am J Cardiol 2006;98:48–53; Woods SE, Narayanan K, Engel A. The influence of gender on colon cancer stage. J Womens Health (Larchmt) 2005;14:502–506; Shames RS. Gender differences in the development and function of the immune system. J Adolesc Health 2002; 30(4, Supplement 1)59–70; Bray F, Atkin W. International cancer patterns in men: geographical and temporal variations in cancer risk and the role of gender. J Mens Health Gend 2004;1:38–46; Adlersberg MA, Burrow GN. Focus on primary care thyroid function and dysfunction in women. Obstet Gynecol Surv 2002;57(3):S1–S7; Buchanan RJ, Wang S, Ju H, Graber D. Analyses of gender differences in profiles of nursing home residents with Alzheimer's disease. Gend Med 2004;1:48–59; Fleming M. Gender differences in schizophrenia: The need for a psychosocial and formulation based analysis? Clin Effect Nurs 2004;8:156–160.

has changed dramatically over the past decade, in striking parallel to changes in the culture of health care.

■ Uterine Artery Embolization

In light of these changes, IR is remarkably well positioned to leverage our skill set in a focused fashion to treat conditions that are either unique to or more prevalent in women. Uterine artery embolization (UAE) is a case in point. Uterine fibroids have been shown to be present in the majority of women aged 35 to 49. In African American women, fibroids are seen in 60% at age 35 and upwards of 80% by age 50.[13] Similarly, in Caucasian women, fibroids are seen in 40% at age 35 and almost 70% by age 50. When symptomatic, they are the leading benign cause of hysterectomy in this patient population. Given the possible morbidity associated with the most commonly performed treatment option (surgery), a less invasive treatment option was needed.

The initial work of Ravina et al[14] and Goodwin et al[15] was published in the mid-1990s and it was not until data was presented at the 1997 meeting of the Society of Cardiovascular and Interventional Radiology (SCVIR) that UAE was widely discussed as a treatment option for this patient population. At that time, most practicing gynecologists believed that UAE was not an effective treatment and had a high probability of leading to significant complications. Patients who elected to seek information about and undergo UAE had to do so without the knowledge and support of their gynecologist, which only fueled the prevailing belief that IR should not be involved in the care of these patients. With time, publications appeared both in the Radiology and Obstetrics and Gynecology literature that supported the success of UAE.

Single-center retrospective analyses have led to multicenter comparative trials and a large-scale prospective registry that consistently has demonstrated that UAE, as a minimally invasive treatment option, could successfully improve health-related quality of life and the severity of symptoms in patients with uterine fibroids.[16–21] With Internet-based forums allowing patients to discuss their own experience, prominent individuals undergoing this procedure, and national newspapers raising questions as to why this procedure is not offered to more patients, UAE has increasingly become part of the discussion held with women with symptomatic fibroids. Today, the American College of Obstetrics and Gynecology (ACOG) has supported UAE as a treatment option that should be discussed with patients considering treatment for fibroids.[22] In addition, and perhaps more telling, researchers in gynecology have conceptually endorsed UAE by attempting to develop their own treatment options that are based on diminishing arterial flow to the uterus and fibroids.[23–25] When it came to uterine fibroids, IR recognized the need for better treatments, developed and researched a new option, and has now worked to increase its acceptance by the medical community at large and its availability to patients in need.

■ Interventional Radiology and Women's Health

Similar stories can be told regarding many if not all of the procedures described within this textbook. UAE procedures to treat postpartum hemorrhage have made it possible to avoid hysterectomy in this situation.[26–29] Vertebroplasty and kyphoplasty procedures have made it possible to provide symptomatic relief to patients with vertebral compression fractures due to osteoporosis, a condition which is well known to affect more women than men.[30] Laser ablation of the greater saphenous vein has provided an effective, minimally invasive alternative to saphenous vein stripping for patients with symptomatic varicose veins, another condition that affects more women than men and prompts women to seek treatment more often than men.[31–33] Even procedures that have been around for a longer period, such as ovarian vein embolization to treat patients with pelvic congestion syndrome or fallopian tube recanalization to treat patients with tubal infertility, continue to remain important in the care of female patients with these conditions. Finally, the area of breast interventions remains a frontier for many interventional radiologists who have the skills necessary to diagnose and treat many forms of breast cancer. These techniques have no doubt revolutionized the care offered to female patients with these conditions. With innovation continuing, the role of IR in the care of these patients will continue to evolve.

The relationship between IR and women's health is not one-sided. Although it is clear that IR has changed women's health, it is equally clear that involvement in the women's health arena has also changed IR. Much of the impetus for this change lies with the patient population now being served by IR.

Women as patients have a unique set of characteristics. Women are more likely than men to seek treatment for most diseases, to report more symptoms, and to place a higher value on preventive behaviors.[2] In addition, it is known that women tend to make most of the health care decisions within families.[12] In the author's experience, these differences between men and women are most evident in the patients seeking care for symptomatic uterine fibroids, infertility, pelvic congestion syndrome, and varicose veins. What these patients share in common is the fact that they are typically healthy and are going through their first significant experience as a patient. By pursuing an interventional option, they are often seeking an alternative to more established treatment options that have been recommended to them by their primary physicians. This is due, in large part, to the decision-making role that these women have taken on within their families together with the accessibility of health care information on the Internet. Therefore, the relationship that they establish with an interventional radiologist is going to go a long way toward easing any concerns that they may have about selecting a particular treatment option, particularly because most women still rely on their health care providers as their primary source of health information.[12]

The patients seeking out an interventional radiologist for these procedures are very different from the typical IR patients. In the past, patients scheduled to undergo an interventional procedure for peripheral arterial disease or end-stage renal disease were, in general, sent to IR by their physicians without much understanding of the conditions they had and the procedures they were scheduled to undergo. Interventional radiologists would meet them on the morning of their procedure and explain to them what they were about to experience. There was never any genuine effort on either the part of the patient or physician to develop any type of relationship. However, without the benefit of a broader doctor–patient relationship, these interactions typically failed to enhance a patient's understanding of the planned interventional procedure, rendering these interactions less than satisfactory.

As the movement into women's health issues began, it quickly became apparent that this typical model of interventional practice was no longer acceptable for these patients. The 40- to 50-year-old patient with symptomatic fibroids presenting for UAE was going to be demanding more from the physician taking care of her than patients presenting to IR have demanded in the past. It was never going to be acceptable for one of these patients to present to the hospital in the morning for a UAE procedure without ever having met the physician and to then be managed after the procedure by a physician who did not have an intimate knowledge of the procedure that was performed. Looking back, it is hard to believe that this style of care was ever acceptable, but this model had never been challenged until UAE came along. Now, for IR to develop an increasing presence within this area of medicine, something had to change.

The concept of interventional radiologists taking on the responsibility of directly managing their patients is not new. In 1968, Charles Dotter remarked that clinical management of patients undergoing IR procedures is an essential component of a successful IR practice.[34] Since then, this sentiment has been echoed by many well-respected interventional radiologists, including Bob White, who said that "a clinic is evidence to both our patients and the referring physicians of our commitment to patient care."[35] This was formally recognized in May 2003, when the American College of Radiology acknowledged that clinical management of patients before and after interventional procedures is crucial for the overall care of the patient.[36] In addition, it was stressed that longitudinal care is necessary to optimize patients' experiences with IR.

Despite these calls for interventional radiologists to provide direct patient care services, this was never widely accepted in practice. Radiology practices, whether community- or university-based, were never set up to afford this opportunity to their interventional radiologists. The physical layout of radiology practices was not exactly conducive to one-on-one physician–patient interaction performed in the setting of a traditional doctor's office. Private patient examination or consultation rooms were not usually part of hospital-based radiology departments or outpatient imaging centers and the potential benefit of developing such a space was never felt to be justified from an economic perspective. In addition, expectations were such (and many cases still are) that interventional radiologists not actively performing procedures were expected to participate in the interpretation of diagnostic radiology studies. Time away from these responsibilities was not seen as improving the care of IR patients as much as it was seen to be a failure to contribute to the overall diagnostic workload of the practice.

■ Model of Care

Once interventional radiologists began their involvement in women's health, it became evident that direct clinical patient management was a necessary ingredient for success. This, more than anything, is where procedures such as UAE and others have revolutionized the field of IR. Now, there was an expectation on the part of the patient that their encounter with an IR team was going to mimic the interactions between patients and physicians providing procedural services, such as surgeons. They would be initially seen in consultation by an interventional radiologist at which time their records would be evaluated, they would be examined, and a determination would be made as to whether or not their clinical condition supported performance of a procedure. Following that, the interventional radiologist would arrange for performance of the procedure and subsequently perform the procedure on the scheduled date. They would then assume the responsibility for managing the patient after the procedure, until the recovery had been completed and the results of the procedure could be assessed. At that time, they would return to their primary care physician if the need for additional care arose in the future.

Today, this is the model of care that these patients expected and as a result, this is the model of care that has been put into place in many IR practices. The barriers described above, which in the past prevented interventional radiologists from providing these services, had to be broken down, and to a large degree, they have. Duszak and Mabry[37] reported that 92% of interventional radiologists provide clinical services to their patients and Khan et al[38] reported increases in the number of evaluation and management codes reimbursed by the Centers for Medicare and Medicaid Services (CMS) to interventional radiologists. Practices today often boast about their outpatient offices, with many either building new facilities or converting existing space into suitable patient care offices. Support staff, as well as nurse practitioners and physician assistants, are being hired into radiology practices to assist interventional radiologists at developing these clinical practices. Even though many of these clinical practices started with providing these services to patients being considered for UAE, they have evolved into a setting in which many of the procedures performed by interventional radiologists can be discussed with patients.

In our own practices, an outpatient office serves as the point of entry for patients being evaluated for UAE, spine interventions (including kyphoplasty and pain injection procedures), endovascular procedures, transjugular portosystemic portosystemic shunts (TIPS), local tumor therapy, and varicose vein interventions. Importantly, there is no doubt that this style of practice began with UAE and has largely evolved concomitantly with our increased involvement with women's health issues. It has also contributed to some crossover care because patients with uterine fibroids frequently have varicose veins that require therapy and certainly a local tumor therapy practice can lead to kyphoplasty and breast procedures. This model, which has enabled all of these patients to be entered into a system providing longitudinal care before, during, and after interventional procedures, has been successful at providing the necessary counseling and follow-up that these patients expect. Most importantly, it has improved the care that we offer to our patients and has sent a message to physicians referring patients to IR that we, as a specialty, are serious in our commitment to take on the responsibility of caring for our patients.

The impact of IR's involvement with women's health has actually extended beyond the clinical practice model that is now in place within many groups. The attention paid to UAE and the amount of research that has gone into optimizing this procedure has had the added benefit of creating a new level of interest in many different applications of embolization. Not since the early to mid-1970s has so much attention been paid to developing new embolic agents and studying new indications for embolization. Spherical embolic agents have been developed with UAE serving as a platform for evaluating these agents. Products have come and gone because of how they perform during UAE. The development of these agents has prompted additional research into drug-loaded embolic agents and how they can be used to optimize pain control after UAE,[39] which has led, in turn, to additional advances in drug-loading embolic agents for use during chemoembolization procedures.[40,41] This is just one example of how the enthusiasm behind developing the UAE procedure has led to an additional level of understanding about embolization in general, which has brought about impressive changes in how embolization is used in today's interventional practice.

■ Conclusions

In conclusion, the partnership between the women's health movement and IR has been one that has benefited everyone involved. As the various procedures in this textbook are reviewed, it will be easy to see how the procedures themselves have positively impacted women. Minimally invasive treatment options offered by IR have almost become the standard of care in many settings with increased penetration still widely felt to be possible. All of medicine has been striving of late for effective, minimally invasive treatment options for a variety of medical conditions. IR has been so successful that other specialties are either developing the skill set to take control of these procedures or developing similar procedures of their own. It is timely that the skills inherent to IR are being directed toward an at-need patient population. More importantly, it is equally satisfying to see the field of IR evolving to maximize the contribution that can be made to this group of patients and to take these lessons and apply them to all areas of contemporary IR practice.

References

1. United States Department of Health and Human Services Office on Women's Health. Mission, history, and functions. Available at: http://www.4women.gov/owh/about/mhf.cfm. Accessed October 3, 2007
2. Brittle C, Bird CE. Literature review on effective sex- and gender-based systems/models of care. Produced for the Office on Women's Health within the U.S. Department of Health and Human Services. Available at: http://www.4women.gov/owh/multidisciplinary/reports/GenderBasedMedicine/FinalOWHReport.pdf. Accessed January 30, 2007
3. Kim JK, Alley D, Seeman T, Karlamangla A, Crimmins E. Recent changes in cardiovascular risk factors among women and men. J Womens Health (Larchmt) 2006;15:734–746
4. Collins TC, Suarez-Almazor M, Bush RL, Petersen NJ. Gender and peripheral arterial disease. J Am Board Fam Med 2006;19:132–140
5. Argulian E, Patel AD, Abramson JL, et al. Gender differences in short-term cardiovascular outcomes after percutaneous coronary interventions. Am J Cardiol 2006;98:48–53
6. Woods SE, Narayanan K, Engel A. The influence of gender on colon cancer stage. J Womens Health (Larchmt) 2005;14:502–506
7. Shames RS. Gender differences in the development and function of the immune system. J Adolesc Health 2002;30(4, Supplement 1)59–70
8. Bray F, Atkin W. International cancer patterns in men: geographical and temporal variations in cancer risk and the role of gender. J Mens Health Gend 2004;1:38–46
9. Adlersberg MA, Burrow GN. Focus on primary care thyroid function and dysfunction in women. Obstet Gynecol Surv 2002;57(3):S1–S7
10. Buchanan RJ, Wang S, Ju H, Graber D. Analyses of gender differences in profiles of nursing home residents with Alzheimer's disease. Gend Med 2004;1:48–59
11. Fleming M. Gender differences in schizophrenia: the need for a psychosocial and formulation based analysis? Clin Effect Nurs 2004;8:156–160
12. Salganicoff A, Ranji UR, Wyn R. Women and Health Care: A National Profile—Key Findings from the Kaiser Women's Health Survey. Menlo Park, CA: Henry J. Kaiser Family Foundation; 2005
13. Parker WH. Etiology, symptomatology, and diagnosis of uterine myomas. Fertil Steril 2007;87:725–736
14. Ravina JH, Herbreteau D, Ciraru-Vigneron N, et al. Arterial embolization to treat uterine myomata. Lancet 1995;346:671–672
15. Goodwin SC, Vedantham S, McLucas B, Forno AE, Perrella R. Preliminary experience with uterine artery embolization for uterine fibroids. J Vasc Interv Radiol 1997;8:517–526
16. Walker WJ, Pelage J. Uterine artery embolization for symptomatic fibroids: clinical results in 400 women with imaging follow-up. BJOG 2002;109:1262–1272
17. Pron G, Bennett J, Common A, et al. The Ontario uterine fibroid embolization trial: part 2. Uterine fibroid reduction and symptoms relief after uterine artery embolization for fibroids. Fertil Steril 2003;79:120–127
18. Spies JB, Bruno J, Czeyda-Pommersheim F, et al. Long-term outcome of uterine artery embolization of leiomyomas. Obstet Gynecol 2005;106:933–939
19. Spies JB, Myers ER, Worthington-Kirsch R, et al. The FIBROID registry: symptom and quality of life status 1 year after therapy. Obstet Gynecol 2005;106:1309–1318
20. Goodwin SC, Bradley LD, Lipman JC, et al. Uterine artery embolization versus myomectomy: a multicenter comparative study. Fertil Steril 2006;85:14–21
21. Spies JB, Cornell C, Worthington-Kirsch R, Lipman JC, Benenati JF. Long-term outcome from uterine fibroid embolization with tris-acryl gelatin microspheres: results of a multicenter study. J Vasc Interv Radiol 2007;18:203–207
22. American College of Obstetricians and Gynecologists. ACOG Practice Bulletin: Alternatives to hysterectomy in the management of leiomyomas. Obstet Gynecol 2008;112(2 Pt 1):387–400
23. Hald K, Langebrekke A, Klow NE, et al. Laparoscopic occlusion of uterine vessels for the treatment of symptomatic uterine fibroids: initial experience and comparison to uterine artery embolization. Am J Obstet Gynecol 2004;190:37–43
24. Liu WM, Ng HT, Wu YC, et al. Laparoscopic bipolar coagulation of uterine vessels: a new method for treating symptomatic uterine fibroids. Fertil Steril 2001;75:417–422
25. Istre O, Hald K, Qvigstad E. Multiple myomas treated with a temporary, noninvasive Doppler-directed transvaginal uterine artery clamp. J Am Assoc Gynecol Laparosc 2004;11:273–276
26. Mitty HA, Sterling KM, Alvarez M, Gendler R. Obstetric hemorrhage: prophylactic and emergency arterial catheterization and embolotherapy. Radiology 1993;188:183–187
27. Palacios Jaraquemada JM. Life-threatening primary postpartum hemorrhage: treatment with emergency selective arterial embolization. Radiology 1999;210:876–878
28. Pelage JP, Soyer P, Repiquet D, et al. Secondary postpartum hemorrhage: treatment with selective arterial embolization. Radiology 1999;212:385–389
29. Ojala K, Perala J, Kariniemi J, Ranta P, Raudaskoski T, Tekay A. Arterial embolization and prophylactic catheterization for the treatment for severe obstetric hemorrhage. Acta Obstet Gynecol Scand 2005;84:1075–1080
30. Taylor RS, Taylor RJ, Fritzell P. Balloon kyphoplasty and vertebroplasty for vertebral compression fractures: a comparative systematic review of efficacy and safety. Spine 2006;31:2747–2755
31. Min RJ, Khilnani N, Zimmet SE. Endovenous laser treatment of saphenous vein reflux: long-term results. J Vasc Interv Radiol 2003;14:991–996
32. Brand FN, Dannenberg AL, Abbott RD, Kannel WB. The epidemiology of varicose veins: the Framingham Study. Am J Prev Med 1988;4:96–101
33. Bergan JJ, Schmid-Schonbein GW, Smith PD, et al. Chronic venous disease. N Engl J Med 2006;355:488–498

34. Becker GJ. 2000 RSNA Annual Oration in Diagnostic Radiology: the future of interventional radiology. Radiology 2001;220:281–292
35. White RI, Denny DF, Osterman FA, Greenwood LD, Wilkinson LA. Logistics of a university interventional radiology practice. Radiology 1989;170:951–954
36. Pentecost MJ. American College of Radiology: Clinical Practice of Interventional Radiology and Neurointerventional Radiology White Paper, May 2003. Reston, VA: ACR; 2003
37. Duszak R, Mabry MR. Clinical services in interventional radiology: results from the National Medicare Database and a Society of Interventional Radiology membership survey. J Vasc Interv Radiol 2003;14:75–81
38. Khan N, Murphy TP, Soares GM, Zahir IS. Clinical services provided by Interventional Radiologists to Medicare beneficiaries in the United States, 2000–2003. J Vasc Interv Radiol 2005;16:1753–1757
39. Borovac T, Pelage JP, Kasselouri A, et al. Release of ibuprofen from beads for embolization: in vitro and in vivo studies. J Control Release 2006;115:266–274
40. Varela M, Real MI, Burrel M, et al. Chemoembolization of hepatocellular carcinoma with drug eluting beads: efficacy and doxorubicin pharmacokinetics. J Hepatol 2007;46:474–481
41. Taylor RR, Tang Y, Gonzalez MV, Stratford PW, Lewis AL. Irinotecan drug eluting beads for use in chemoembolization: in vitro and in vivo evaluation of drug release properties. Eur J Pharm Sci 2007;30:7–14

2 Radiation Safety

R. Torrance Andrews and Todd L. Kooy

The increased availability and acceptance of fluoroscopically guided minimally invasive procedures has significantly altered the management of such disparate women's health concerns as osteoporotic vertebral fractures, breast masses, uterine fibroids, fertility, and chronic pelvic pain. Conditions that once required major surgery and prolonged recovery for their treatment can now be managed on an outpatient basis with little or no morbidity. However, even as these techniques have reduced the risks associated with traditional surgical alternatives, they have introduced the new and often underappreciated risk of radiation injury.

Exposure to ionizing radiation can cause local injury ranging from erythema to skin necrosis, can increase the long-term risk of malignancy, and can both reduce fertility by damaging ovarian function and increase the risk of genetic damage to a patient's future children. Although the likelihood of such outcomes is low, the risk is nonetheless infinitely higher than would be the case if no radiation were utilized. Furthermore, there is neither a visible nor a sensory indication to the patient or the operator that an injury is being induced: radiation damage is painless in the acute phase. For these reasons, it is imperative that the operator be aware of, and observe, all available precautions for reducing radiation exposure.

■ Radiation Effects

Radiation effects can be divided into two broad categories: stochastic and nonstochastic (also referred to as deterministic). Stochastic effects are those that can occur at any radiation dose, without a finite safety threshold.[1] The likelihood of a stochastic effect rises with increasing exposure, but the effect itself is binary – it either occurs or it does not – and the amount of radiation has no impact upon its severity. Examples of these chance events include genetic damage leading to cancer and chromosomal defects in future children, either of which could theoretically occur at very low doses, but might not occur even at very high doses.[1,2] Nonstochastic or deterministic radiation effects, in contrast, occur only once a specific threshold exposure value has been reached and increase in severity with increased dose. Skin injury at the beam entry site and radiation-mediated ovarian failure are examples of nonstochastic events: clinically significant skin injury at the beam entry site does not occur below a threshold of 200 cGy and ovarian failure does not occur below a threshold of 400 cGy.[2–4]

Radiation-induced skin damage is the most commonly observed injury following interventional procedures. As indicated, the severity of a skin injury is dependent upon the radiation dose (that is, it is a nonstochastic, or deterministic, event). Both the degree of skin injury and its progression over time follow a predictable course (**Table 2.1**). The first sign of injury is erythema, which can be seen within just a few hours of exposure to a dose of 200 cGy; temporary or permanent epilation follows within 3 to 4 weeks of doses of 300 to 700 cGy, respectively; a dose of 1000 cGy can cause desquamation after 4 to 5 weeks; and skin necrosis can occur within 10 weeks of an 1800 cGy dose. Unfortunately, once these injuries have occurred, there are few options for treatment other than palliative support and, in severe cases, skin grafting. Avoiding injurious doses is thus the most important factor in patient outcome.

Stochastic effects are also of great concern in interventional procedures that utilize ionizing radiation. Uterine fibroid embolization (UFE) and ovarian vein embolization, for instance, are procedures that specifically seek to conserve the organs of reproduction. Beyond simply retaining these organs, many women are hoping to preserve or even

Table 2.1 Radiation Dose and Time Course for Radiation-Induced Skin Injuries

Effect	Dose (Gray)	Onset	Peak
Early transient erythema	2	Hours	24 Hours
Temporary epilation	3	3 Weeks	NA
Permanent epilation	7	3 Weeks	NA
Dry desquamation	10	4 Weeks	5 Weeks
Moist desquamation	15	4 Weeks	5 Weeks
Dermal necrosis	18	>10 Weeks	NA
Dermal atrophy phase 1	10	>14 Weeks	NA
Dermal atrophy phase 2	10	>1 Year	NA
Skin cancer	Unknown	>5 Years	NA

Abbreviation: NA, not applicable.
Source: Adapted from Wagner LK, Archer BR. Minimizing risks from fluoroscopic x-rays. 2nd ed. Houston, TX: Partners in Radiation Management, 1998.

Table 2.2 Relative Radiation Sensitivity of Different Organs

Organ or Tissue	Relative Sensitivity
Gonads	20
Red bone marrow	12
Colon	12
Lung	12
Stomach	5
Bladder	5
Breast	5
Liver	5
Esophagus	5
Thyroid	5
Skin	1
Bone	1

Source: Adapted from Brateman L. Radiation safety considerations for diagnostic radiology personnel. Radiographics 1999;19(4):1037–1055. Adapted by permission.

improve their fertility, with the goal of becoming pregnant. An injury that induced malignant degeneration in the reproductive tract or caused chromosomal damage in as-yet unfertilized oocytes would be devastating. However, by definition, stochastic events are a matter of chance and are therefore impossible to predict with certainty. Furthermore, the likelihood of such events is known to vary by tissue type, with some organs, like the ovaries, being more "radiation-sensitive" than others (**Table 2.2**). Because the likelihood of these events increases with dose and because, again, there is no outward indication of injury, the only mechanism for protecting patients is to minimize their radiation exposure.

■ Dose Monitoring

Continuous, real-time monitoring of radiation dose during interventional procedures is critical and serves several purposes. An unexpectedly high dose rate may be the operator's best indication that otherwise occult technical or procedural factors are negatively impacting a given case. Having this information immediately available may allow for immediate corrective action. It also allows the operator to avoid a nonstochastic injury: as the dose approaches the 200 cGy threshold for a skin burn, for example, he or she can consider terminating the procedure or taking other steps (as discussed below) to stay below this threshold. If the threshold is exceeded, this fact must be recognized so that the patient can be followed appropriately for the development of clinical manifestations. Knowing a specific dose is less useful for predicting stochastic injuries, but a relative risk can be estimated.

Unfortunately, reliable dose monitoring is difficult, and all of the techniques in current use have significant limitations.

Fluoroscopic Time

Recording the number of minutes during which the imaging beam is active is quite simple. By law, all fluoroscopic equipment sold in the United States must be equipped with a mechanism for recording the fluoroscopic time, along with an alarm that sounds as each 5-minute increment passes. As a result, fluoroscopic time has become the most widely used tool for tracking patient dose. Unfortunately, this measure does not account for the dose delivered during image acquisitions, which is significantly higher than that delivered during fluoroscopy. A single recorded image can generate a dose equivalent to over 40 seconds of fluoroscopy,[5] and the dose delivered during a typical angiographic sequence of 20 to 40 images can therefore far exceed the amount of radiation being "measured" by fluoroscopic time. In addition, fluoroscopic time fails to reflect such factors as beam collimation, filtration, magnification, and other aspects of imaging technique that can critically impact the dose rate. These factors are discussed in detail later in this chapter.

Dose Area Product

Dose area product (DAP) is a calculated value derived by multiplying the actual dose delivered to the patient by the area over which the radiation is experienced. This value, which is calculated by the fluoroscopic equipment in units of $Gy \cdot cm^2$, includes both the dose from fluoroscopic observation and that from image acquisition; it also reflects the use of collimation, filtration, magnification, and other techniques used to reduce patient exposure. DAP is therefore a much better tool than fluoroscopic time for monitoring overall patient exposure, and thus the risk for stochastic injury. Unfortunately, it provides only a general estimate of dose at the entry site: a small region exposed to a large amount of radiation might have the same DAP as a large region exposed to a small dose, but would have a much greater risk for local injury.

In Situ Dosimeters

A direct measurement (rather than a calculation) of dose can be made at a specific point in or on a patient's body with a personal dosimeter placed at that point. This device can be a thermoluminescent dosimeter, a radiolucent probe, or, over a larger treatment area, radiation verification film. The primary advantage of such an approach is its high degree of accuracy. It is completely independent of all techniques utilized during a procedure and gives a very reliable indication of the actual dose being absorbed at the point where it is placed. Unfortunately, this information is not available until the dosimeter has been read, a process that can take several days; therefore, no real-time feedback is provided to the operator. In addition, placement of the device into a body cavity is, by definition, invasive, and may create complications independent of the procedure being performed.

■ Risk-Reduction Techniques

The most important factor in reducing the risk of radiation-induced injuries is to limit radiation exposure. This concept is referred to as the ALARA principle: keeping radiation dose as low as reasonably achievable. It is accomplished by reducing the time during which radiation is being delivered and also reducing the energy deposited per unit time.

Variables Beyond Operator Control

Some of the factors that influence patient dose are inherent in radiographic imaging and cannot be directly manipulated. An awareness of these issues is nonetheless useful and they are briefly discussed in the next several paragraphs.

Imaging Equipment

The conversion efficiency of the imaging chain – its ability to convert radiant energy to a useful fluoroscopic image – has a direct impact upon patient dose. To maximize safety, the radiographic equipment used for interventional procedures must be well maintained and regularly inspected by qualified personnel.

Area of Interest and Body Habitus

As the body part being studied increases in density, more radiation is required to penetrate the tissues and generate a useful image. Therefore, procedures in the abdomen and pelvis, which contain mostly solid organs, require more radiation for imaging than do those in the chest. In addition, patients who are physically larger experience a greater exposure than do patients of smaller size. Accordingly, a prospective review of 25 patients undergoing UFE found a positive correlation between radiation and body mass index.[6] Another study showed than an increase in anteroposterior chest diameter from 23 to 28 cm resulted in a dose increase of 50% during cardiac catheterization.[7]

Operator Experience

Any interventional procedure requires operator experience before it can be performed quickly and efficiently. Until one reaches this level of experience, it is likely that he or she will rely more heavily upon imaging guidance and thus expose the patient to more radiation per case. In a prospective trial of patients undergoing UFE, Pron et al[8] found that fluoroscopy time decreased with operator experience from a mean of 21.3 minutes to mean of 16.2 minutes. Andrews and Brown[5] reported a similar decrease in a retrospective analysis of their first 35 cases, noting a reduction in mean fluoroscopic time from 27 minutes for the first 16 cases to 14.8 minutes for the subsequent 19, with a reproducibly short fluoroscopic time seen after the 20th procedure. It is important to note that both studies involved operators who were already proficient in image-guided catheter techniques. Longer exposure times and a more protracted training period can be assumed for those who lack such previous experience.

Variables That Can Be Controlled

Careful attention to the operation of fluoroscopic equipment during interventional procedures can reduce a patient's radiation exposure by several orders of magnitude.[5] Most of the techniques described below apply to all fluoroscopic units, but there are variations among manufacturers. A discussion with the equipment vendor or onsite radiation physicist may be required to determine the applicability of the following recommendations to each unit.

Table Configuration

Patient dose can be reduced by more than 50% if the operator positions the x-ray tube, the patient, and the image detector correctly (**Fig. 2.1**).[5,9] Radiation decreases as the square of the distance between the radiation source and the object being irradiated. If the source-object distance (SOD) is doubled, the dose is reduced to one-fourth. Therefore, one should always raise the patient table as far from the imaging tube as possible without compromising the operator's work. Having passed through the patient, the x-ray beam continues to lose energy as it travels to the radiographic detector for conversion to an image. If the distance between the patient (the object) and the imaging unit (the object-image distance [OID]) is excessive, the overall efficiency of the imaging chain is reduced and the fluoroscopic unit responds by increasing its dose rate. For this reason, the imaging detector should always be as close to the patient as possible.

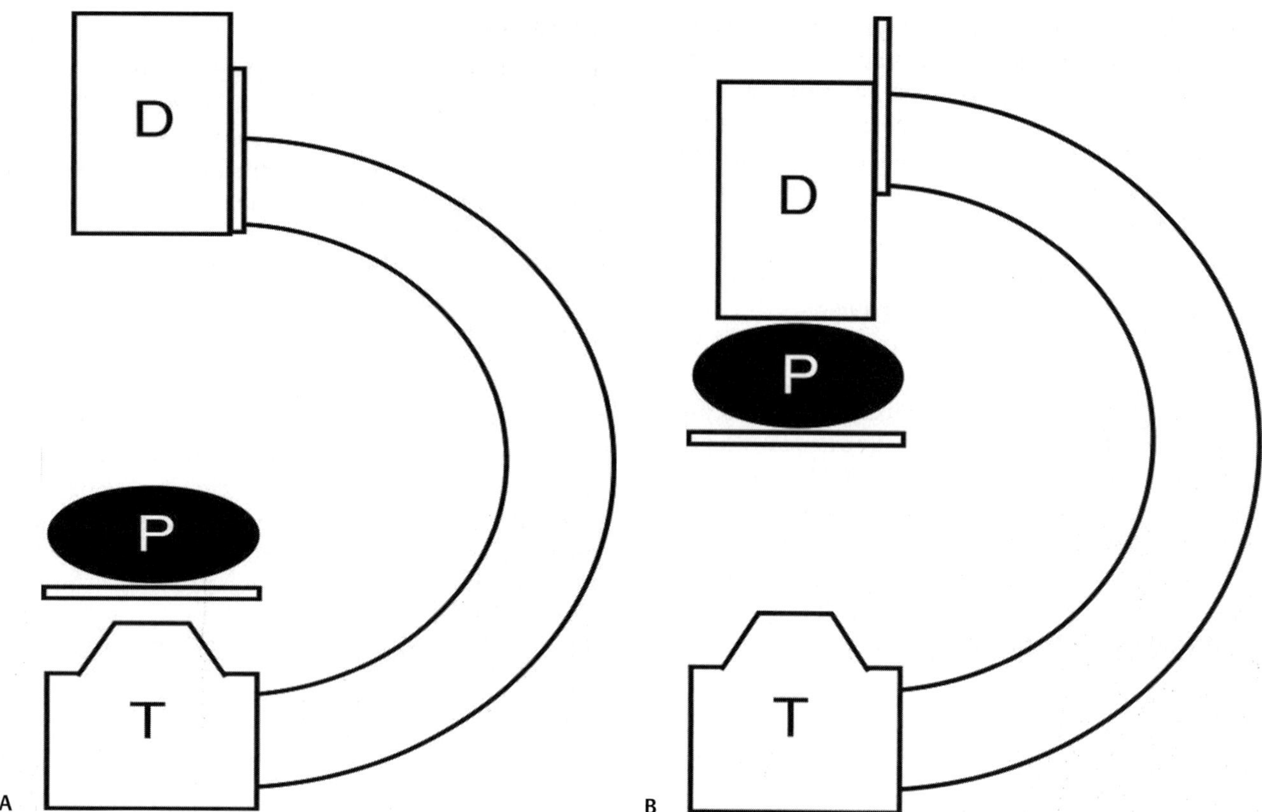

Fig. 2.1 Table configuration. An unfavorable configuration of the imaging chain, as shown in **(A)** places the patient (P) in close proximity to the fluoroscopic tube (T) and has the image detector (D) far away from the patient. Dose can be dramatically reduced if, as in **(B)**, the patient is moved away from the tube and the detector is brought close to the patient's body.

In a dedicated angiographic suite, table height and imaging detector position can usually be controlled independently. In contrast, both table height and tube position are fixed in overhead fluoroscopy units of the type often used for general radiography and endoscopy. With such units, the only variable is the position of the image detector, which should be kept as low as possible. Portable C-arm units often have a fixed distance between the radiographic source and the imaging detector (the source-image distance [SID]), but this entire assembly can generally be raised or lowered. With such machines, the table should be as high as possible within the gap of the imaging unit. If the C-arm can be moved vertically but the table is fixed, then the C-arm should be as low as possible. If, on the other hand, the table can be moved but the C-arm cannot, then the table should be raised.

It should be noted that increasing the source-object distance (between the tube and the patient) will also increase under-table radiation scatter to the operator. When SOD is maximized, the operator should consider using floor-level shielding for personal protection.[10]

Collimation and Filtration

Collimation is the process of reducing the imaging field to show only the target area: the operator can electronically move lead shields inside the x-ray tube housing into and out of the beam. Collimation "crops" the image, reducing the area being irradiated and thereby reducing the amount of radiation being absorbed.

Filtration does not reduce the area being irradiated, but does reduce the amount of radiation that reaches the target. Filters, like collimators, are located within the tube housing and controlled electronically, but are less radio-opaque. By partially limiting radiation to less-dense areas of the imaging field (such as the lung when imaging over the chest), their use increases the homogeneity and visibility of the image and improves imaging efficiency.

Fluoroscopic Mode

The nature of the radiographic beam can be altered to reduce its dose rate in either or both of two ways. A low-dose beam is created by interposing various filters into the beam within the tube housing. This process blocks the radiation that is most likely to be absorbed by skin, thus preventing injury to the skin. A pulsed beam results from interrupting power to the tube at rates of 4 to 30 pulses per second (PPS). In addition to lowering the patient's radiation dose, pulsed fluoroscopy also reduces motion-related blur. Low-dose and pulsed fluoroscopy modes can be activated by the operator and can reduce the fluoroscopic dose by more than 50%.[5,9,11]

In some cases, very high-frequency (30 PPS) pulsed fluoroscopy can actually generate a higher patient dose than a continuous beam.[5] In addition, dedicated angiographic machines often have a "high dose" mode that can be activated when additional energy is required to generate a useful image (as might be required in an extremely large patient). The associated radiation is generally much higher than standard fluoroscopy. Therefore, before one begins to employ high-frequency pulsed or high-dose fluoroscopy in a given angiography suite, it may be useful to have these features specifically evaluated by a radiation physicist.

Image Projection

One of the great advantages of imaging equipment that can be angled is that it allows the operator to see target structures in the orientation that is most useful to him or her. Unfortunately, angling the beam can increase the amount of tissue through which it must travel and thus increase the deposition of energy into the patient. For example, the use of oblique imaging during pelvic angiography has been shown to increase dose by up to 30% over that of direct frontal projection imaging.[12] Although it is important to use whatever image projection is required to perform a procedure safely and efficiently, oblique imaging should be limited to only those portions of the procedure for which it is required.

Roadmapping

Some angiographic units allow a previously stored image of the vasculature to be superimposed over the live fluoroscopic image. This "roadmap" feature is intended to facilitate the catheterization of branch vessels; as such, it has the potential to reduce procedural (and fluoroscopic) time. In most cases, activation of the roadmap feature does not alter the radiation dose. However, in some machines, doing so simultaneously disables the pulsed and low-dose fluoroscopic modes. For such units, activation of the roadmap feature might increase dose by a factor of 200%.[5] This change in beam quality may not be indicated to the operator, leaving him or her unaware that dose has been increased. As with other features discussed here, the use of roadmapping and its effect upon dose should be discussed with the vendor of the specific fluoroscopic unit in question and tested by a radiation physicist if there is any uncertainty.

Magnification

Like angling the imaging beam and roadmapping, magnifying the live image can facilitate a procedure and thus reduce the procedural and fluoroscopic time required to perform it. Like these other options, magnification may have a cost in radiation dose. Traditional fluoroscopic machines use an image intensifier to create a fluoroscopic image. For these units, magnification is an analog process that increases dose by 31 to 154%.[5,9,12] When using an image intensifier, the operator should avoid magnification except as necessary to accomplish specific aspects of their procedures. In newer machines, the image intensifier has been replaced by a digital detector. With these units, magnification is a postprocessing function that simply projects a larger pixel. The enlarged image is slightly less sharp (though not to a degree that can be appreciated by the naked eye), but is made without an increase in dose.

Image Acquisition

Even with high-efficiency imaging equipment, the amount of radiation required to create permanent images (that is, "spot" films or angiographic "runs"), is significantly greater than that required for fluoroscopy: a single radiographic image can expose the patient to the same amount of radiation as 50 seconds of fluoroscopy.[5] Not surprisingly, the total patient dose associated with a procedure can be dramatically reduced simply by limiting the number of images acquired.

Most modern fluoroscopic machines will allow one to digitally save or film the fluoroscopic image – the single "last image" or up to several seconds' worth of live fluoroscopy. In most cases, this information is adequate for documentation purposes. When dedicated acquisition sequences cannot be avoided, these studies should be performed with the slowest acceptable imaging rate (0.5 to 1 frame per second rather than the usual 3 to 4) and performed for the shortest acceptable time. It may also be possible to image more than one target simultaneously, thereby reducing multiple sequences to just one. An example of this was described by Nikolic et al,[11] who performed a simultaneous bilateral uterine arteriography with a single filming sequence.

Dose Spreading

During most fluoroscopically guided procedures, the imaging beam is directed continually at a single region of interest. If the tube position is held constant, all of the incident radiation passes through the same entry site and, over time, increases the likelihood of an injury at that site. However, if one periodically reorients the beam, angling it through different entry sites, one can markedly reduce the peak skin dose or maximum skin dose. Of course, this approach results in a continually varying image orientation, which can be distracting. In addition, as described above, an oblique angle increases dose when compared with a direct angle. Nonetheless, the resulting distribution of dose over a larger area may well balance out this risk. Another alternative is to invert the imaging chain (that is, rotate the gantry such that the x-ray tube is above the table and the detector below). This distributes the entry dose without changing the apparent orientation of the image, but greatly increases scatter radiation to the operator's head and upper body.

■ Specific Procedures

Radiation doses associated with fluoroscopically guided interventions vary widely by procedure (**Table 2.3**). Dose reduction techniques should be used during all fluoroscopic procedures; however, they are of particular importance when the target lies within the female pelvis. As discussed earlier, the ovaries are among the most radiation sensitive tissues in the female body. The most common of such procedures are UFE, ovarian vein embolization, and fallopian tube recanalization.

Uterine Fibroid Embolization

Few image-guided minimally invasive interventions have so dramatically altered the patient's care experience as has UFE (also known as uterine artery embolization [UAE]). Patients with symptomatic uterine fibroids who, in the past, would have required open abdominal hysterectomy under general anesthesia and 6 to 8 weeks of recovery can now be treated on an outpatient basis and return to their usual level of activity within days. Ironically, UFE may also be the image-guided intervention that represents the greatest radiation risk to patients: the uterus and ovaries – the very organs intended to be spared by this nonsurgical approach – lie directly in the path of the x-ray beam throughout the treatment and cannot be shielded without compromising the procedure.

Table 2.3 Reported Radiation Exposures for Selected Interventional Radiology Procedures

Procedure Description	Total Cases	Fluoroscopy Time (min)		Dose Area Product ($Gy \cdot cm^2$)		Cumulative Dose (mGy)	
		M	Range	*M*	Range	*M*	Range
Nephrostomy							
Obstruction	79	10.5	1.3–56.9	25.5	0.41–212.25	257	3–2,169
Stone access	64	17.6	3.0–79.4	45.1	0.47–418.5	611	10–6,178
IVC Filter placement only	279	2.8	0.7–11.4	44.5	1.70–203.27	166	9–680
Renal/visceral angioplasty							
No stent	53	16.5	3.1–106.6	157.4	26.19–1040.75	1,183	157–5,482
Stent	103	21.6	4.1–86.9	190.0	9.83–724.2	1,605	104–7,160
Iliac angioplasty							
No stent	24	13.4	3.3–25.4	163.5	20.6–300.99	885	189–1,562
Stent	93	18.4	4.6–66.4	212.8	11.48–886.5	1,335	211–4,567
Hepatic chemoembolization	126	16.8	2.1–69.5	282.3	17.12–904.15	1,406	61–6,198
Pelvic arterial embolization							
Trauma	18	20.1	5.7–61.7	316.2	92.91–623.58	1,705	455–4,797
Tumor	19	28.4	8.6–91.9	302.8	110.02–838.11	1,846	493–4,133
Fibroids	90	29.5	2.0–101.4	298.2	4.16–815.75	2,460	15–6,990
AVM	12	38.4	16.1–61	484.2	218.42–980.28	2,818	1,071–6,149
Aneurysm	4	24.4	11.5–36.5	223.8	164.97–279	2,599	808–3,885
Ovarian vein embolization	6	44.5	23.4–64	413.5	122.17–1026.05	2,838	1,628–5,406
Other tumor embolization	91	21.7	2.5–89.7	274.8	16.68–1520.05	1,579	24–7,986
Peripheral AVM embolization	17	23.8	3.4–60	119.1	3.3–541.29	990	16–4,606
GI Hemorrhage: diagnosis/therapy	94	25.8	3.5–93.7	347.5	27.13–1294.65	2,367	105–7,160

Abbreviations: AVM, arteriovenous malformation; GI, gastrointestinal; IVC, inferior vena cava.

Source: Adapted from Miller DL, Balter S, Cole PE, et al. Radiation doses in interventional radiology procedures: The RAD-IR Study Part I: Overall Measures of Dose. J Vasc Interv Radiol 2003; 14:711–728. Copyright 2003 Elsevier. Adapted by permission.

The radiation exposure during fibroid embolization can vary markedly. A prospective observational study of 90 UFE procedures at seven institutions demonstrated fluoroscopy times ranging from 2 to 101 minutes, number of images acquired from 15 to 991, and DAP values between 4.16 and 81.6 Gy • cm^2.[13] In a different study, the mean DAP for UFE at a single center was reduced from 211.4 to 30.6 Gy • cm^2 through the aggressive application of the dose-control techniques described above.[5]

Ovarian Vein Embolization

Much of the imaging required for ovarian vein embolization is directed into the upper abdomen rather than the pelvis. However, pelvic imaging is also required and can be extensive, especially if the operator also performs embolization of the internal iliac vein branches.

Radiation exposure during gonadal vein embolization was evaluated in the multicenter study just discussed. Among six ovarian embolization procedures reported, total fluoroscopic time ranged from 23.4 to 64 minutes, images acquired from 63 to 187, and DAP from 12.2 to 102 Gy • cm^2. Among 14 male varicocele embolization procedures (which are identical in technique to ovarian embolization, with the exception that internal iliac vein embolization is never performed) fluoroscopy time ranged from 6.4 to 40.5 minutes, images acquired from 6 to 127, and DAP from 7.4 – 19 Gy • cm^2.

Fallopian Tube Recanalization

No fluoroscopically guided intervention is as closely associated with the issue of genetic damage to oocytes as fallopian tube recanalization. By definition, all patients who undergo this procedure do so with the specific goal of becoming pregnant. That being the case, there is surprisingly little (and no current) data regarding radiation exposure with this procedure. A study of 29 patients, published in 1991, measured radiation exposure associated with fluoroscopically guided fallopian tube recanalization by placing TLDs in the posterior vaginal fornix.[14] The authors reported fluoroscopic time of 8.5 minutes, an average of 14 images acquired, and an average ovarian absorbed dose of 8.5 mGy. DAP was not recorded.

■ Conclusions

All fluoroscopically guided interventions carry some risk of radiation injury to the patient. This risk, while it cannot be eliminated, can be reduced significantly if the operator follows the ALARA principle. Doing so requires that the operator be familiar with the specific operational features of the equipment under his or her control and that these features be applied as appropriate throughout a given case. The real-time tracking of patient dose is also critical in providing operational feedback to the operator so that he or she can modify an ongoing procedure as necessary to maximize safety.

References

1. Radiogenic cancer at specific sites. In Committee on the Biological Effects of Ionizing Radiation (Ed): health effects of exposure to low levels of ionizing radiation (BEIR-V). Washington, DC: National Academy Press; 1990: 242–351
2. Genetic effects of radiation. In Committee on the Biological Effects of Ionizing Radiation (Ed.): health effects of exposure to low levels of ionizing radiation (BEIR-V). Washington, DC: National Academy Press; 1990: 65–134
3. Wagner LK, Eifel PJ, Geise RA. Potential biological effects following high x-ray dose interventional procedures. J Vasc Interv Radiol 1994;5(1):71–84
4. Dembo AJ, Thomas GM. The ovary. In: Moss WT, Cox JT (Eds.), Radiation Oncology: rational, technique, results. St. Louis: Mosby; 1994: 712–713
5. Andrews RT, Brown PH. Uterine embolization: factors influencing patient radiation exposure. Radiology 2000;217:713–722
6. White AM, Banivac F, Spies JB. Patient radiation exposure during uterine fibroid embolization and the dose attributable to aortography. J Vasc Interv Radiol 2007;18:573–576
7. Cusma JT, Bell MR, Wondrow MA, Taubel JP, Holmes DR. Real time measurement of radiation exposure to patients during diagnostic coronary angiography and percutaneous intererventional procedures. J Am Coll Cardiol 1999;33:427–435
8. Pron G, Bennett J, Common A, et al. Technical results and effects of operator experience on uterine artery embolization for fibroids: the Ontario uterine fibroid embolization trial. J Vasc Interv Radiol 2003;14: 545–554
9. Wagner LK, Archer BR, Cohen AM. Management of patient skin dose in fluoroscopically guided interventional procedures. J Vasc Interv Radiol 2000;11:25–33
10. Brateman L. Radiation safety considerations for diagnostic radiology personnel. Radiographics 1999;19(4):1037–1055
11. Nikolic B, Spies JB, Campbell L, Walsh SM, Ababa S, Lundsten MJ. Uterine artery embolization: reduced radiation with refined technique. J Vasc Interv Radiol 2001;12(1):39–44
12. Nikolic B, Abbara S, Levy E, et al. Influence of radiographic technique and equipment on absorbed ovarian dose associated with uterine artery embolization. J Vasc Interv Radiol 2000;11(9):1173–1178
13. Miller DL, Balter S, Cole PE, et al. Radiation doses in interventional radiology procedures: The RAD-IR Study Part I: Overall measures of dose. J Vasc Interv Radiol 2003;14:711–728
14. Hedgpeth PL, Thurmond AS, Fry R, Schmidgall JR, Rösch J. Radiographic fallopian tube recanalization: absorbed ovarian radiation dose. Radiology 1991;180(1):121–122
15. Wagner LK, Archer BR. Minimizing risks from fluoroscopic x-rays. 2nd ed. Houston, TX: Partners in Radiation Management; 1998.

3 Female Physicians in Interventional Radiology

Meridith Englander

What justifies a chapter in this book about women in interventional radiology? What makes us so special? It is unlikely that anybody has ever been asked to write a chapter entitled "Male Physicians in Interventional Radiology" or that one even needs to be written? Yet one about women seems timely and necessary. Who are we? How did we get here? Where are we going? Only 8% of the people practicing interventional radiology (IR) today are women and only 2% of practicing women radiologists list themselves as interventional radiologists. That is 400 women in the United States.[1] This number is so small that it is quite possible that one practicing female interventionalist may not even know another practicing female interventionalist. What we share in common is that we have all chosen a career that is challenging, exciting, demanding, and very satisfying. We are researchers, clinicians, and teachers. Importantly, we are also daughters, mothers, wives, and partners. So again, why do we need a chapter about women in IR? This chapter was written to give a voice to all of the women in IR and to all women thinking about a career in IR.

When the Society of Cardiovascular and Interventional Radiology (SCVIR) was founded in 1973, there were 57 founding fellows. Three of these individuals were women, including Helen Redman, Ethel Finck, and Renate Soulen. They loved their jobs, yet faced many challenges because of their gender. They were different because they were women in a field dominated by men. In the early days of SCVIR, gender was not a significant issue. Everyone was involved in a revolutionary career, which was defining a new specialty. Therefore, individuals were valued based on their contribution to the field. At home institutions, however, the environment was not as accepting. Male colleagues earned more money for similar work, doctors' bathrooms were for men only, and child care responsibilities were not understood. Despite these challenges, the early female interventionalists had productive careers and subsequently served as important role models for the next generation, including Arina van Breda, who served as the first female president of SCVIR in 1992.

It seems that as a medical specialty, IR is quite accepting of women. This may be due to the unique nature of this field. Just past its infancy, the old boy network within IR is actually not that old. Also, because the current Society of Interventional Radiology (SIR) is small, many women have access to the network of people that are at its center. SIR is relatively blind to a member's gender and in fact, does not track gender on any membership materials. Despite the fact that women attend national society meetings and genuinely feel that they are active contributors to the specialty of interventional radiology, they are still often facing difficulties in the comfort of their own practices.

When trying to understand why there are so few women entering IR, one only has to look at the issues facing women today and wonder why, at this time, issues that should not be issues are issues. Women interventional radiologists face challenges including pregnancy and child rearing, social issues, and occupational issues such as salary inequity, obstacles to promotion, and relationships with patients and staff. Some of these challenges are unique to IR; nevertheless, some are shared by female physicians from many different specialties. In this chapter, I will discuss these challenges and others that may be serving as a barrier to women considering entering the field of IR.

■ Pregnancy Issues

Women get pregnant and men do not. This clear, single fact underlies many of the different work-related issues facing men and women. Childbearing is a woman's responsibility and it is being pregnant, having children, and raising them that create a great deal of gender-related tension in the workplace. During pregnancy, there are many potential threats to a woman and her fetus in the IR suite, including exposures to radiation, chemicals, and blood-borne pathogens. Despite the rumors and misconceptions, the risks to a pregnant interventionalist are minimal and should not prompt a woman with plans for a future pregnancy from avoiding IR as a career.

Radiation Exposure

To put the risk of radiation exposure into perspective, one must first consider the normal background exposure in our environment that all people are exposed to on a regular basis. Radon alone contributes a mean exposure of ~200 millirem (mrem)/year; some areas have considerably higher levels. Cosmic radiation contributes an additional 100 mrem/year. Consumer products including building materials, luminous watches, and smoke detectors contribute ~9 mrem/year. A single cross-country flight from New York to Seattle exposes an individual to 6 mrem.[2,3]

The difference between living in Miami and living in Denver adds ~50 mrem/year. When one considers this normal exposure, it is estimated that the average fetal dose over the course of a pregnancy approaches 75 mrem from these background sources.

Radiation risks fall into two categories: stochastic and nonstochastic. Nonstochastic risks are predictable and include miscarriage, mental retardation, congenital malformations, and growth restriction. The dose threshold for these effects is much higher than 2 rem. This dose is assumed, but there has been no definitive data demonstrating fetal harm at radiation dose levels below 2 rem. The stochastic risks occur unpredictably and later in life. Cancer, and specifically childhood leukemia, is the concerning outcome from fetal radiation exposure. Unfortunately, there are no clear threshold doses for these effects. The U.S. Nuclear Regulatory Commission Regulatory Guide (NRCP) has issued guidelines, setting the limit for occupational exposure to ionizing radiation for pregnant women at 500 mrem for the duration of the pregnancy, with a one monthly equivalent dose of 50 mrem (0.5 millisievert [mSv]).[4]

Table 3.1 is helpful for estimating the additional risk from occupational exposure to radiation. There is an increased probability of malformation or childhood cancer with a significant radiation dose to the fetus. From the data in this table, there is a 4.07% chance of childhood cancer or congenital defect. With radiation exposure, this percentage chance increases to 4.12%, which translates to a risk of 0.05%. Wagner et al[5] considered the above data and offered the opinion that irrational exaggeration of the potential effects of prenatal radiation will significantly alter the contribution that women will make to the radiologic profession, and it could conceivably be used as a basis for reproachable practices of job discrimination. Wagner et al[5] also evaluated the gonadal dose associated with standard radiologic procedures, as outlined in **Table 3.2**. The conceptus dose is assumed to be one-half the gonadal dose based on literature examining computed tomography (CT), which shows internal radiation to be one-half of skin dose. Faulkner et al[6] used phantom data to show that actual fetal dose is about one-half of underapron exposures.

Table 3.1 Risk of Malformation or Cancer from Occupational Exposure to Radiation[5]

Dosage	Chance of No Malformation (%)	Chance of No Cancer (%)	Chance of No Cancer or Malformation (%)
With no dose above background	96.00	99.93	95.93
At 500 mrem	95.99	99.89	95.88

Table 3.2 Gonadal Radiation Dose Associated with Common Interventional Procedures[5]

Procedure	Radiation Exposure
Cardiac catheterization	0.2–10 mrem
Renal angiogram	<0.12 mrem
Cerebral angiogram	0.20 mrem
Venogram	0.33 mrem

Marx et al[7] performed a prospective study looking at radiation exposure in 30 interventional radiologists over a 2-month period. The mean projected yearly dose (PYD) overlead was 49.1 mSv. For radiologists performing more than 1,000 cases per year, this dose increased to 66.6 mSv. The underlead PYD was 0.9 mSv on average. For radiologists wearing 0.5-mm-thick lead, the underlead PYD was 1.3 mSv. For those wearing 1.0-mm-thick lead, the underlead PYD was only 0.4 mSv. When converted to mrem, the average underlead exposure in this population was 40 mrem. This study demonstrates that wearing an extra layer of lead significantly reduces the underapron radiation exposure.

Nikalson et al[8] further evaluated Marx's data in 28 interventional radiologists, looking at the effective dose resulting from exposure to radiation. Their evaluation showed that the mean annual effective dose is 3.16 mSv (316 mrem), far below the NCRP limits. The maximum dose received by one of the study subjects was 10.1 mSv (1010 mrem). Assuming that these evaluations can be projected onto the general population of interventional radiologists, it is clear that radiation doses are generally small. Even so, there are outliers. Individuals should therefore keep careful track of their own exposures, before and during a pregnancy.

Other than monitoring exposure, there are proactive ways to minimize radiation exposure, which are well known to most interventional radiologists. Schueler et al[9] evaluated operator exposure during IR procedures. She found that operator dose is largely a factor of scatter, which increases with input dose and the use of image filters. Patient size is most important as the scatter dose is 2 to 4 times higher with an obese patient. Decreasing the pulse rate directly lowers radiation exposure. The use of undertable skirts and ceiling shields, as well as increasing the distance from the beam decrease operator dose.

Adler et al[10] authored a position article for the American Association of Women Radiologists (AAWR) in 1986. The authors stated that radiation risk for a conceptus is theoretical, but they recommended counseling for all women entering radiology as a profession and that they should be willing to accept the theoretical risks involved in fluoroscopy.

Although shielding is foremost in importance at reducing radiation exposure, the most obvious way for an interventional radiologist to reduce his or her exposure is to limit fluoroscopy time. Fortunately, today's IR practice typically utilizes multiple modalities for imaging guidance. The use of ultrasound and CT guidance essentially eliminates the operator's radiation exposure, and therefore provides pregnant interventional radiologists with many opportunities to limit fluoroscopy time and remain productive.

Methylmethacrylate Exposure

For women performing vertebroplasty and kyphoplasty procedures, methylmethacrylate exposure may be concerning due to its potential harmful effects during pregnancy. Polymethylmethacrylate (PMMA) is a volatile acrylic monomer. It has proven to be toxic to many organ systems of laboratory animals exposed to extremely high doses.

In the early 1970s, Singh et al[11] studied the effects of intraperitoneal exposure of methacrylic acid in gestational rats. These rats showed slightly worse outcomes than those exposed to saline. McLauglin et al[12] exposed pregnant mice to PMMA vapor for 2 hours twice daily from day 6 to day 15 of their pregnancy. No statistically significant difference between the two groups was detected. There was no increase in miscarriage rate or rate of subsequent malformations. Despite these conflicting studies, pregnant women have been virtually banished from operating rooms when PMAA is being mixed and used during surgical procedures. The Occupational Health and Safety Administration (OSHA) has set standards for occupational exposure. For any 8-hour work shift, exposure shall not exceed 100 ppm. Cloft et al[13] measured methylmethacrylate (MMA) vapors in the room during the mixing of 20 mL of PMMA for vertebroplasty procedures. Ten samples were obtained during five procedures and all values were below detectable levels of 4.8 ppm.

Linehan looked at the serum and breast milk concentrations in orthopaedic surgeons after exposure to PMMA during a hip arthroplasty.[14] No serum or breast milk samples demonstrated evidence of methacrylic acid at the 0.5-part-per-million level and no levels were higher than in the control group without immediate PMMA exposure. PMMA is rapidly cleared from blood through the lungs. Despite this, these authors reported the results of a survey of female orthopedic surgeons showed that 38% left the operating room during the cement phase of surgery while pregnant and 16% left while breastfeeding.

So what does this mean to an interventional radiologist? Again, there is a very low risk to a fetus if an interventional radiologist is involved in a vertebroplasty or kyphoplasty procedure during pregnancy.

General Anesthesia Gases Exposure

The gases used in general anesthesia can pose a threat to a pregnant woman who is occupationally exposed. Nitrous oxide is a known teratogen. This is based on studies that have shown a significantly higher rate of miscarriages in operating room nurses as compared with general duty nurses and in anesthesiologists as compared with pediatricians.[15,16]

Today, all anesthesia carts are installed with scavenging devices. These are filters on the outgoing ventilation tube that capture the exhaled anesthetic gases. The result is significantly decreased exposure for personnel in the room. In fact, the levels of toxic anesthetic gases can be brought to essentially nothing. However, there are many factors that undermine the effectiveness of these devices. If the endotracheal tube cuff is not inflated, gases will leak out. This is almost always the case with pediatric patients. In addition, there are a few times during a case when the inflow gases are disconnected from the patient, but the anesthetics are not turned off. This most often happens when the patient is being moved, if the patient needs to be manually ventilated, or when a case has been completed.

Fortunately, exposure to an interventional radiologist working with a general hospital population should be minimal and occasional. To minimize exposures, pregnant women should make sure that the anesthesiologist knows that she is pregnant and does not leave the nitrous oxide on if there is a chance for someone other than the patient to be exposed. Many anesthesiologists will avoid caring for pediatric patients when pregnant. Therefore, when feasible, it may be a good practice for a pregnant interventionalist to avoid general anesthesia cases on pediatric patients.

Blood-borne Pathogen Exposure

Exposure to blood-borne pathogens is a risk that physicians assume every time they work with a needle that is entering or has entered a patient. Human immunodeficiency virus (HIV) and hepatitis B and C viruses (HBV and HCV) are documented to be spread from patient to health care provider through needle sticks. The risk of transmission of HIV from a percutaneous exposure is estimated to be 0.3%. An increased risk is associated with large bore needles, whether the needle had been in a blood vessel, the depth of penetration of the needle, and the patient's viral load. Postexposure prophylaxis is recommended for health care workers exposed to infected or potentially infected patients, with two or three agents for a course of 4 weeks. The most common side effects of these agents include nausea and vomiting, fatigue, and serious drug interactions.

The data regarding the safety of antiretroviral agents used during pregnancy are limited. Some agents are documented teratogens. Others are associated with increased risks of hyperbilirubinemia and renal stones, in the mother and fetus. Neurologic disease and death has been reported in uninfected children whose mothers had taken antiretrovirals to prevent perinatal transmission.[17]

The best protection against HBV is vaccination. This vaccine has been available for years as a series of three or four injections. Antibody titers should be checked to confirm immunity. There is currently no vaccine or postexposure prophylaxis for exposure to HCV. Although most interventionalists have had a needle stick during their careers, the potential implications are often disregarded. It is much more difficult to dismiss a needle stick when pregnant or nursing due to the implications of a possible infection and the possible risks associated with therapy.

■ Social Issues

Are the issues facing women interventionalists different from those facing other female physicians? Jennifer Gould, MD, an interventional radiologist, conducted an informal survey of women interventional radiologists attending the 2007 annual meeting of the SIR. The women responding to the survey represented only a small percentage of all women attending the conference. Nonetheless, this survey showed that women interventional radiologists are not much different than other female physicians. Our demographics are similar. Most of us are married to working men, have children, and practiced medicine while we were pregnant.

Our perceived differences from men are similar. Fortunately, most women did not report discrimination from their partners. But there are perceived differences in the treatment from nursing and technical staff. Referring physicians treat us differently as well. Many women described being repeatedly overlooked by referring physicians wandering through the department looking for an IR to discuss a case with. Women report that they are excluded from the social networking that occurs casually. Male partners tend to be friendlier with their male colleagues. Sharing lunches and playing tennis or golf are subtle things which are not intentionally excluding women, but are effectively keeping them separate.

Surveys of physicians in other specialties show interesting patterns as well. All of these generally lead to the conclusion that male and female physicians are different. A survey of male and female cardiologists from 1998 in many ways mirrors the issues facing women in IR.[18] Fewer women were married (71% versus 90% of men), fewer women had children (64% versus 88% of men), and fewer women had a spouse that provided all child care (8% versus 55% of men). Thirty-nine percent of women (versus 25% of men) felt that their family responsibilities interfered with their ability to accomplish their professional work. Despite this, most women were moderately or very satisfied with their family life. Finally, 70% of women (versus 21% of men) experienced discrimination during their career; 81% of respondents said this was based on gender and 8% said this was based on parenting responsibilities (versus 4% and 1%, respectively, in men).

Similar information has been revealed in surveys of otolaryngologists and plastic surgeons.[19,20] Women ear, nose, and throat (ENT) physicians were more likely to be divorced and had fewer children than their male counterparts. Only 8% of female physicians identified their spouse as having responsibility for running the household compared with 49% of males. Although 89% of men reported that their wives cared for their children's minor illnesses, only 14% of women claimed the same about their husbands. Thirty percent of women (versus 24% of men) believed that their career interfered with their personal life. Thirty-one percent of women said sexual discrimination had hindered career development or advancement. Among the plastic surgeons, fewer women than men were married (65% versus 89%), and fewer women had children (52% versus 86%). Married women were most often married to professionals (82%) whereas only 50% of men's spouses had a professional career. Thirty-four percent of men were married to homemakers. Forty-three percent of women and 22% of men reported that their career had been slowed or markedly slowed by having children. Eighty-nine percent of women (versus 27% of men) experienced gender discrimination or sexual harassment at some point during training or practice.

Based on these studies, performed across many specialties, the demographic information summarizing female physicians are similar. Women are married less often than men, have fewer children and have children later than men, and have greater responsibility for child care than men. This may be the result of choice, but it may also be the result of circumstances facing female physicians. Encouragingly, having children is not a predictor of work burnout. Indeed, some psychologists think that having multiple roles helps to mitigate against stress. Crosby wrote of the unexpected advantages of balancing career and family.[21] She found that women were able to juggle their many responsibilities successfully, while thriving professionally and having a happy home life.

■ Occupational Issues

Physical Hurdles

During the preparation of this chapter, my partners were asked if they could suggest some issues that they thought were faced by women in IR. Some thought that the lead apron was so heavy that women must have back problems from wearing it. But actually, a woman's lead apron weighs less because it tends to be smaller. At the present time, there is no medical literature reporting an increased incidence of back problems in women interventional radiologists than in men. Personally, I have found that the Autofill syringes (Vascular Solutions, Minneapolis, MN) are bulky for my hands, but otherwise I have not had problems using any equipment. It was suggested that it might be a problem for a short woman to scrub in with a taller man. That might have been a problem during my residency and fellowship, but as an attending, that problem belongs to whoever is scrubbing in with me.

Inequity in Salary and Promotions

A review of the literature discussing physician salary is at the very least eye-opening. Weeks and Wallace compiled data from the American Medical Association (AMA).[22–25] When adjusted for physician work effort, provider characteristics, and practice characteristics, there are startling trends seen across many fields of medicine, including radiology. Women earn considerably less then men. A sample of this data is presented in **Table 3.3**. These trends have been reinforced by the research of others as well. Grandis et al[19] reported that female ENTs earned 15 to 20% less when controlled for type of practice, years in practice, and hours worked in the operating room. Female psychiatrists' incomes were 33% less than the incomes of their male counterparts when adjusted for work setting, hours worked, and patient load.[26]

A review of this topic in the *Annals of Internal Medicine*[27] demonstrates that even when adjusted for specialty, hours worked, productivity, and achievement (number of publications), women earned significantly less money than men did. This salary differential increased as seniority increased. Women were also less likely to reach the highest ranks of department chair and dean. Despite women sacrificing earning power for greater work flexibility, women still earn less when the numbers are adjusted.

Women are also not promoted at the same rate as men. In a cohort analysis, women and men appointed to faculty position in 1980 were tracked for 11 years. Eighty-three percent of men and 59% of women had achieved the title of professor or associate professor; 23% of men and only 5% of women were a full professor. This is despite the fact that women and men had the same board certifications, advanced degrees, and research during fellowship training. Women were less likely to have office or laboratory space, protected time for research or to have begun their careers with grant support. Women worked ~10% fewer hours a week than men, but even when adjusted for this, they were substantially less likely to be promoted.[28]

Table 3.3 Salary Differences Between Male and Female Physicians[21–25]

	Actual Average Salary Difference between Men and Women	Percentage (%) Difference between Men's and Women's Actual Salary
Radiology	$80,090	23
General surgery	$63,856	21
Obstetrics-gynecology	$47,409	16
Internal medicine	$36,609	19

In an editorial remark on these findings, Laine and Turner believe that this data are due to the fact that women are poor negotiators at determining compensation and promotions.[29] Women are less likely to initiate salary negotiations and more likely to accept whatever their employer offered. They concluded that women need to develop negotiation skills and learn how to advocate for themselves. Yet they even hypothesize that there may be an element of blatant sexism. Everyone has heard the story that women do not need to earn as much as men because they often belong to two-income families. Therefore, compensation should therefore be less of a concern for women than for their male colleagues who are often the sole breadwinners for their families. Clearly, this type of thinking still serves as a barrier to many women when it comes to salary equity.

The American Association of Medical Colleges (AAMC) investigated barriers to the advancement of women in academic medicine.[30] A survey of department chairs acknowledged barriers to the advancement of women including the constraints of traditional gender roles, manifestations of sexism in the medical environment and lack of effective mentors. Women chairs also felt that men did not respond well to women in positions of power. They reported a lack of recognition, inappropriate attention paid to them, resistance in reporting to them, and constraints on their leadership and decision-making styles. Women are perceived as not being tough enough for positions of power, but when they exhibit power, they are perceived as being a "bitch."

Is this applicable to radiology? Radiologists responding to a 1986 survey about women in radiology noted that although female diagnostic radiologists felt that they could function in any practice, their male counterparts stated that women were better for general radiology.[31] Only 26% of respondents saw women as completely equal and would encourage women to enter radiology. The authors concluded that "women are viewed as valuable colleagues in radiology but often not as true equals." They further hypothesized that men who perceived a threat from women might respond differently if they had greater contact with women in the field. This survey is now over 20 years old, but many of these issues still seem relevant today.

Job Satisfaction

It has been shown in recent years that women are not entering radiology in greater numbers than they have in the past. Over the past 10 years, the number of women in radiology residency slots has remained relatively stable at 23 to 27%.[32] Women who choose radiology for specialty training cite "the intellectual challenge" and "their talent for the skill characteristics of the specialty." Women are actually less likely to use life-style, work hours, call hours, or salary as reasons for choosing a specialty.[33] The influence that women in a medical specialty have on other women considering entering that specialty is significant. When looking at women entering surgery, a correlation has been found between the numbers of women entering the field of surgery to the number of women on the surgical faculty at their medical school. If the number of women in practice stays constant, it can be expected that the number of applicants will also remain constant.

Are there other factors influencing women away from radiology? Ewa Kuligowski, MD, a past president of the American Association of Women Radiologists believes that women are underrepresented in radiology because there is a misperception about the role of radiologists in the care of patients. As a general rule, women in medicine tend to strive for the feeling of being able to make a difference in the lives of their patients. They think that radiologists are in the background. Unfortunately, most medical students are not typically exposed to patient interaction in radiology, especially in the subspecialties such as ultrasound and IR.[34]

In a survey by Frank et al[35] women radiologists believe that they have less control, work too much, and have more stress at work compared to female physicians in other specialties. It is possible that this dissatisfaction is being transmitted to interested medical students as they are exposed to radiology during the course of their training. If the women in field are not happy, why would a prospective applicant be happy?

Women who report a high degree of work satisfaction tend to have a high degree of control of their daily work.[36] Female pediatric surgeons surveyed have confirmed this.[37] It is when we feel that our lives are out of our control that we feel stress.

Given this, women in IR are uniquely positioned among other radiologists. As the practice of an interventional radiologist becomes more clinically oriented, there is greater control of our patients and our case load. The days of waiting for referring physicians to send the patients are over. Although this model of practice comes with new pressures, the control that interventional radiologists now have over their practice has the potential to improve levels of job satisfaction.

Sexual Harassment

Unfortunately, sexual harassment needs to be mentioned as an issue in today's world. In a survey of 4501 women physicians, 48% reported gender-based harassment at some point in their career; 37% specifically reported sexual harassement.[38] In radiology, harassment is seen at all levels: medical school, training, and in practice. Harassment is associated with fatigue, depression, anger, fear, alienation, and vulnerability. Women who felt that they had less control of their work environment and are dissatisfied with their career choice are more likely to report gender-based harassment. Harassment may cause feelings of helplessness, worthlessness, and guilt.

Radiologists were somewhat more likely to report gender-based discrimination while in medical school and postgraduate training. In addition, they were more likely to report sexual harassment while in practice than were other women physicians. Forty-eight percent of all women physicians and 54% of women radiologists reported gender-based harassment. Thirty-seven percent of all physicians and 45% of radiologists reported sexual harassment. This is not a problem in medicine that is unique to physicians. Fifty-four percent of nurses responding to a survey felt they had been sexually harassed during their career.[39]

How can we overcome this? It is unrealistic to think it will go away as our numbers increase. Sexual harassment is about power, and not so much about sex. As long as there is a hierarchy in medicine, this will be an issue. However, it doesn't have to be tolerated. Institutions and practices need to be firm with a no tolerance policy. Women physicians must support each other to move toward optimizing the work environment for women.

Staff Relationships

Within the specialty of IR, the relationship between a physician and the nurses and technologists is always an important component of day-to-day life in an IR suite. There is no doubt that a good working relationship with the staff in the suites makes life much easier. Is it harder for a woman interventional radiologist to have a good relationship with nurses and technologists?

Gjerberg et al[40] studied the doctor–nurse relationship in Norway. The doctor–nurse relationship has historically been a male–female interaction. There are expectations about gender roles that male doctors and female nurses easily and comfortably satisfy. The dilemma for those interacting with a woman physician is having to choose between treating her primarily as "a member of the medical profession" or as "a woman." The female physician must also try to fulfill the expectations of being both "a doctor" and "a woman." In surveys of male and female physicians, there is a clear difference. Male doctors said that female nurses act differently toward female doctors in respect and confidence and in the degree of assistance they offer in practical situations. Nurses provided less help and assistance to female physicians and questioned medical decisions made by women physicians. This lessened as female physicians gained seniority. The authors hypothesized about the causes of these differences. They questioned whether female nurses were trying to minimize the status differences between them and female physicians. It is also possible that female physicians have a hard time giving clear orders. Some female doctors may leave supportive work to the nurses as a strategy to separate the relationship between the two, and to confirm the doctor's autonomy. There is also the element of sexual tension and flirtation that may make helping a male physician more exciting than helping a female. Flirting and the sexualization of the doctor–nurse relationship have often been regarded as improving working relations.

Is it possible for a woman interventional radiologist to overcome these obstacles and have good and productive working relationships in the suites? Often, women will establish friendships with the nurses and technologists. Other women will try and carry out support tasks themselves (such as setting trays, cleaning up after cases, etc.) to help foster relationships in the suites by minimizing conflict and creating a collaborative work environment. There are also women who will clearly define their authority and demand respect from the support staff in the interventional suites without attempting to make friends with the support staff. Despite our similarities, we are different, after all.

■ The Effect of Mentoring

In a review of the literature using the keyword, mentor, Sambunjak et al[41] found that mentors are important in choosing a career, staying in academic medicine, and in research. Medical students, residents, and attending staff identified having a mentor as a positive experience that was important in specialty choice, promotions, and research grant success. Not having a mentor might even be a barrier to promotion and a serious obstacle to a successful academic career. It is clear that mentors are needed to optimize the professional socialization process.

In a survey of cardiologists, 70% of respondents reported having a mentor.[18] Mentors were listed as being important for providing introductions in the field, promoting participation in research, career encouragement, and acting as a career and noncareer role model. Women in particular found mentors to be helpful for job placement, but less helpful for career planning. In this survey, only 14% of women's mentors were women. The fact is that most mentors are men. Having a mentor of the same sex is not necessarily important; 80% of women faculty surveyed did not think so. However, 41% of female residents surveyed thought that a same sex mentor would be more understanding. In addition, it has been found that some men have difficulty effectively mentoring women and ethnic minorities. The most important thing, however, is having a mentor. This relationship provides the social capital and essential information to advance a career. When lacking, it can result in isolation and a reluctance to pursue professional goals.

At Johns Hopkins (Baltimore, MD), multiple interventions to encourage career development in its female faculty were able to increase the number of women at the associate professor level by 550% over 5 years. Their program reassessed retention, promotion, mentoring, and salary equity policies. Strategies to decrease isolation and integrate women into the scientific community were successful.[42]

This data all leads to one conclusion. Mentoring is important. It is important to the field of medicine: strong mentors build strong practitioners and researchers. It is just as important for an individual choosing a career and maintaining a successful career. It is impossible to expect to attract women to a specialty if they feel unwelcome or ill at ease. For this reason, women with successful careers in IR will help to increase the amount of women entering this specialty in the future because of the opportunity to identify role models and build relationships with mentors of the same gender.

Most people are comfortable in acknowledging that women are different than men; therefore, women physicians are different from male physicians. An interesting question to ask, however, is whether these differences give women an advantage in performing their job as a physician. The differences between men and women probably do not give one group an advantage over another, but they do give us a different perspective. For example, women communicate in a more democratic style, using collaboration with their patients. This can enhance patient compliance and satisfaction. A woman's leadership style is also more collaborative, encouraging a team approach. Although this has been alluded to negatively, in a small office, this can potentially empower staff and encourage effectiveness.[43]

The differences can also manifest themselves in patient preferences when it comes to choosing a physician. Do patients prefer female physicians? In some settings, the answer is yes. It has been shown that women prefer female endoscopists.[44] Similarly for urology, infertility/gynecology, and colorectal issues, patients prefer a physician of the same gender.[45] Patients prefer a physician of the same gender when undergoing procedures that are perceived as more intimate in nature.[46] This obviously creates a niche for the female interventional radiologist. There are many procedures, many of which are discussed in later chapters within this book, which can be considered intimate, including uterine fibroid intervention, fallopian tube recanalization or occlusion, ovarian vein embolization, and treatment of varicose veins. Women patients may seek out female physicians to perform these interventions. However, women do not blindly choose their physicians based solely on their gender. Physician bedside manner, hospital affiliation, and recommendations from physicians or friends are also important to women in choosing a physician.[47]

In the future, it is certainly possible and perhaps likely that the old-boys network can and will become the old-girls network. There are plenty of female referring physicians out there who would love to send their patients to other female physicians, especially one who is skilled in the minimally invasive procedures inherent to our specialty. However, this may be harder to capitalize on for a woman. We tend not to get together to play golf or tennis or cards and we do not go to the gym as often as men. These are the places where a lot of informal networking occurs. As women, we have to use the opportunities available to us. We should not be bashful about promoting the good work that we do. Even when sharing a quick cup of coffee with a colleague, time together with other female physicians should be used wisely to encourage referrals. Women doctors often get together at the pool, at the spa, at school functions, and even at soccer games. All of these are great times to let others know what you do. Women tend to shy away from these opportunities, but we cannot and we should not.

■ Conclusions

In 1998, Joan Cassell,[48] a sociologist, wrote a book about female surgeons. She interviewed and shadowed numerous women and concluded that female surgeons should unite. By uniting, they would be able to share knowledge concerning how they have balanced their careers and family, how they have dealt with difficult colleagues, and how they have addressed the challenges they have faced in developing their practices. This would make approaching these situations less stressful to a female surgeon entering the profession because there is comfort in knowing that others have common experiences. She quoted Benjamin Franklin by saying, "we must hang together, or assuredly we will all hang separately."

The same can be said for women interventional radiologists. As our numbers grow, it will become increasingly important to continue raising and discussing the unique issues facing us as a group. Creating a forum for these discussions and for developing strategies to address these issues will be integral to both attracting more women into the specialty of IR and for preserving the level of job satisfaction presently experienced by female interventionalists. There is strength in unity.

In conclusion, women interventionalists are a diverse group. As individuals, we have different skills and interests. Yet, we are united by our gender. That our patients expect quality care and our undivided attention, our families expect our time, and our partners expect our commitment also unite us. With these demands, it can be easy to feel overwhelmed. Yet we thrive. Our many roles are our strength. We have selected a profession that is exciting and rewarding. We are the lucky ones.

References

1. Lewis RS, Bhargavan M, Sunshine JH. Women radiologists in the United States: results from the American college of radiology's 2003 survey. Radiology 2007;242(3):802–810
2. U.S. Nuclear Regulatory Commission Regulatory Guide 8.29 rev.1. Washington, DC: U.S. Nuclear Regulatory Commission; 1996
3. Barish RJ. In-flight radiation exposure during pregnancy. Obstet Gynecol 2004;103(6):1326–1330
4. U.S. Nuclear Regulatory Commission Regulatory Guide 8.13 rev. 3. Washington, DC: U.S. Nuclear Regulatory Commission; 1999
5. Wagner LK, Hayman LA. Pregnancy and women radiologists. Radiology 1982;145:559–562
6. Faulkner K, Marshall NW. Personal monitoring of pregnant staff in diagnostic radiology. J Radiol Prot 1993;13(4):259–265
7. Marx MV, Niklason L, Mauger EA. Occupational radiation exposure to interventional radiologists: a prospective study. J Vasc Interv Radiol 1992;3(4):597–606
8. Niklason LT, Marx MV, Chan HP. Interventional radiologists: occupational radiation doses and risks. Radiology 1993;187:729–733
9. Schueler BA, Vrieze TJ, Bjarnason H, et al. An investigation of operator exposure in interventional radiology. Radiographics 2006;26:1533–1541
10. Adler YT, Fernbach SK, Hayman LA, Redman HC, Rumack C. The impact of maternity on radiologists: the AAWR position and its acceptance by women. AJR Am J Roentgenol 1986;146:415–417
11. Singh AR, Lawrence WH, Autian J. Embryonic-fetal toxicity and teratogenic effects of a group of methacrylate esters in rats. J Dent Res 1972;51:1632–1638
12. McLaughlin RE, Reger SI, Barkalow JA, Allen MS, Dafazio CA. Methylmethacrylate: a study of teratogenicity and fetal toxicity of the vapor in the mouse. J Bone Joint Surg Am 1978;60:355–358
13. Cloft HJ, Easton DN, Jensen ME, et al. Exposure of medical personnel to methylmethacrylate vapor during percutaneous vertebroplasy. AJNR Am J Neuroradiol 1999;20:352–353
14. Linehan CM, Gioe TJ. Serum and breast milk levels of methymethacrylate following surgeon exposure during arthroplasty. J Bone Joint Surg Am 2006;88:1957–1961
15. Cohen EN, Bellville JW, Brown BW. Anesthesia, pregnancy, and miscarriage: a study of operating room nurses and anesthetists. Anesthesiology 1971;35(4):343–437
16. Spence AA, Cohen EN, Brown BW Jr, Knill-Jones RP, Himmelberger DU. Occupational hazards for operating room-based physicians. Analysis of data from the United States and the United Kingdom. JAMA 1977;238(9):955–959
17. US Public Health Service. Updated U.S. Public Health Service. Guidelines for the Management of Occupational Exposures to HIV and Recommendations for Postexposure Prophylaxis. MMWR Morb Mortal Wkly Rep 2005;54:1–52

18. Limacher MC, Zaher CA, Walsh MN, et al. The ACC professional life survey: career decisions of women and men in cardiology. A report of the Committee on Women in Cardiology. J Am Coll Cardiol 1998;32:827–835
19. Grandis JR, Gooding WE, Zamboni BA, et al. The gender gap in a surgical subspecialty. Arch Otolaryngol Head Neck Surg 2004;130:695–702
20. Capek L, Edwards D, Mackinnon S. Plastic surgeons: a gender comparison. Plast Reconstr Surg 1997;99(2):289–299
21. Crosby FJ. Juggling. New York: The Free Press;1991
22. Weeks WB, Wallace AE. Race and gender differences in general internists' annual incomes. J Gen Intern Med 2006;21:1167–1171
23. Weeks WB, Wallace AE. Association of race and gender with general surgeons' annual incomes. J Am Coll Surg 2006;203:558–567
24. Weeks WB, Wallace AE. The influence of physician race and gender on obstetrician-gynecologists's annual income. Obstet Gynecol 2006;108:603–611
25. Weeks WB, Wallace AE. Gender differences in diagnostic radiologists' annual incomes. Acad Radiol 2006;13(10):1266–1273
26. Dial TH, Grimes PE. Sex differences in psychiatrists' practice patterns and incomes. Am J Psychiatry 1994;151:96–101
27. Ash AS, Carr PL, Goldstein R, et al. Compensation and advancement of women in academic medicine: is there equity? Ann Intern Med 2004;141:205–212
28. Laine C, Turner BJ. Unequal pay for equal work: the gender gap in academic medicine. Ann Intern Med 2004;141:238–240
29. Tesch BJ, Wood HM, Helwig AL, et al. Promotion of women physicians in academic medicine. Glass ceiling or sticky floor? JAMA 1995;273(13):1022–1025
30. Bickel J, Wara D, Atkinson BF, et al. Increasing women's leadership in academic medicine: Report of the AAMC Project Implementation Committee. Acad Med 2002;77(10):1043–1061
31. Martin CA, Wooding JH. Attitudes toward women in radiology. J Am Med Womens Assoc 1986;41:50–53
32. Baker SR, Barry M, Chaudhry H, et al. Women as radiologists: are there barriers to entry and advancement? J Appl Commun Res 2006;3:131–134
33. Potterton VK, Ruan S, Sunshine JH, et al. Why don't female medical students choose diagnostic radiology? A review of the current literature. J Appl Commun Res 2004;1:583–590
34. Kuhar J. Searching for the garden of equality. RT Image 2004;17(22)
35. Frank E, Vydareny K. Characteristics of women radiologists in the United States. AJR Am J Roentgenol 1999;173:531–536
36. McMurray JE, Linzer M. The work lives of women physicians. Results from the physician work life study. J Gen Intern Med 2000;15:372–380
37. Caniano DA, Soccino RE, Paolo AM. Keys to career satisfaction: insights from a survey of women pediatric surgeons. J Pediatr Surg 2004;39:984–990
38. Frank E, Brogan D, Schiffman M. Prevalence and correlates of harassment among US women physicians. Arch Intern Med 1998;158:352–358
39. Fiedler A, Hambry F. Sexual harassment in the workplace. Nurse's perceptions. J Nursing Admin 2000;30(10):497–503
40. Gjerberg E, Kjolsrod L. The doctor-nurse relationship: how easy is it to be a female doctor co-operating with a female nurse? Soc Sci Med 2001;52:189–202
41. Sambunjak D, Straus SE, Marusic A. Mentoring in academic medicine. A systematic review. JAMA 2006;296:1103–1115
42. Fried LP, Francomano CA, MacDonald SM, et al. Career development for women in academic medicine: multiple interventions in a department of medicine. JAMA 1996;276:898–905
43. Levinson W, Lurie N. When most doctors are women: what lies ahead? Ann Intern Med 2004;141:471–474
44. Menees SB, Inadomi J, Korsnes S, et al. Women patients' preference for women physicians is a barrier to colon cancer screening. Gastrointest Endosc 2005;62(2):219–223
45. Barden LS, Teutsch CB, Barden RS. The role of gender in patient preferences and satisfaction with the patient-physician relationship. J Am Med Womens Assoc 2000;55(1):39
46. Kerssens JJ, Bensing JM, Andela MG. Patient preferences for genders of health professionals. Soc Sci Med 1997;44(10):1531–1540
47. Plunkett BA, Kohli P, Milad MP. The importance of physician gender in the selection of an obstetrician or a gynecologist. Am J Obstet Gynecol 2002;186:926–928
48. Cassell J. The woman in the surgeon's body. Cambridge, MA: Harvard University Press;1998

II Uterine Interventions

4 Clinical Review: Uterine Leiomyomas

Richard Shlansky-Goldberg, Mark Rosen, and Ann Honebrink

The term fibroids was introduced by Karl von Rokitansky in 1860 and M. M. Klob in 1863.[1] Virchow demonstrated that these neoplasms were derived from smooth cells and introduced the word *myoma*.[1] These benign neoplasms are composed of smooth muscle cells arranged in a whorl-like pattern with a variable amount of collagen, extracellular matrix, and fibrous tissue. They are the most common gynecologic tumor. Leiomyomata are also known as myomas, fibroids, fibromyomas, leiomyofibromas, and fibroleiomyomas.[2] The term fibroid is used based on the fibrous tissue demonstrated in these tumors along with the smooth muscle tissue.[2] Clinical studies of women during their reproductive age demonstrate a prevalence of 20 to 25%.[3] The prevalence is three to nine times higher in black women as compared with white women.[4] The data are not as available for other groups, but the rates are similar in white, Hispanic, and Asian women.[4] Twenty to fifty percent of uterine leiomyomas are thought to produce symptoms.[5–7] Leiomyomas may develop in multiple locations (**Fig. 4.1**). The severity of symptoms depends on the number, size, and location of these benign tumors.[5–7]

It is difficult to predict the biological behavior of uterine smooth muscle tumors. Myomas appear to arise from a single myometrial cell mutation and are often described as clonal.[8,9] The vast majority of these neoplasms follow a benign course, but a small number will behave aggressively, exemplified by metastatic disease or recurrence after surgery. Patients after myomectomy have demonstrated a 10-year clinical recurrence rate of 27% using life-table analysis.[10] One concern is that if there is rapid growth, there may be an increased risk for malignancy. More recent studies have shown that even with rapid growth, the chance of developing a malignancy in preexisting fibroids remains very low.[3,11] The incidence of leiomyosarcoma is

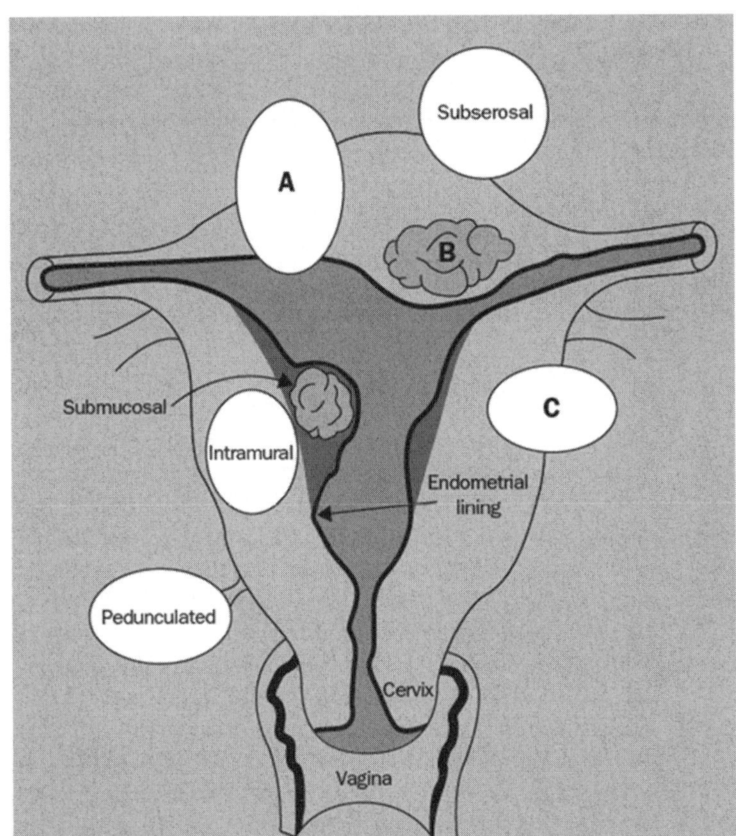

Fig. 4.1 Leiomyomas may be located in multiple different locations within the uterus. Submucosal leiomyomas extend into the cavity, intramural leiomyomas are contained within the wall of the uterus, and subserosal leiomyomas extend from the uterus surface. Most leiomyomas are mixed such as A, B, and C. Leiomyomas in position A are transmural extending from the submucosa into the serosa. Pedunculated submucosal leiomyomas are intracavitary. (From Stewart EA. Uterine fibroids. Lancet 2004;357:293–298. Reprinted with permission.)

estimated to be 0.23% in premenopausal women and peaks at <2% in postmenopausal women.[12]

The genetic differences between leiomyomas and sarcomas suggest that they develop from different origins and that sarcomas do not result from malignant degeneration of an existing leiomyoma.[13] Benign and malignant uterine smooth muscle tumors are cytogenetically distinct.[14] More than half of leiomyomas have no discernible karyotypic abnormalities on conventional cytogenetic analysis. With the remainder of these benign tumors having simple karyotypes that have been characterized into, at least, six cytogenetic subgroups, suggesting that multiple genes and mechanisms are involved in the development of these tumors.[14] In contrast, leiomyosarcomas have frequent structural and numerous chromosomal abnormalities and karyotypes vary widely among metaphase cells.[15]

A majority of classification schemes prognosticates the biological behavior of a myoma and relies on mitotic behavior.[16] In 1970, Kempson and Bari[17] developed a scheme on nuclear atypia and mitotic rate. Although other markers have been evaluated, these seem like the two that are the most useful criteria to establish the aggressiveness of the tumor.[16] There are unusual forms of leiomyomas that have both malignant and benign features. These include benign metastasizing leiomyomas (BML), which is characterized by leiomyoma-like lesions in the lungs or abdomen in patients with uterine leiomyomas (**Fig. 4.2**). Lymphangioleiomyomatosis, similar to BML, has a characteristic lung lesion that originates from benign renal angiomyolipomas.[18] Intravenous leiomyomatosis are hormonally responsive lesions that have vermiform extensions from the uterus, which may extend to the heart but do not metastasize.[19]

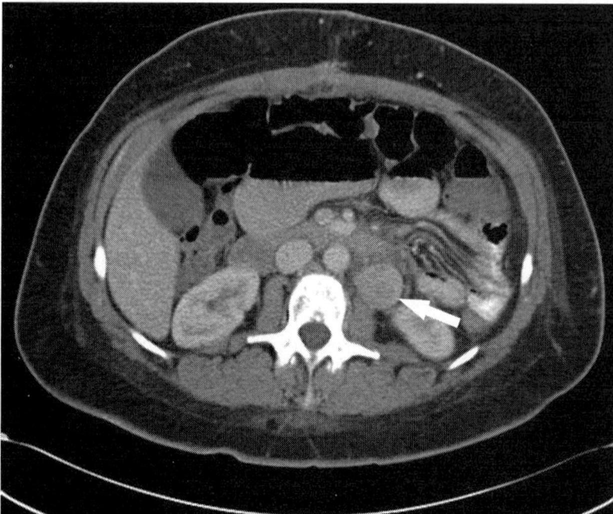

Fig. 4.2 Benign metastasizing leiomyoma. A forty-one year-old woman with prior hysterectomy for leiomyomata, presenting with multiple retroperitoneal masses. Computed tomography (CT) scan at the level of the lower kidneys demonstrates a round uniformly enhancing mass in the paraaortic region (*arrow*). On biopsy, pathology demonstrated benign metastasizing leiomyoma. Remaining mass was stable at 6-month follow-up imaging.

■ Racial Demographics and Risk Factors

Investigating the racial differences in the incidence of leiomyomas, Kjerulff et al[20] reviewed the hysterectomy data for noncancerous diseases for 409 black and 836 white women in 28 hospitals in Maryland. They found that 89% of the black women, compared with only 59% of white women, had leiomyomas. The black women had larger and more numerous leiomyomas. They were also more symptomatic, despite being diagnosed at an earlier age than whites. In reviewing the risks of uterine leiomyomas in black women, Wise et al[25] found the presence of leiomyomas were inversely associated with age at menarche, parity, and age at first birth, and positively associated with years since last birth. Increased weight or obesity appeared to attenuate the inverse association between parity and uterine leiomyomas. In general, greater parity decreases the risk of developing leiomyomas.[21,22]

The use of oral contraceptives in patients with leiomyomas has been controversial in the past. Initially, oral contraceptive therapy was felt to be contraindicated because it was thought that it might stimulate the tumors resulting in an increase in size and numbers. Recent data suggests that oral contraceptives may protect against leiomyoma formation.[22-24] Ross et al[22] reported a 31% risk reduction in women who had used oral contraceptives for more than 10 years. Some investigators did demonstrate an increase in risk associated with the use of oral contraceptive. Marshall et al[4] demonstrated that, when used between the ages of 13 to 16, there was an increased risk of leiomyoma formation. Wise et al[25] found an inverse relationship with progestin-only pills when compared with no hormone use and no other consistent patterns of increased growth for other forms of hormonal control. Lower dose oral contraceptives are commonly used currently to treat the heavy bleeding that is often associated with fibroids.

Other environmental factors may impact the risk of developing leiomyomas. Smoking has been associated with decreasing the risk of developing leiomyomas.[21,22] Consumption of beef and ham has been shown to increase the risk whereas eating green vegetables may decrease the risk.[26] Wise and colleagues[25] demonstrated an increased risk for women consuming alcohol, but no increase seen in cigarette smokers or caffeine drinkers. There is no evidence that changing dietary habits impacts the growth of fibroids once diagnosed or the risk of developing symptoms.[27]

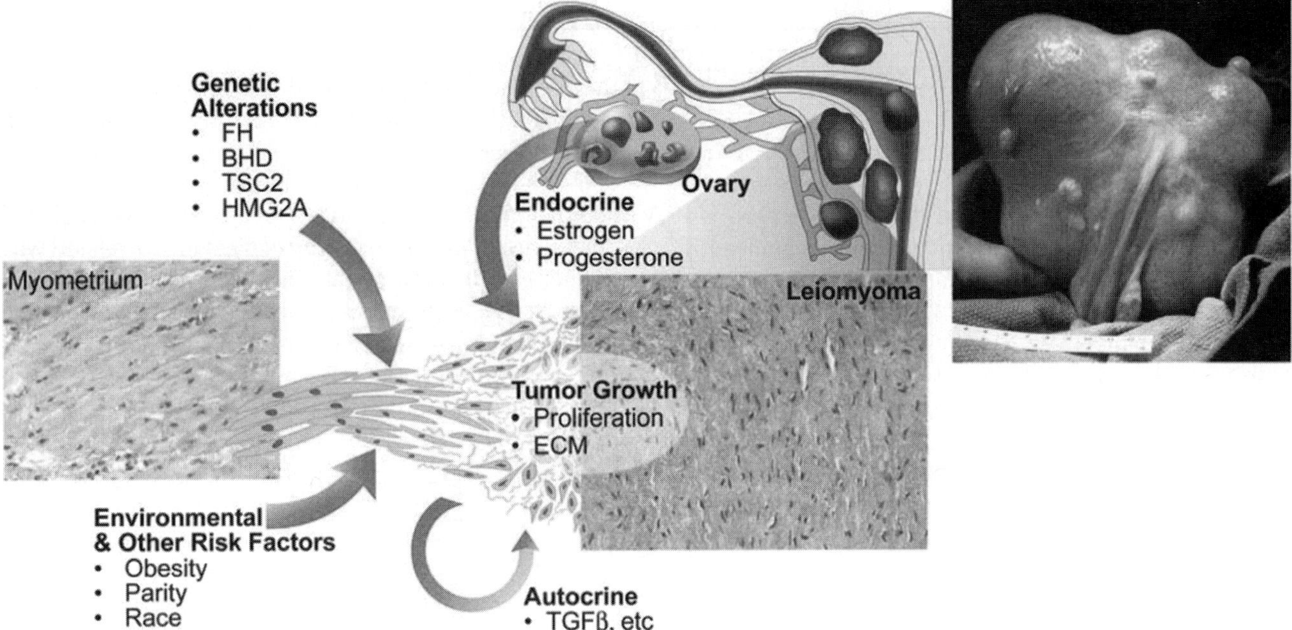

Fig. 4.3 The development of uterine leiomyomas is variable in their natural history and etiology. Hereditary genetic defects in several genes (fumarate hydratase (FH); Birt–Hogg–Dubé syndrome (BHD), and tuberous sclerosis 2 (TSC2), as well as somatic changes in the high mobility group AT-hook 2 (HMGA2) genes and risk factors such as obesity, parity, and race participate in the development of leiomyomas. Tumor growth takes place due to an increase in number of cells and extracellular matrix and is influenced by endocrine and autocrine growth factors. (From Walker CL, Stewart EA. Uterine fibroids: the elephant in the room. Science 2005; 308:1589–1592. Reprinted with permission from AAAS.)

■ Genetics

Historically, leiomyomas have not been considered a genetic disorder; however, clinical evidence suggests that there may be some genetic component in their etiology.[28] Having a first-degree relative with the disease increases the risk of an individual developing leiomyomas and identical twins have a higher concordance than fraternal twins.[29–31] Also, patients with the autosomal dominant disease, hereditary leiomyomatosis, and renal cell carcinoma have genetic defects in the fumarate hydratase (FH) gene, which may be involved in the development of these tumors.[32,33] Approximately 40% of leiomyomas have an abnormal karyotype with some consistent patterns suggesting that the genetic abnormality may be located in these disrupted regions.[8,34,35] Other genes include the tuberous sclerosis 2 (TSC2) gene and the Birt–Hogg–Dube syndrome (BHD) gene due to the increase in leiomyomas in these patients.[28] The HMGI-C gene, now called the high mobility group AT-hook 2 (HMGA2) gene, was the first gene identified in chromosomal rearrangements in the development of uterine leiomyomas.[36] Potentially, the recognition of different phenotypes and genotypes of specific leiomyomas may have an impact on deciding what therapy to offer patients, if risks such as sarcoma or recurrence can be seen to be associated with specific genetic findings.[28]

■ Pathophysiology

The risk factors associated with leiomyomas are important through their contribution to the initiation or promotion of tumorigenesis. As mentioned above, genetics play an important role. Estrogen and progesterone act as important promoters of uterine leiomyoma growth.[37] This is substantiated by the fact that fibroids have not been reported in girls prior to puberty. Most women are diagnosed in their 30s and 40s when their symptoms begin or when fibroids are found incidentally during a routine pelvic exam.[27] Estrogen upregulates both the estrogen and progesterone receptors in leiomyomas during the follicular phase of the menstrual cycle, followed by progesterone-induced mitogenesis during the luteal phase.[37] In addition, several growth factors are involved in the development of these tumors including transforming growth factor beta (TGF-β), basic fibroblastic growth factor (bFGF), epidermal growth factor (EGF), platelet-derived growth factor (PDGF), vascular endothelial growth factor (VEGF), and insulin-like growth factor (IGF).[37] TGF-β and bFGF may be partiality important given their combined mitogenic effect and promotion of extracellular matrix.[37] EGF and TGF-β3 are important factors because both have elevated expression during the luteal phase when leiomyoma mitotic activity is greatest. IGF-I has a potent mitogenic effect because both the peptide and its receptors are overexpressed in leiomyomas.[37] A summary of the multiple factors involved in the development of leiomyomas can be seen in **Fig. 4.3**.

■ Symptoms

Most patients with leiomyomas are asymptomatic. When symptoms occur, they are variable, but generally the published data on health-related quality of life (HRQOL) associated with uterine leiomyomas report significantly lower HRQOL scores for women with leiomyomas than for women without this disorder.[38] In addition, the health care costs for patients with symptomatic leiomyomas are almost four times higher than those who do not have leiomyomas.[39] Symptoms include bleeding, infertility, pain, pressure, urinary frequency, and constipation. As previously mentioned, the degree of symptoms is influenced by the location, size, and number of leiomyomas. In a literature review by Buttram and Reiter, [3] in 1698 patients prior to myomectomy, the incidence of menorrhagia and pain was 30% and 34%, respectively. In a more recent study of patients undergoing uterine artery embolization by Myers et al, the distribution of the predominant symptoms of bleeding, pain, and bulk related was 64.7%, 10.5%, and 23.3%, respectively.[40]

Several causes of bleeding due to leiomyoma have been suggested. The severity of bleeding may be impacted by the presence of submucosal leiomyomas; the incidence of bleeding is not dependant on this location.[3] Sehgal and Haskins[41] suggested that the surface area of the endometrium is increased by the presence of submucosal leiomyomas, which provides a greater area to bleed. They demonstrated that the severity of bleeding correlated with the increase in surface area. This hypothesis does not explain the cause of increased bleeding in patients with intramural or subserosal leiomyomas.[3] Another mechanism that may explain the cause of bleeding is that leiomyomas may interfere with uterine contraction, which is thought to play a role in the regulation of bleeding.[42,43] This theory has not been proven.[3] The theory that may best explain the mechanism for bleeding involves the changes in venous structures in the endometrium and myometrium causing venule ectasia.[44] This concept was originally described by Sampson in 1912[45] and supported by Faulkner[42] in 1945. Later, light microscopy studies by Farrer-Brown et al demonstrated the venous ectasia.[43,46] The original concept was that the leiomyomas compress the venous drainage resulting in the ectasia (**Fig. 4.4**).[3] Current data suggests that the venous ectasia is due to vasoactive growth factors such as bFGF and VEGF.[44] These studies also implicate arterial

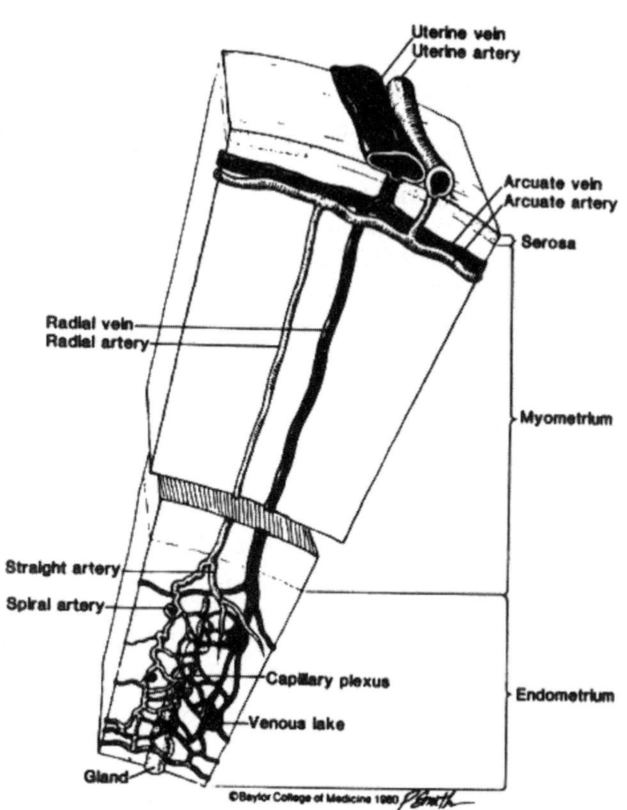

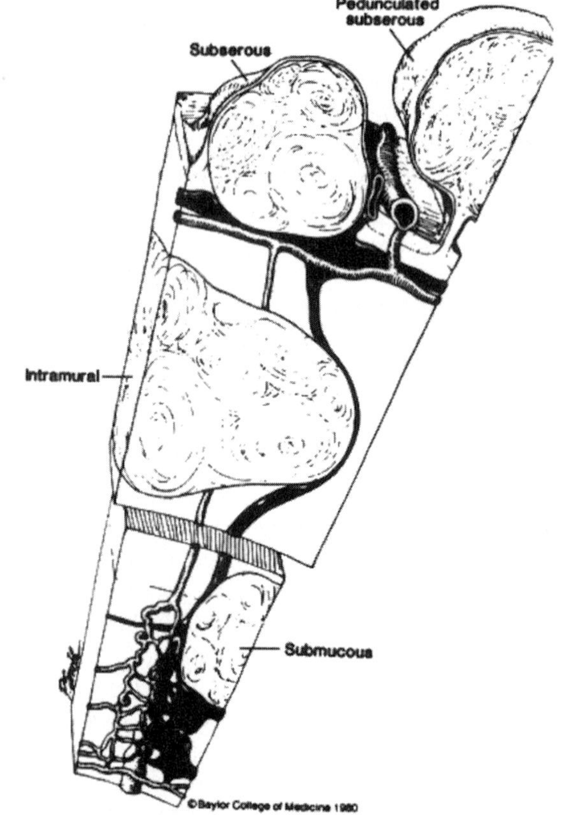

Fig. 4.4 Anatomical causes of uterine bleeding due to the presence of leiomyomas. **(A)** Diagram demonstrates the vascular structures of a normal uterus. **(B)** Diagram of the venule ectasia found in the endometrium caused by the physical obstruction by leiomyoma in the myometrium as proposed by Farrer-Brown.[43,46] (From Buttram VC, Jr., Reiter RC. Uterine leiomyomata: etiology, symptomatology, and management. Fertil Steril 1981; 36:433-445. Reprinted by permission.)

changes that result in an increase in arterial supply to the leiomyomas.[44]

Fibroids are felt to be the cause of infertility in less that 1 to 3% of infertile women. However, their role remains a subject of debate.[3,47] The primary suspected mechanisms include interference of implantation by altering the endometrial contour, enlargement and deformity or obstruction of the uterine cavity, altered contractility of the uterine inhibiting sperm transport, obstruction of the tubal ostia, and persistence of intrauterine blood or clots.[48] In patients with infertility due to leiomyomas, pregnancy rates may be improved by surgical resection.[49] In a meta-analysis of 46 articles by Donnez and Jadoul, they determined the pregnancy rate after myomectomy to be 48%, without any significant difference between hysteroscopic myomectomy (45%) and laparoscopic and abdominal myomectomy (49%). Pregnancies occurred quite soon after myomotomy, 7.5 ± 2.6 months.[50] Leiomyomas are also associated with an increased risk in placental abruption if the placenta implants over the leiomyoma.[51] In addition, in pregnancies occurring in patients with coexisting fibroids, pain and premature labor are directly related to the size of the leiomyoma.[51]

■ Imaging

In patients with suspected leiomyomas, endovaginal or transabdominal ultrasound typically is the initial modality utilized for imaging.[52,53] It is the most readily available technique and the least costly. One potential problem with ultrasound is that it can be limited by field of view, especially in patients with a large body habitus or with distorted anatomy due to large leiomyomas.[52,54] Ultrasound may also miss leiomyomas less than 2 cm in diameter as well as comorbid conditions such as adenomyosis, which may be contributing to the patient's symptoms. Magnetic resonance imaging (MRI) is very good at differentiating leiomyomas from adenomyosis.[55] MRI can also better characterize the origin of pelvic masses.[56] Sonohysterography is also very useful for detecting submucosal and endometrial abnormalities. In addition, sonohysterography can be used to distinguish a small submucosal leiomyoma from a polyp because polyps may demonstrate a classic central feeding artery. MRI is extremely useful when there is a need for a more thorough evaluation or ultrasound findings are unclear.[54,56,57]

Magnetic resonance imaging is the most accurate imaging method for diagnosing leiomyomas especially in delineating their location and number. MRI is performed best on a high-field strength magnet with a phased array coil. Gadolinium is often used to demonstrate vascularity of the leiomyomas, especially helpful when considering uterine artery embolization. Standard approach includes the use of both T1- and T2-weighted sequences. Leiomyomas are best seen on T2-weighted images as sharply marginated, low signal masses relative to the myometrium.[58] Leiomyomas as small as 0.5 cm are routinely imaged (**Fig. 4.5**). Leiomyoma location may be submucosal, intramural, or subserosal (**Fig. 4.6**). They also may be pedunculated and extend into the peritoneal cavity or into the endometrial cavity (**Fig. 4.7**). Large leiomyomas may also be transmural, extending through the uterine wall from the submucosal region to the subserosa. Many intramural or subserosal leiomyomas may be circumscribed by a high signal intensity rim that represents a combination of dilated lymphatics, veins, and/or edema.[59] Leiomyomas >3 cm are often heterogeneous due to varying degrees of infarction.[57,60] Those with hemorrhagic degeneration demonstrate high signal intensity T1-weighted images and do not enhance with gadolinium (**Fig. 4.8**).[57] Advanced hyaline degeneration when accompanied with fatty degeneration may be confused with a benign mixed müllerian tumor or lipoadenofibroma.[57,61] There may also be cystic degeneration.[60] Differentiating types of degeneration by MRI may be extremely difficult except for hemorrhagic or fatty degeneration. Cellular leiomyomas, characterized by having densely packed smooth muscle cells with little connective tissue, will have high signal intensity on T2-weighted images. These leiomyomas are reported to respond better with greater volume loss to both uterine artery embolization and gonadotropin-releasing hormone therapy.[60]

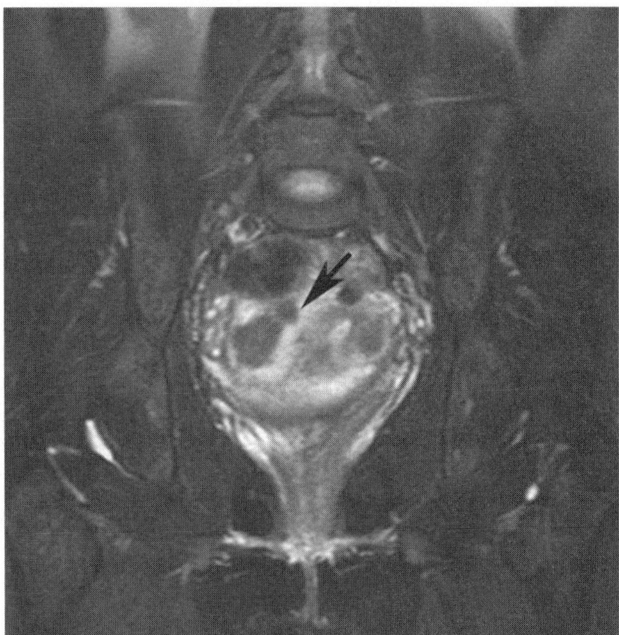

Fig. 4.5 Coronal T2-weighted magnetic resonance image of the uterus demonstrates multiple fibroids as dark uniform masses within the intermediate signal intensity uterine myometrium. Fibroids as small as 5 mm (*arrow*) are easily depicted by this technique.

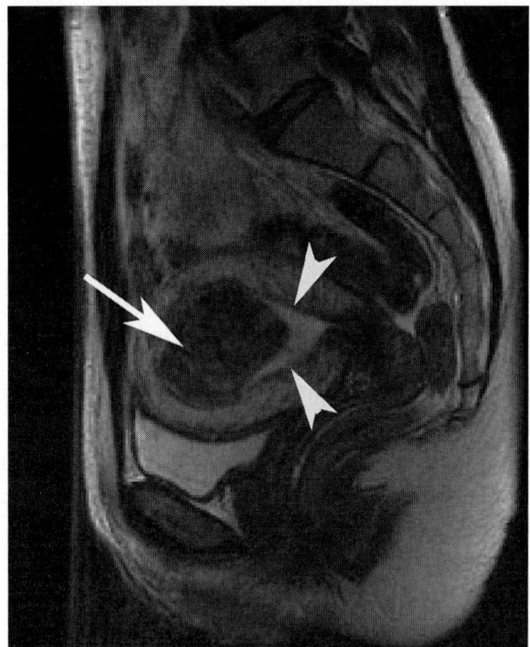

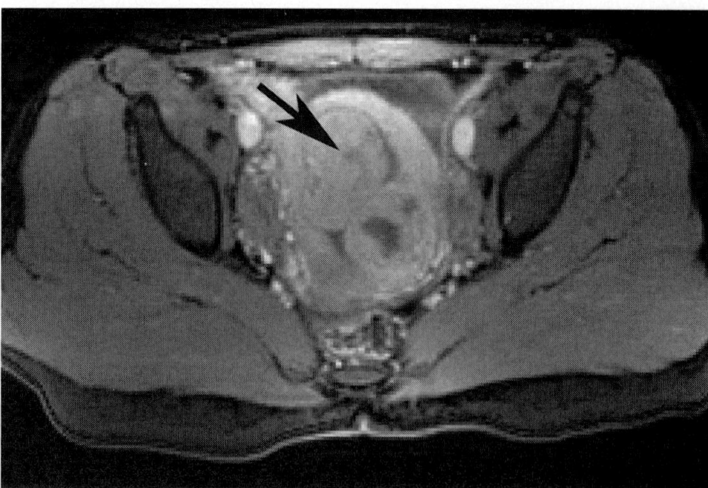

Fig. 4.6 (A) Category T:II submucosal fibroid. Sagittal T2-weighted magnetic resonance image (MRI) demonstrates a large fundal fibroid (*white arrow*) with roughly 30% coverage by the distended bright endometrial stripe (*white arrowheads*). MRIs in any one plane can be deceptive for grading the degree of submucosal extension, and multiplanar imaging should be used to observe fibroid from all projections in the course of planning therapy. **(B)** Category T:II submucosal fibroid. Axial post-gadolinium T1-weighted MRI shows the submucosal portion of the fibroid (*arrow*) en face, apparently 100% surrounded by endometrium.

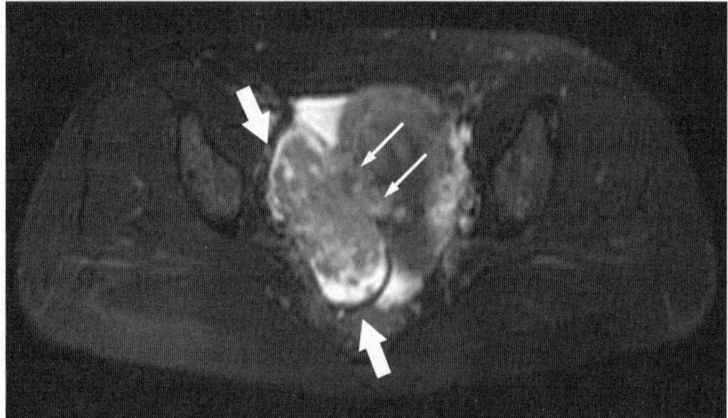

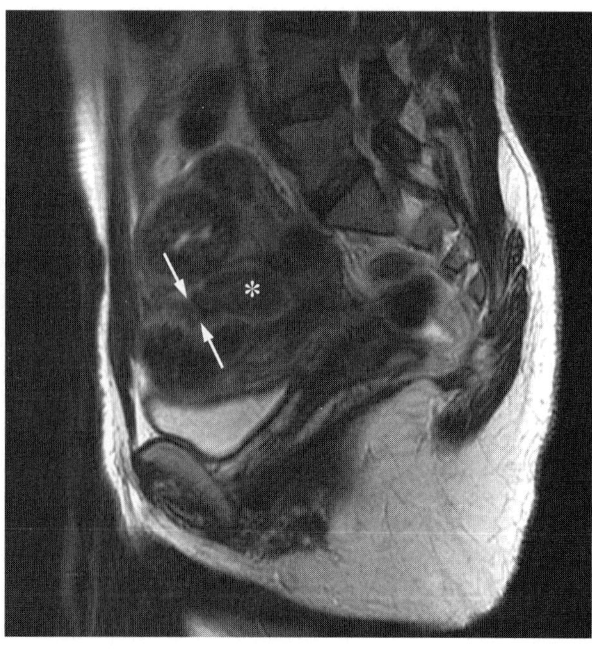

Fig. 4.7 (A) Pedunculated fibroid. Axial T2-weighted magnetic resonance image (MRI) demonstrates a large exophytic fibroid (*large white arrows*) with a broad flat stalk (*small white arrows*) projecting from the uterine surface. **(B)** Sagittal postgadolinium T1-weighted MRI shows an oblong intracavitary mass (*asterisk*) projecting from a stalk emanating from the endometrial surface (*arrowheads*).

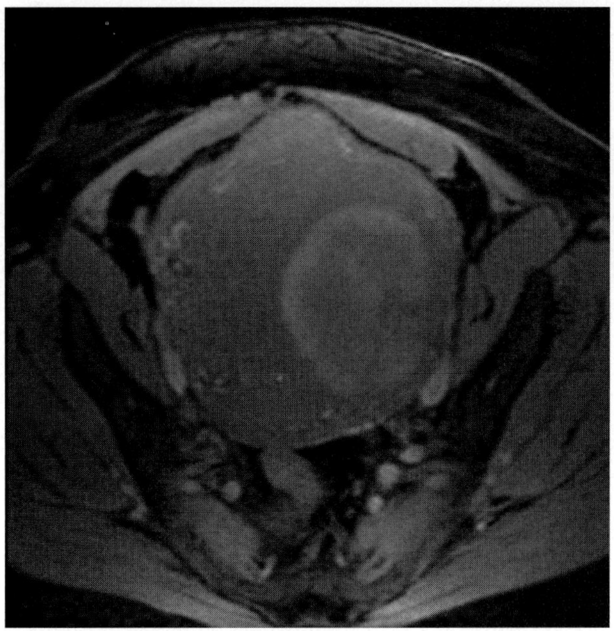

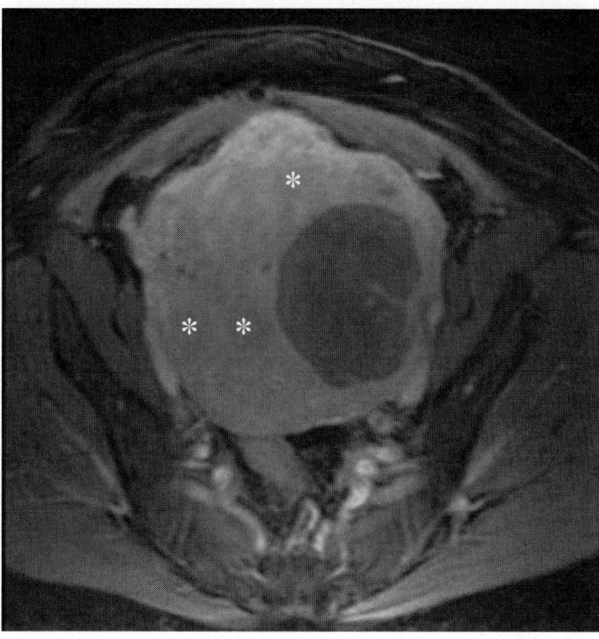

Fig. 4.8 (Auto) infarcted fibroid. Axial T1-weighted magnetic resonance image (MRI) **(A)** before and **(B)** after administration of gadolinium contrast in a woman prior to uterine artery embolization. **(A)** A single heterogeneous bright intramural mass is seen. Spontaneous, fibroid necrosis can be documented by MRI. These masses typically show internal bright T1-weighted signal intensity due to the presence of hemorrhagic degeneration. **(B)** This mass is shown to be largely nonenhancing; multiple additional fibroids (*asterisks*) are vaguely seen.

■ Treatment

Conventional management of leiomyomas involves either medical hormonal therapy or a surgical procedure such as myomectomy or hysterectomy. Myomectomy for serosal or intramural fibroids may be performed via open or a laparoscopic route whereas submucous fibroids may be resected hysteroscopically. The choice of therapy and route of surgery depends on the location of the fibroids in addition to the degree of symptoms and the desire of the patient for future fertility. Although leiomyomas may impact a woman's quality of life, they less commonly cause clinically significant health problems. Severe anemia due to bleeding and hydronephrosis due to ureteral obstruction are the most likely clinically significant medical problems. Because leiomyoma growth and symptomatology are unpredictable, preemptive intervention is usually not justified. In addition most symptoms can often be medically managed with hormonal intervention.[62]

Medical Treatment

Gonadotropin-releasing hormone agonist (GnRH-a) therapy produces a decrease in uterine volume, leiomyoma volume, and bleeding. The benefits are typically short lived after discontinuation and long-term use is limited by the risks and side effects.[62] Gonadotropin-releasing hormone (GnRH) is secreted by the hypothalamus in a pulsatile fashion and stimulates production of luteinizing hormone (LH) and follicle-stimulating hormone (FSH) by the pituitary.[63] GnRH-a works by having a long half-life and a high affinity for the GnRH receptor. This receptor binding results in a downregulation of the gonadotropin receptors and a decrease in LH and FSH production, which results in decreased ovarian activity. This ultimately produces a hormonal state resembling menopause, which results in the shrinkage of the leiomyomas and a cessation in menstruation.[64] Individual leiomyomas have a variable response to GnRH-a due to the variability in composition of the leiomyomas (e.g., fibrous or calcified leiomyomas may not respond).[64] Studies in women being treated with GnRH-a have demonstrated between 35 to 61% reduction of both leiomyomas and uterine volumes after 3 to 6 months of therapy. The maximal effect of therapy on reduction in uterine and leiomyoma volume is seen after the third or fourth month of therapy.[64] Therapy is usually limited by the pseudomenopausal side effects such as osteopenia, vasomotor symptoms, hair loss, irregular vaginal bleeding, vaginal dryness, headaches, and depression. Add-back therapy in the form of low doses of estrogen and/or progesterone has been utilized in attempts to counteract the adverse side effects of GnRH-a.[62,64]

After discontinuation of therapy with a GnRH-a, the uterus rapidly returns to its pretreatment volume within weeks. Treatment is usually reserved for patients who are perimenopausal with the hope that the patient will become menopausal while on GnRH-a.[64] It also can be used for younger patients to modify the route of surgery necessary for treatment, such as converting an abdominal to vaginal hysterectomy because of decreased uterine size after GnRH-a agonist therapy. In addition, because bleeding is decreased or absent during treatment, patients with anemia have the opportunity to recover and enter surgery with higher hemoglobin levels without the need for transfusion.[65] When GnRH-a is utilized prior to planned myomectomy, there is some concern that treatment may cause small leiomyomas to become more difficult to find and thus increase their recurrence rate after surgery. In addition, there may be an associated fibrotic response that may make definition of surgical planes during myomectomy more difficult. Tibolone, a synthetic steroid that has estrogenic, androgenic, and progestogenic properties, has been successful in controlling the adverse effects of GnRH-a. It has been used in Europe, but has not been approved in the United States.[66,67] Newer gonadotropin-releasing hormone antagonists are being developed such as ganirelix. This class of steroid has been shown to rapidly reduce the size of leiomyomas with only minor side effects as compared with GnRH agonists.[68]

Mifepristone (RU-486) is an oral progesterone receptor modulator that antagonizes progesterone and results in the reduction of leiomyoma size. Various mechanisms for this action have been suggested, including reduction in the number of progesterone receptors within the leiomyoma, abolishing the ovarian hormonal cycle, and decreasing blood flow to the leiomyoma by a direct vascular effect.[69–71] An analysis by Steinauer et al[72] concluded that mifepristone demonstrated a reduction in leiomyomas size and improvement in symptoms, but also has the adverse effect of causing endometrial hyperplasia. Mifepristone is not currently available for this use in the United States.

A levonorgestrel-releasing intrauterine system (LNG-IUS) has also been used to reduce menstrual bleeding.[73] Review of existing literature on the use of LNG-IUS in women with fibroids revealed that contraceptive efficacy is high and menstrual blood loss is reduced.[74] LNG-IUS expulsion rates may be higher in women with fibroids compared with women with normal uteri. In addition, studies of LNG-IUS in women with fibroids have not demonstrated any reduction in fibroid size associated with their use.[74]

Oral contraceptives and long-acting progesterones, as well as cyclic oral progesterones are often utilized as first-line therapy in an attempt to control fibroid associated symptoms of both menorrhagia and dysmenorrhea. Long-acting progesterones (Depo-Provera; Pfizer, Inc., New York, NY) have been shown to both reduce bleeding and fibroid size in symptomatic women.[75] The use of oral contraceptives in women with abnormal uterine bleeding refractory to cyclic medroxyprogesterone acetate treatment has been compared with hysterectomy in a clinical trial. Hysterectomy was associated with a higher cost, but also with improvement in quality of life scores when compared with medical management.[76]

Surgical Treatment

Hysterectomy is the definitive treatment for leiomyomas and has traditionally been the option offered to women with symptomatic fibroids, especially when leiomyosarcoma or other uterine malignancy is suspected. Recent surveillance of hysterectomy in the United States shows that fibroids were the indication for 27% of hysterectomies done in 2004 to 2005.[77] There are several different approaches to hysterectomy including abdominal, vaginal, laparoscopically assisted vaginal, and laparoscopically assisted supracervical hysterectomy. The appropriate route is determined by the uterine size, the patient's prior surgical history, and the type of pathology that is expected, as well as patient preference and the physician's experience and training.[78]

All routes of hysterectomy pose some risk both intraoperatively and postoperatively. In a 1998 review of surgical complications of hysterectomy in Finland, Harkki-Siren found a rate of 1/1000 ureteral injuries and a vesicovaginal fistula occurrence of 1.3/1000. Rates for all types of urinary tract injury were higher with the laparoscopic than abdominal or vaginal approach.[79] In patients with previous pelvic surgery, there is an increase in the risk of bowel and urinary tract injuries with repeated surgeries. In one multicenter trial involving 1851 women, the risk of death was 0.1% for abdominal and 0.2% for vaginal hysterectomy. In another large multicenter study of 3928 patients, the major complication rate for laparoscopic hysterectomy was 2.2% with one death from pulmonary embolism.[80] When done for the indication of fibroids, vaginal hysterectomy is often more difficult because of uterine size or may be impossible in some patients. Recently, laparoscopic hysterectomy has become feasible for women with leiomyomas offering less postoperative pain, shorter hospital stay, and faster recovery.

A surgical alternative to hysterectomy for the treatment of fibroids is myomectomy where the leiomyomas are individually resected from the myometrium. In general, myomectomy is performed when preservation of fertility is desired or if the patient wants to retain her uterus. The success in controlling symptoms is ~80%. The recurrence rate of leiomyomas is estimated to range from ~4 to 30%.[3] As previously mentioned, the 10-year recurrence rate is 27% and is significantly lower in women who have given birth after myomectomy as compared to those who have not given birth.[10] Recurrences appear to be less common following removal of a single myoma as compared with removal of multiple ones.[81] Resection can be performed abdominally or laparoscopically. Laparoscopic resection was once thought to have a higher recurrence rate due to the difficulty in observing smaller myomas; other studies have disputed this suggestion.[82] Myomectomy was thought to have a greater surgical risk as compared with hysterectomy, but this also has not been seen in recent studies.[83,84] In addition, West et al[83] demonstrated no greater risk of myomectomy, even in large uteri equal to or larger than 16 weeks. Although there is a risk of a myomectomy resulting in hysterectomy, this complication was not reported.

Submucosal leiomyomas can also be removed with a hysteroscopic approach. Submucosal leiomyomas can be classified by the degree of the fibroid within the cavity as can be seen in **Fig. 4.9**.[85] Category T:O and T:I leiomyomas are more pedunculated and less intramural, whereas T:II leiomyomas have >50% intramural extension. The depth of extension of submucosal fibroids into the myometrium increases the chance of surgical complications with hysteroscopic resection.[2] Long-term follow-up studies have shown that 20% of patients who undergo hysteroscopic resection will require additional therapy within the next several years. This may be secondary to both recurrence of fibroids and incomplete removal of the initial leiomyoma.[2] In addition, when submucous fibroids are >5 cm in diameter, hysteroscopic resection is deferred because there is a higher risk of systemic intravasation of the fluid, and potential fluid overload caused by the fluid used in distending the uterus during the procedure.[86]

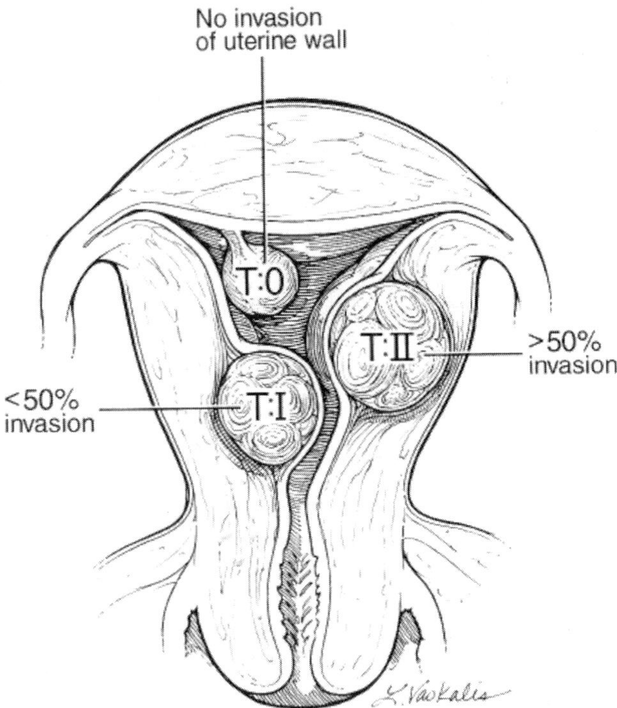

Fig. 4.9 Classification of submucosal leiomyomas depending on the percentage of leiomyoma within the uterine cavity by Cohen et al. Type 0 is intracavitary. (From Cohen LS, Valle RF. Role of vaginal sonography and hysterosonography in the endoscopic treatment of uterine myomas. Fertil Steril 2000; 73:197–204. Reprinted by permission.)

Uterine artery embolization is a technique familiar to interventional radiologists that is discussed in more detail in later chapters within this text. Operative techniques include myolysis, which includes thermomyolysis, cryomyolysis, or laser therapies to ablate the leiomyomas that are discussed in more detail as well. To date, these ablative techniques have met with very limited success in the treatment of symptomatic fibroids.[62,87] Endometrial ablation using varying devices to resect the endometrium was originally thought not to work well in patients with leiomyomas due to the distortion of the uterine cavity.[88] Recently, studies have demonstrated success with these patients depending on the device used.[88] Ablation does improve the outcome of patients after hysteroscopic resection of submucosal fibroids.[89]

■ Conclusions

Leiomyomas are very commonly found in women of reproductive age. Contemporary management of fibroids is limited to observation unless symptoms arise. Heavy and/or prolonged bleeding as well as pelvic pressure and dysmenorrhea are symptoms commonly associated with leiomyoma. Although the definitive treatment for symptomatic leiomyoma is hysterectomy, there are many other options available for management, some of which allow preservation of fertility. Options range from medical hormonal treatment to uterine artery embolization to myomectomy or hysterectomy. Emerging data comparing different treatment options will hopefully allow additional clinical guidance when treating an individual woman with symptomatic fibroids.

References

1. Sutton CJ. Historical curiosities in the surgical management of myomas. J Am Assoc Gynecol Laparosc 2004;11:4–7
2. Wallach EE, Vlahos NF. Uterine myomas: an overview of development, clinical features, and management. Obstet Gynecol 2004;104:393–406
3. Buttram VC Jr, Reiter RC. Uterine leiomyomata: etiology, symptomatology, and management. Fertil Steril 1981;36:433–445
4. Marshall LM, Spiegelman D, Goldman MB, et al. A prospective study of reproductive factors and oral contraceptive use in relation to the risk of uterine leiomyomata. Fertil Steril 1998;70:432–439
5. Babaknia A, Rock JA, Jones HW Jr. Pregnancy success following abdominal myomectomy for infertility. Fertil Steril 1978;30:644–647
6. Hunt JE, Wallach EE. Uterine factors in infertility–an overview. Clin Obstet Gynecol 1974;17:44–64
7. Ingersoll FM. Fertility following myomectomy. Fertil Steril 1963;14: 596–602
8. Rein MS, Friedman AJ, Barbieri RL, Pavelka K, Fletcher JA, Morton CC. Cytogenetic abnormalities in uterine leiomyomata. Obstet Gynecol 1991;77:923–926
9. Townsend DE, Sparkes RS, Baluda MC, McClelland G. Unicellular histogenesis of uterine leiomyomas as determined by electrophoresis

by glucose-6-phosphate dehydrogenase. Am J Obstet Gynecol 1970; 107:1168–1173
10. Candiani GB, Fedele L, Parazzini F, Villa L. Risk of recurrence after myomectomy. Br J Obstet Gynaecol 1991;98:385–389
11. Parker WH, Fu YS, Berek JS. Uterine sarcoma in patients operated on for presumed leiomyoma and rapidly growing leiomyoma. Obstet Gynecol 1994;83:414–418
12. Guarnaccia MM, Rein MS. Traditional surgical approaches to uterine fibroids: abdominal myomectomy and hysterectomy. Clin Obstet Gynecol 2001;44:385–400
13. Walker CL, Stewart EA. Uterine fibroids: the elephant in the room. Science 2005;308:1589–1592
14. Quade BJ, Wang TY, Sornberger K, Dal Cin P, Mutter GL, Morton CC. Molecular pathogenesis of uterine smooth muscle tumors from transcriptional profiling. Genes Chromosomes Cancer 2004;40:97–108
15. Fletcher JA, Morton CC, Pavelka K, Lage JM. Chromosome aberrations in uterine smooth muscle tumors: potential diagnostic relevance of cytogenetic instability. Cancer Res 1990;50:4092–4097
16. Layfield LJ, Liu K, Dodge R, Barsky SH. Uterine smooth muscle tumors: utility of classification by proliferation, ploidy, and prognostic markers versus traditional histopathology. Arch Pathol Lab Med 2000;124:221–227
17. Kempson RL, Bari W. Uterine sarcomas. Classification, diagnosis, and prognosis. Hum Pathol 1970;1:331–349
18. Henske EP. Metastasis of benign tumor cells in tuberous sclerosis complex. Genes Chromosomes Cancer 2003;38:376–381
19. Dal Cin P, Quade BJ, Neskey DM, Kleinman MS, Weremowicz S, Morton CC. Intravenous leiomyomatosis is characterized by a der(14)t(12;14)(q15;q24). Genes Chromosomes Cancer 2003;36:205–206
20. Kjerulff KH, Langenberg P, Seidman JD, Stolley PD, Guzinski GM. Uterine leiomyomas. Racial differences in severity, symptoms and age at diagnosis. J Reprod Med 1996;41:483–490
21. Parazzini F, Negri E, La Vecchia C, et al. Uterine myomas and smoking. Results from an Italian study. J Reprod Med 1996;41:316–320
22. Ross RK, Pike MC, Vessey MP, Bull D, Yeates D, Casagrande JT. Risk factors for uterine fibroids: reduced risk associated with oral contraceptives. Br Med J (Clin Res Ed) 1986;293:359–362
23. Chiaffarino F, Parazzini F, La Vecchia C, Marsico S, Surace M, Ricci E. Use of oral contraceptives and uterine fibroids: results from a case-control study. Br J Obstet Gynaecol 1999;106:857–860
24. Borgfeldt C, Andolf E. Transvaginal ultrasonographic findings in the uterus and the endometrium: low prevalence of leiomyoma in a random sample of women age 25–40 years. Acta Obstet Gynecol Scand 2000;79:202–207
25. Wise LA, Palmer JR, Harlow BL, et al. Reproductive factors, hormonal contraception, and risk of uterine leiomyomata in African-American women: a prospective study. Am J Epidemiol 2004;159:113–123
26. Chiaffarino F, Parazzini F, La Vecchia C, Chatenoud L, Di Cintio E, Marsico S. Diet and uterine myomas. Obstet Gynecol 1999;94:395–398
27. Stewart EA. Uterine fibroids. Lancet 2001;357:293–298
28. Stewart EA, Morton CC. The genetics of uterine leiomyomata: what clinicians need to know. Obstet Gynecol 2006;107:917–921
29. Treloar SA, Martin NG, Dennerstein L, Raphael B, Heath AC. Pathways to hysterectomy: insights from longitudinal twin research. Am J Obstet Gynecol 1992;167:82–88
30. Van Voorhis BJ, Romitti PA, Jones MP. Family history as a risk factor for development of uterine leiomyomas. Results of a pilot study. J Reprod Med 2002;47:663–669
31. Vikhlyaeva EM, Khodzhaeva ZS, Fantschenko ND. Familial predisposition to uterine leiomyomas. Int J Gynaecol Obstet 1995;51:127–131
32. Alam NA, Rowan AJ, Wortham NC, et al. Genetic and functional analyses of FH mutations in multiple cutaneous and uterine leiomyomatosis, hereditary leiomyomatosis and renal cancer, and fumarate hydratase deficiency. Hum Mol Genet 2003;12:1241–1252
33. Kiuru M, Launonen V, Hietala M, et al. Familial cutaneous leiomyomatosis is a two-hit condition associated with renal cell cancer of characteristic histopathology. Am J Pathol 2001;159:825–829
34. Mark J, Havel G, Grepp C, Dahlenfors R, Wedell B. Cytogenetical observations in human benign uterine leiomyomas. Anticancer Res 1988;8:621–626
35. Meloni AM, Surti U, Contento AM, Davare J, Sandberg AA. Uterine leiomyomas: cytogenetic and histologic profile. Obstet Gynecol 1992;80:209–217
36. Schoenberg Fejzo M, Ashar HR, Krauter KS, et al. Translocation breakpoints upstream of the HMGIC gene in uterine leiomyomata suggest dysregulation of this gene by a mechanism different from that in lipomas. Genes Chromosomes Cancer 1996;17:1–6
37. Flake GP, Andersen J, Dixon D. Etiology and pathogenesis of uterine leiomyomas: a review. Environ Health Perspect 2003;111:1037–1054
38. Williams VS, Jones G, Mauskopf J, Spalding J, DuChane J. Uterine fibroids: a review of health-related quality of life assessment. J Womens Health (Larchmt) 2006;15:818–829
39. Lee DW, Ozminkowski RJ, Carls GS, Wang S, Gibson TB, Stewart EA. The direct and indirect cost burden of clinically significant and symptomatic uterine fibroids. J Occup Environ Med 2007;49:493–506
40. Myers ER, Goodwin S, Landow W, et al. Prospective data collection of a new procedure by a specialty society: the FIBROID registry. Obstet Gynecol 2005;106:44–51
41. Sehgal N, Haskins AL. The mechanism of uterine bleeding in the presence of fibromyomas. Am Surg 1960;26:21–23
42. Faulkner R. The blood vessels of the myomatous uterus. Am J Obstet Gynecol 1945;47:185–197
43. Farrer-Brown G, Beilby JO, Tarbit MH. The vascular patterns in myomatous uteri. J Obstet Gynaecol Br Commonw 1970;77:967–975
44. Stewart EA, Nowak RA. Leiomyoma-related bleeding: a classic hypothesis updated for the molecular era. Hum Reprod Update 1996;2:295–306
45. Sampson JA. The blood supply of uterine myomata. Surg Gynecol Obstet 1912;14:215
46. Farrer-Brown G, Beilby JO, Tarbit MH. Venous changes in the endometrium of myomatous uteri. Obstet Gynecol 1971;38:743–751
47. Donnez J, Jadoul P. What are the implications of myomas on fertility? A need for a debate? Hum Reprod 2002;17:1424–1430
48. The Practice Committee of the American Society for Reproductive Medicine. Myomas and reproductive function. Fertil Steril 2006;86: S194–S199
49. Garcia CR, Tureck RW. Submucosal leiomyomas and infertility. Fertil Steril 1984;42:16–19
50. Dessolle L, Soriano D, Poncelet C, Benifla JL, Madelenat P, Darai E. Determinants of pregnancy rate and obstetric outcome after laparoscopic myomectomy for infertility. Fertil Steril 2001;76:370–374
51. Rice JP, Kay HH, Mahony BS. The clinical significance of uterine leiomyomas in pregnancy. Am J Obstet Gynecol 1989;160:1212–1216
52. Gross BH, Silver TM, Jaffe MH. Sonographic features of uterine leiomyomas: analysis of 41 proven cases. J Ultrasound Med 1983;2:401–406
53. Karasick S, Lev-Toaff AS, Toaff ME. Imaging of uterine leiomyomas. AJR Am J Roentgenol 1992;158:799–805
54. Dudiak CM, Turner DA, Patel SK, Archie JT, Silver B, Norusis M. Uterine leiomyomas in the infertile patient: preoperative localization with MR imaging versus US and hysterosalpingography. Radiology 1988;167:627–630
55. Mark AS, Hricak H, Heinrichs LW, et al. Adenomyosis and leiomyoma: differential diagnosis with MR imaging. Radiology 1987;163:527–529
56. Weinreb JC, Barkoff ND, Megibow A, Demopoulos R. The value of MR imaging in distinguishing leiomyomas from other solid pelvic masses when sonography is indeterminate. AJR Am J Roentgenol 1990;154:295–299
57. Hricak H, Tscholakoff D, Heinrichs L, et al. Uterine leiomyomas: correlation of MR, histopathologic findings, and symptoms. Radiology 1986;158:385–391
58. Ascher SM, Jha RC, Reinhold C. Benign myometrial conditions: leiomyomas and adenomyosis. Top Magn Reson Imaging 2003;14:281–304

59. Mittl RL Jr, Yeh IT, Kressel HY. High-signal-intensity rim surrounding uterine leiomyomas on MR images: pathologic correlation. Radiology 1991;180:81–83
60. Yamashita Y, Torashima M, Takahashi M, et al. Hyperintense uterine leiomyoma at T2-weighted MR imaging: differentiation with dynamic enhanced MR imaging and clinical implications. Radiology 1993;189:721–725
61. Horie Y, Ikawa S, Kadowaki K, Minagawa Y, Kigawa J, Terakawa N. Lipoadenofibroma of the uterine corpus. Report of a new variant of adenofibroma (benign müllerian mixed tumor). Arch Pathol Lab Med 1995;119:274–276
62. Parker WH. Uterine myomas: management. Fertil Steril 2007;88:255–271
63. Knobil E. The neuroendocrine control of the menstrual cycle. Recent Prog Horm Res 1980;36:53–88
64. Chavez NF, Stewart EA. Medical treatment of uterine fibroids. Clin Obstet Gynecol 2001;44:372–384
65. Stovall TG, Ling FW, Henry LC, Woodruff MR. A randomized trial evaluating leuprolide acetate before hysterectomy as treatment for leiomyomas. Am J Obstet Gynecol 1991;164:1420–1423 discussion 1423–1425
66. Palomba S, Affinito P, Tommaselli GA, Nappi C. A clinical trial of the effects of tibolone administered with gonadotropin-releasing hormone analogues for the treatment of uterine leiomyomata. Fertil Steril 1998;70:111–118
67. Modelska K, Cummings S. Tibolone for postmenopausal women: systematic review of randomized trials. J Clin Endocrinol Metab 2002;87:16–23
68. Flierman PA, Oberye JJ, van der Hulst VP, de Blok S. Rapid reduction of leiomyoma volume during treatment with the GnRH antagonist ganirelix. BJOG 2005;112:638–642
69. Murphy AA, Kettel LM, Morales AJ, Roberts VJ, Yen SS. Regression of uterine leiomyomata in response to the antiprogesterone RU 486. J Clin Endocrinol Metab 1993;76:513–517
70. Murphy AA, Morales AJ, Kettel LM, Yen SS. Regression of uterine leiomyomata to the antiprogesterone RU486: dose-response effect. Fertil Steril 1995;64:187–190
71. Reinsch RC, Murphy AA, Morales AJ, Yen SS. The effects of RU 486 and leuprolide acetate on uterine artery blood flow in the fibroid uterus: a prospective, randomized study. Am J Obstet Gynecol 1994;170:1623–1627 discussion 1627–1628
72. Steinauer J, Pritts EA, Jackson R, Jacoby AF. Systematic review of mifepristone for the treatment of uterine leiomyomata. Obstet Gynecol 2004;103:1331–1336
73. Grigorieva V, Chen-Mok M, Tarasova M, Mikhailov A. Use of a levonorgestrel-releasing intrauterine system to treat bleeding related to uterine leiomyomas. Fertil Steril 2003;79:1194–1198
74. Kaunitz AM. Progestin-releasing intrauterine systems and leiomyoma. Contraception 2007;75:S130–S133
75. Venkatachalam S, Bagratee JS, Moodley J. Medical management of uterine fibroids with medroxyprogesterone acetate (Depo Provera): a pilot study. J Obstet Gynaecol 2004;24:798–800
76. Showstack J, Lin F, Learman LA, et al. Randomized trial of medical treatment versus hysterectomy for abnormal uterine bleeding: resource use in the medicine or surgery (MS) trial. Am J Obstet Gynecol 2006;194:332–338
77. Merrill RM. Hysterectomy surveillance in the United States, 1997 through 2005. Med Sci Monit 2008;14:CR24–CR31
78. Parker WH. Total laparoscopic hysterectomy and laparoscopic supracervical hysterectomy. Obstet Gynecol Clin North Am 2004;31:523–537 viii.
79. Harkki-Siren P, Sjoberg J, Tiitinen A. Urinary tract injuries after hysterectomy. Obstet Gynecol 1998;92:113–118
80. Harkki-Siren P, Sjoberg J, Kurki T. Major complications of laparoscopy: a follow-up Finnish study. Obstet Gynecol 1999;94:94–98
81. Malone LJ. Myomectomy: recurrence after removal of solitary and multiple myomas. Obstet Gynecol 1969;34:200–203
82. Rossetti A, Sizzi O, Soranna L, Cucinelli F, Mancuso S, Lanzone A. Long-term results of laparoscopic myomectomy: recurrence rate in comparison with abdominal myomectomy. Hum Reprod 2001;16:770–774
83. West S, Ruiz R, Parker WH. Abdominal myomectomy in women with very large uterine size. Fertil Steril 2006;85:36–39
84. Sawin SW, Pilevsky ND, Berlin JA, Barnhart KT. Comparability of perioperative morbidity between abdominal myomectomy and hysterectomy for women with uterine leiomyomas. Am J Obstet Gynecol 2000;183:1448–1455
85. Cohen LS, Valle RF. Role of vaginal sonography and hysterosonography in the endoscopic treatment of uterine myomas. Fertil Steril 2000;73:197–204
86. Indman PD. Hysteroscopic treatment of submucous myomas. Clin Obstet Gynecol 2006;49:811–820
87. Zupi E, Sbracia M, Marconi D, Munro MG. Myolysis of uterine fibroids: is there a role? Clin Obstet Gynecol 2006;49:821–833
88. Loffer FD. Endometrial ablation in patients with myomas. Curr Opin Obstet Gynecol 2006;18:391–393
89. Loffer FD. Improving results of hysteroscopic submucosal myomectomy for menorrhagia by concomitant endometrial ablation. J Minim Invasive Gynecol 2005;12:254–260

5 Uterine Fibroid Embolization

Gary P. Siskin

Ravina et al and Goodwin et al have been credited with introducing uterine fibroid embolization (UFE) to interventional radiology (IR).[1–3] Since their respective publications in the mid-1990s, UFE has enjoyed growing acceptance as an alternative to the surgical resection of symptomatic uterine fibroids.[4,5] In fact, Jacobson et al[6] recently demonstrated the growing role that UFE is playing as a uterine-conserving option for these patients. In their review of patients in northern California, they found that though the total rate of invasive treatment for fibroids has stayed constant in recent years, the rate of hysterectomies decreased from 2.13 per 1000 patients to 1.91 per 1000 patients. At the same time, the rate of UFE procedures increased from less than 0.1 per 1000 patients to 0.24 per 1000 patients. Hence, UFE alone is responsible for decreasing the hysterectomy rate in this population; the effect is likely similar wherever UFE is being offered.

■ Indications and Contraindications

The UFE procedure is indicated for the treatment of symptomatic uterine fibroids. The symptoms that are associated with uterine fibroids that might prompt a patient to discuss treatment options with her physician include abnormal uterine bleeding, pelvic pain, dyspareunia, abdominal distension, and frequent urination. Infertility and pregnancy-related concerns may also lead to discussions regarding treatment options for uterine fibroids. It is important to address the issue of performing this procedure in patients without symptoms as simply a way to address the "presence" of a fibroid within the uterus. This has not yet been established as an indication for UFE; therefore, although exceptions can be made on a case-by-case basis, UFE is probably best utilized as a treatment for patients with symptomatic fibroids as opposed to asymptomatic fibroids.

As an angiographic procedure, some possible relative contraindications must be considered prior to performing a UFE procedure. Because iodinated contrast is utilized during this procedure, a patient's renal status must be considered prior to the procedure. Although most of the patients undergoing UFE are young and healthy individuals, some patients may have or be at risk for renal insufficiency and an evaluation of renal function is recommended in these individuals prior to the use of iodinated contrast. Similarly, patients felt to be at risk for bleeding complications relating to performance of an arterial puncture into the common femoral artery should have their hematologic status evaluated prior to performance of the procedure. Finally, patients with an allergy to iodinated contrast material will likely have difficulty undergoing this angiographic procedure; however, performing this procedure without the use of iodinated contrast material has been described.[7,8]

There are uterine or fibroid issues that may serve as relative contraindications for the performance of a UFE procedure. Some patients will present with pedunculated fibroids, which are connected to the uterus via a stalk (**Fig. 5.1**). Pedunculated subserosal fibroids have generally been recognized as a relative contraindication for UFE.[9] It is felt by some that embolization may lead to necrosis and disruption of the stalk, causing the fibroid to separate from the uterus and be free within the peritoneal cavity. There are cases that have been reported where hysterectomy and bowel resection have been performed after septic necrosis of pedunculated subserosal fibroids.[10,11]

Therefore, recent recommendations have been made to assess the diameter of the stalk relative to the diameter of the fibroid before performing a UFE procedure on a patient with a pedunculated fibroid. Katsumori et al[12] reported the safety of performing UFE in patients with pedunculated subserosal fibroids that have a stalk diameter of 2 or more centimeters. In their series, they encountered no serious complications, such as separation of septic necrosis of pedunculated fibroids, torsion of the tumor, infection, or increased tumor size caused by liquefied change as reported by Walker et al.[13] Margau et al[14] reported no unique complications after UFE of pedunculated subserosal fibroids with stalk diameters ranging from 0.7–7.8 cm. Others have discussed the safety of performing UFE if the diameter of the stalk is greater than one-third the width of the diameter of the fibroid. If the diameter of the stalk is less than one-third the width of the diameter of the fibroid then consideration should be given toward recommending laparoscopic resection of the fibroid. In the case of pedunculated submucosal fibroids, Verma et al[15] evaluated the relationship between the fibroid and endometrium and determined the ratio between the largest endometrial interface and the maximum dimension of the fibroid. A stalk diameter >45% was found to decrease the risk of endocavitary migration after UFE. Thinner stalks should necessitate consideration of a hysteroscopic myomectomy.

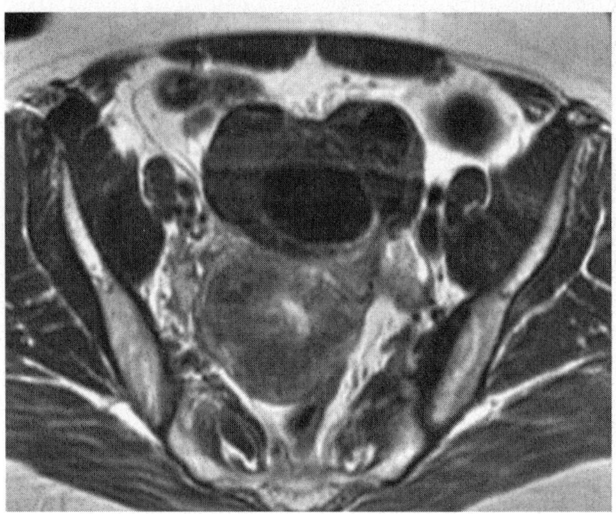
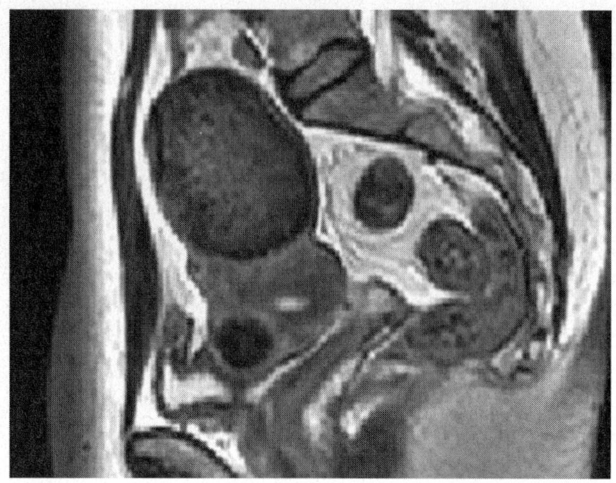

Fig. 5.1 (A) Axial and **(B)** sagittal T2-weighted magnetic resonance images of the pelvis demonstrating pedunculated subserosal fibroids with a broad-based attachment to the uterus (>50% of the diameter of the fibroid).

The presence of adenomyosis within the uterus is considered controversial within the IR community as to whether or not this actually is a contraindication to UFE. Adenomyosis is a disorder that is characterized by the presence of endometrial islets within the myometrium. By definition, they pathologically consist of epithelial as well as stromal elements and are situated at least 2.5 mm below the endometrial–myometrial junction.[16] Clinically, adenomyosis can result in abnormal bleeding, pain, and bulk-related symptoms that may be similar to those seen in patients with uterine fibroids. On magnetic resonance imaging (MRI), T2-weighted images are useful in identifying a junctional zone with a thickness >12 mm and oftentimes containing subendometrial cysts (**Fig. 5.2**).

Initially, cases of treatment failure after UFE were attributed to the presence of adenomyosis; therefore, adenomyosis was felt to be a contraindication to this procedure.[17,18] Later studies, in the form of small retrospective case series, demonstrated the potential for patients with adenomyosis, with or without the presence of uterine fibroids, to benefit from embolization.[19–21] Additional data has been published over the course of the last several years, which continue to support the use of embolization in this population of patients, albeit with expectations regarding success that are less than that seen with embolization in patients with fibroids without adenomyosis.[22–25] This is especially true when adenomyosis exists alone within the uterus, without the presence of uterine fibroids. For example, Lohle et

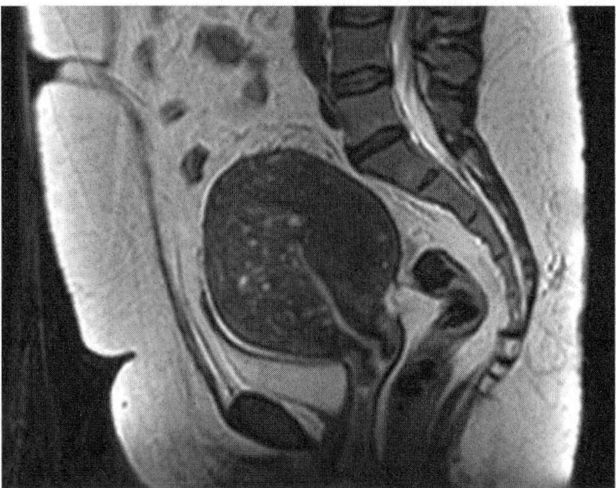
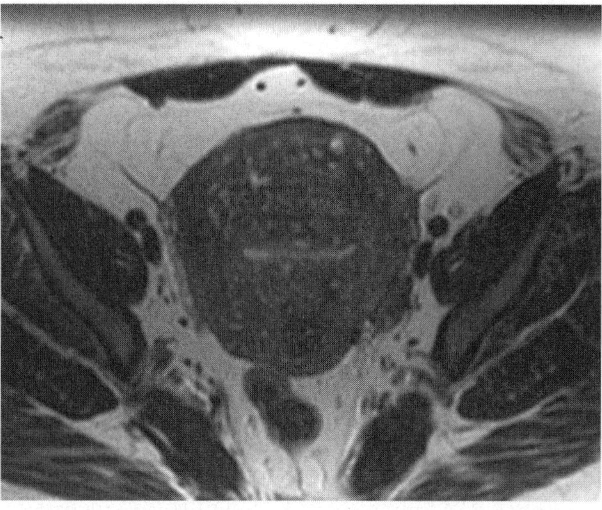

Fig. 5.2 (A) Sagittal and **(B)** axial T2-weighted magnetic resonance images of the pelvis demonstrating a thickened junctional zone containing subendometrial cysts seen as punctuate foci of high signal. These findings are consistent with diffuse adenomyosis.

al[23] studied 38 patients with symptomatic adenomyosis with or without fibroids. After a median follow-up of 16.5 months, 84.2% of patients were satisfied with the clinical improvement they experienced after embolization.

On the other hand, Pelage et al[25] published a prospective study of 18 patients with adenomyosis and no fibroids. In this study, embolization resulted in good short-term control of symptoms with 94% of patients reporting improvement or resolution at 6 months. This number, however, decreased with time and only 55% were clinically improved after 2 years of follow-up. Similarly, Kim et al[24] studied 54 patients with adenomyosis and no fibroids who underwent UAE and had a minimum of 3 years of follow-up. In this patient population, 57.4% of patients had long-term success documented as improvement in menorrhagia and dysmenorrhea scores. The remaining patients had a mean of 17.3 months between embolization and symptom recurrence. These results have been viewed as suboptimal in the IR community, but interestingly are viewed positively within the gynecology community as possible evidence that embolization can be considered as a nonsurgical option for this difficult patient population.[26] Therefore, with such discrepant interpretations offered for these results it seems fair to say that UAE can be considered as treatment for patients with symptomatic fibroids and adenomyosis. The results seem only slightly inferior to those seen in patients with fibroids and no evidence for adenomyosis. In addition, results in patients with adenomyosis and no evidence for uterine fibroids seem to leave approximately one-half of patients with recurrent symptoms over time. Therefore, the decision to perform embolization should be made on a case-by-case basis because a success rate of 50% of patients may be appropriate in some patients and not appropriate in others.

The presence of extremely large fibroids has been considered by some to be a contraindication to the performance of UFE. The literature supporting this has been mixed. Prollius et al[27] reported on the outcomes of UFE in patients with a uterus greater than the size of a 24-week gestation (volume >780 cm^3) and compared them to patients with smaller uteri. There was no difference in the complication rate, in the degree of symptomatic improvement, and satisfaction after the procedure between the two groups of patients. However, Spies et al, in their study describing long-term outcomes after UFE, demonstrated that patients with very large uteri and large dominant leiomyomata are among those that are more likely to have recurrence and subsequent intervention.[28] Therefore, patients with large uteri and dominant fibroids need to be counseled regarding the uncertainty of their clinical outcome after UFE.

Additional contraindications include the presence of a viable intrauterine pregnancy for obvious reasons. An active, untreated infection represents a contraindication due to the risk of abscess formation and related septic complications.[9] Similarly, chronic endometritis, hydrosalpinx, or partially treated pelvic infections represent contraindications as well.[29] The question of whether or not UFE is appropriate to perform in a patient with a desire to have children in the future is one that frequently arises in the course of today's IR practice and is addressed in Chapter 7.

■ Preprocedure Patient Evaluation

Prior to the performance of a UFE procedure, patients should be seen and evaluated in an outpatient setting, preferably in an office-based setting that is conducive to performing patient assessments and maintaining continuity of care.[9,30] The purpose of this visit is to determine if the embolization procedure is indicated and to determine if it is the best and most appropriate option for the patient. During this visit, the patient's history is reviewed (including the results of her most recent gynecologic examination, which should be within the last 12 months) and a physical examination is performed. All prior tests, including the results of a recent Papanicolaou (Pap) test, endometrial biopsy, and blood test results should be reviewed. The patient should have a normal Pap test result within 12 months before embolization is performed.[9] Patients who present with a history of continuous bleeding, very prolonged menstrual periods, significant intermenstrual bleeding, or bleeding after menopause should undergo an endometrial biopsy prior to UFE due to their risk for endometrial hyperplasia or endometrial malignancy; postmenopausal patients with bulk-related symptoms have been shown to benefit from UFE.[31] Old imaging studies should be reviewed as well. From the perspective of a radiologist, films rather than reports should be reviewed when it comes to previously performed imaging studies. Only after that is completed can a physician provide the patient with an appropriate recommendation regarding treatment.[9]

For most patients, routine blood work is not necessarily indicated. Certainly if a patient is at risk given their medical history for bleeding issues associated with a femoral puncture or renal failure secondary to the use of iodinated contrast, then blood work should be obtained to assess their coagulation status (platelet count, activated partial thromboplastin time, prothrombin time, and international normalized ratio) or baseline renal function (blood urea nitrogen and creatinine levels). It is helpful for comparative purposes to obtain a complete blood count (CBC) in patients with a history of abnormal bleeding.

Some of the most interesting investigative work concerning UFE has been surrounding the role of imaging in the pre- and postprocedure assessment of patients undergoing this procedure. There is certainly consensus that preprocedure imaging is required to both confirm the diagnosis of uterine fibroids and to exclude the presence of coexisting pathology. When hysterectomies were routinely being performed for patients requiring treatment for fibroids, great imaging was not necessarily needed prior to surgery. The uterus and possibly the ovaries were going to be removed, and the rest of the pelvis was going to be explored. It was therefore going to be the responsibility of a pathologist to determine what problems existed within the uterus that caused the patient's presenting symptoms. With an organ-sparing philosophy now more prevalent, especially when it comes to UFE, the interventional radiologist performing this procedure has the obligation to obtain the best possible images to make the final determination as to whether or not UFE is the most appropriate treatment to address a patient's presenting symptoms.

The question that then comes up is which modality best serves this purpose and can best answer these questions. In most gynecology practices, the standard of care is to utilize ultrasound to evaluate patients with symptomatic uterine fibroids. This modality has been shown to effectively demonstrate the presence of fibroids and can be utilized to determine their size and their location within the uterus (**Fig. 5.3**). Ultrasound can also be used to characterize the endometrium and the ovaries (which may be difficult in the presence of uterine fibroids). It has also been established that ultrasound is operator dependent, may be limited by the patient's body habitus, may not be able to depict coexistent pelvic disease (such as endometriosis), and may be less sensitive at diagnosing adenomyosis.[31–34]

Spielmann et al[35] retrospectively reviewed the imaging studies of 49 women who were referred for consultation for UFE. They found that MRI discovered additional fibroids in 31 of 49 patients when compared with ultrasound. In addition, they found that fibroids were diagnosed in error on ultrasound in five patients; no fibroids were found on MRI in these patients. Importantly, they found that MRI significantly affected the evaluation of fibroid size and location within the uterus as well. Therefore, this further supports the fact that ultrasound may not be able to supply all of the information an interventional radiologist needs to determine if a patient is an appropriate candidate for UFE.

Magnetic resonance imaging has been shown to be the most effective modality for evaluating a patient prior to UFE. Because of soft tissue characterization, multiplanar imaging capabilities, and enhancement, MRI not only accurately detects and characterizes uterine fibroids, but also may predict who will benefit from embolization.[36] In addition, the ability of MRI to detect coexistent uterine or pelvic pathology may change the diagnosis and treatment plans for patients being evaluated for UFE. The use of MR angiography may be useful in assessing pelvic vascular anatomy before the procedure and in identifying collateral vessels to the uterus.[37]

Omary et al[38] effectively studied the effect of preprocedural MRI on the diagnosis and treatment of patients being evaluated for UFE. In this study, MRI changed the initial diagnosis in 18% of patients. A significant number of patients (19%) who were initially referred for UFE were felt to no longer be appropriate candidates for this procedure after the MRI was performed for reasons such as large fibroids, adenomyosis, pedunculated submucosal fibroids, endometrial lesions, etc. Instead, these patients were referred for surgery, clinical management, or biopsy rather than UFE. Nikolaidis et al[39] expanded upon the previous study by assessing the incidence of nonviable fibroids in patients referred for UFE. In their study, they found that 6% of patients had nonviable dominant fibroids based on a lack of

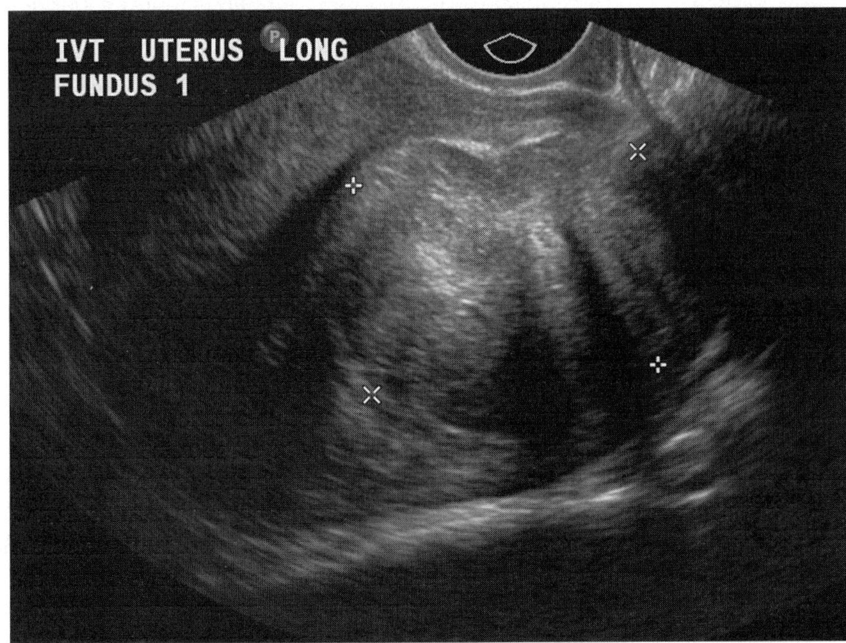

Fig. 5.3 Longitudinal image of the uterus from a transvaginal pelvic ultrasound demonstrating an intramural intrauterine mass consistent with a uterine fibroid.

enhancement on postcontrast images. Given the fact that vascularity is intuitively necessary for embolization to be effective, fibroids without significant vascularity will likely not respond to embolization. Therefore, this information was valuable to these investigators because the decision was then made to not offer UFE to these patients. This once again demonstrates that the information obtained on an MRI has a significant likelihood of altering the treatment plan for a patient being considered for UFE.

There have been some reports at using the findings on a preprocedure MRI to predict outcome after UFE. Harman et al[40] found that the signal characteristics and contrast-enhancement patterns of fibroids before embolization can predict the degree of tumor volume after UFE. Volume reduction was more prominent in fibroids that had high signal intensity on T2-weighted images and a marked contrast enhancement on T1-weighted images. However, the volume reduction was insufficient in fibroids with high signal characteristics on precontrast T1-weighted images. Burn et al[41] found that before embolization, high signal intensity on T1-weighted images was predictive of a poor response, whereas high signal intensity on T2-weighted images was predictive of a good response. The degree of gadolinium enhancement did not correlate with fibroid volume reduction. Jha et al[42] also identified pretreatment MRI features that may be predictive of successful UFE. In this study, a submucosal location was a strong positive predictor of fibroid volume reduction after UFE.

■ Technique

Prior to beginning the procedure, patients are reevaluated in a preprocedure holding area. Informed consent is obtained. An intravenous line is placed to enable the patient to be hydrated and to receive medication for conscious sedation during the procedure (such as midazolam and fentanyl in most centers). In most centers, prophylactic antibiotics are given, but this is not universal among centers performing UFE.[43] Although evidence from randomized controlled trials is lacking, most centers choosing to use prophylactic antibiotics select cefazolin, based on the fact that the most likely source of pathogens during solid organ embolization is contamination by skin pathogens (*Staphylococcus* or *Streptococcus*).[43]

As an angiographic procedure, arterial access is typically gained via the right common femoral artery and unilateral access is maintained throughout the entire procedure. Spies et al has described use of bilateral common femoral artery access with two operators to reduce fluoroscopic exposure (by performing the right and left UAE at the same time) and to allow for bilateral contralateral catheterizations of the uterine artery instead of one contralateral and one ipsilateral catheterization.[28]

The embolization procedure itself is performed using standard angiographic technique. Seldinger technique is used to gain access into the right common femoral artery (assuming unilateral access). A 5-French sheath is used to maintain access within the common femoral artery. At my institution, a 5-French Cobra Glide (Terumo Medical Corporation, Somerset, NJ) catheter is used to catheterize the left internal iliac artery. A pelvic arteriogram is performed to evaluate the left-sided pelvic arterial anatomy and to localize the origin and course of the left uterine artery (**Fig. 5.4A**). Under road-mapping guidance, a microcatheter with a 0.027-inch inner luminal diameter is then introduced into the 5-French Cobra catheter using coaxial technique. This catheter, together with a 0.018-inch guidewire, is advanced into the left uterine artery, which classically arises as the first or second branch of the anterior

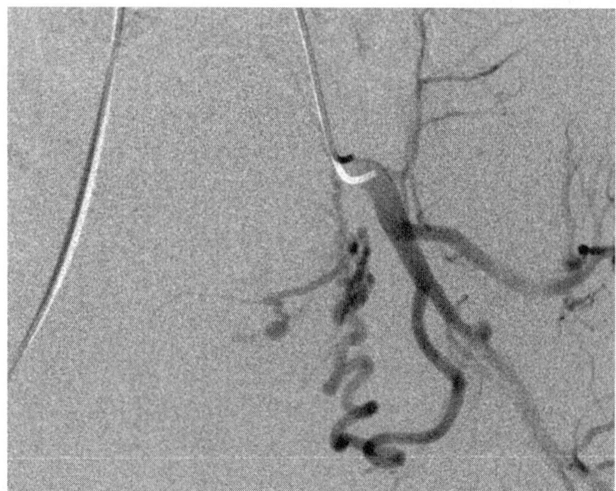
A

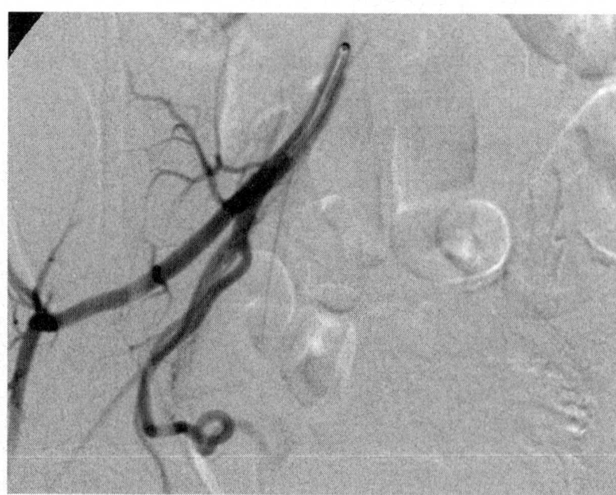
B

Fig. 5.4 **(A)** 30-degree left anterior oblique and **(B)** right anterior oblique images from selective left and right internal iliac artery angiograms demonstrating the origin of the uterine artery from the anterior division of the internal iliac artery.

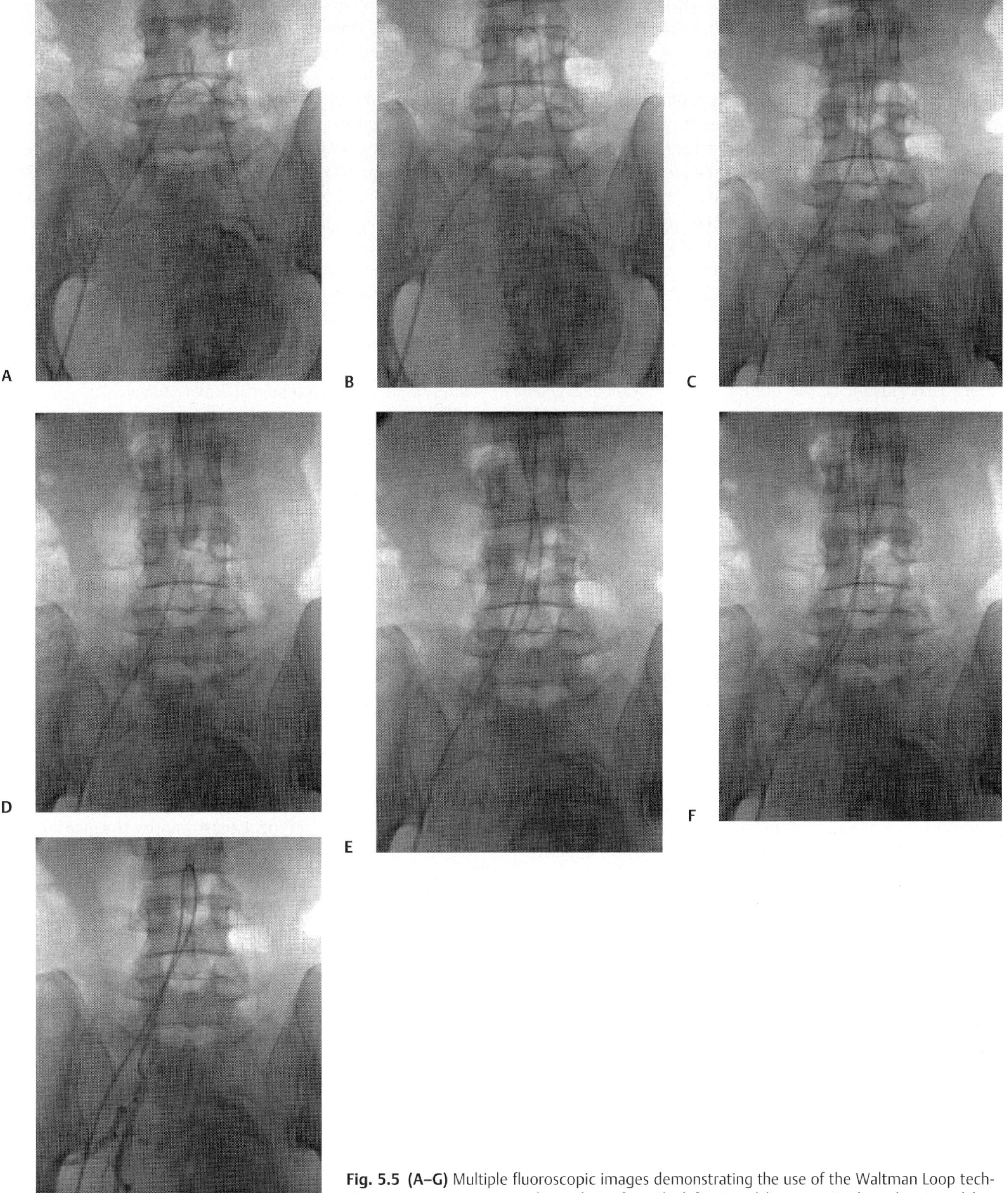

Fig. 5.5 (A–G) Multiple fluoroscopic images demonstrating the use of the Waltman Loop technique to move an angiographic catheter from the left internal iliac artery to the right internal iliac artery prior to selective catheterization of the right uterine artery.

division of the internal iliac artery.[44] If the cervicovaginal branch of the uterine artery, which typically arises from the mid to distal portion of the transverse segment of the uterine artery, is visualized, then the tip of the microcatheter is positioned beyond the origin of that artery.[45] This is done to reduce the possible occurrence of sexual dysfunction following UFE, a complication which has been attributed to embolization of this branch of the uterine artery.[46]

Once the microcatheter is in an appropriate position, the embolic agent selected for use is administered into the uterine artery until the endpoint signifying an appropriate reduction in blood flow has been reached. The most common endpoint to use with particulate polyvinyl alcohol (PVA) is complete stasis of flow within the uterine artery. If a spherical embolic agent, such as tris-acryl gelatin microspheres, is used, then embolization is stopped when there is occlusion of the uterine arterial branches with slow antegrade flow in the main uterine artery.[43] This slow flow can be characterized by visualizing contrast within the main uterine artery for 5 to 10 heartbeats following injection into the uterine artery. At this point, the microcatheter is removed and the Cobra catheter is repositioned into the right internal iliac artery, using the Waltman Loop technique (**Fig. 5.5**).[47] The right uterine artery is then selectively catheterized with the microcatheter and embolization of the right uterine artery is performed (**Fig. 5.4B**).

The question as to whether or not both uterine arteries need to be embolized is a fair one to ask. Even in Goodwin's initial article on UFE in the United States, the utility of bilateral embolization was discussed.[3] The one patient in this limited series that failed after UFE underwent only a unilateral embolization. Recently, Nicholson[48] reported mixed results when unilateral embolization is performed due to technical reasons. In addition, Gabriel-Cox et al[49] reported that unilateral uterine artery embolization predicted subsequent hysterectomy for patients undergoing UFE. Other factors such as age, indication for UFE, uterine volume, embolic agent utilized, and radiologist experience did not predict subsequent hysterectomy for this patient population. This once again demonstrated the importance of a bilateral uterine artery embolization during UFE.

Once both uterine arteries have been embolized, it is fairly typical for a completion abdominal aortogram to be performed. This aortogram can be used to confirm that flow is slowed or stagnant within both uterine arteries. It is also helpful to potentially determine if significant collateral vessels are present to the uterus and the fibroids.[50,51] Specifically, it can help determine if dilated ovarian arteries are present, which are contributing to the arterial supply of the fibroids, especially once the uterine arteries have been embolized (**Fig. 5.6**).

The utility of a completion aortogram is not universally agreed upon. White et al[52] retrospectively reviewed 1072 UFE patients to identify patients in whom ovarian arteries were identified and contributed significantly to pelvic arterial flow. They found that on aortography, only 0.8% of patients had ovarian arteries identified, which supplied arterial flow to >10% of the uterus. When the ovarian arteries identified were selectively catheterized and angiograms were performed, 5.8% of patients were felt to have significant ovarian artery collateral supply to the uterus. Therefore, the sensitivity of aortography was only 18%. This fact, together with the findings that aortography contributes a substantial amount of radiation (>20% of total) to the overall exposure experienced during UFE,[53] has led some to believe that the routine performance of postembolization aortography may be of limited utility and should possibly be reconsidered. In fact, some are now advocating that magnetic resonance angiography (MRA) be used prior to UFE procedures to evaluate for the possibility of significant ovarian arterial collateral flow to fibroids.[54]

The determination as to whether or not a prominent ovarian artery should be embolized is one that may have to be made in response to the findings on an abdominal aortogram or selective ovarian arteriogram. Abbara et al[55] recommended that selective ovarian arteriography be performed if large ovarian arteries with rapid flow extending into the pelvis are identified on aortography. This allows one to determine if the ovarian arteries are responsible for some of the arterial supply of the treated fibroid. It is known that ovarian artery supply can result in treatment failure after UFE, which is why ovarian artery embolization has been used with success in these patients.[55,56] A classification system developed by Razavi et al[57] can potentially help with deciding if an ovarian artery needs to be embolized. In this article, three types of anastomoses were identified. In type I anastomoses, flow from the ovarian artery to the uterus was through anastomoses with the main uterine artery. In type II anastomoses, the ovarian artery supplied the fibroids directly. In type III anastomoses, the major blood supply to the ovary was from the uterine artery. Given this system, identification of a type II anastomoses would likely warrant ovarian artery embolization to be certain that the entire blood supply to the fibroid(s) is addressed.

■ Embolic Agent Selection

Particulate PVA was the agent used historically and was the agent that when used, provided the success of UFE as a treatment option for this patient population. Its ability to address the symptoms of a patient with uterine fibroids and decrease uterine and fibroid volume has been well documented.[3,58–62] As a result, during the early years of UFE, there was virtual agreement that particulate PVA was the most appropriate agent to use for this procedure. In addition, the endpoint of stasis of flow within the uter-

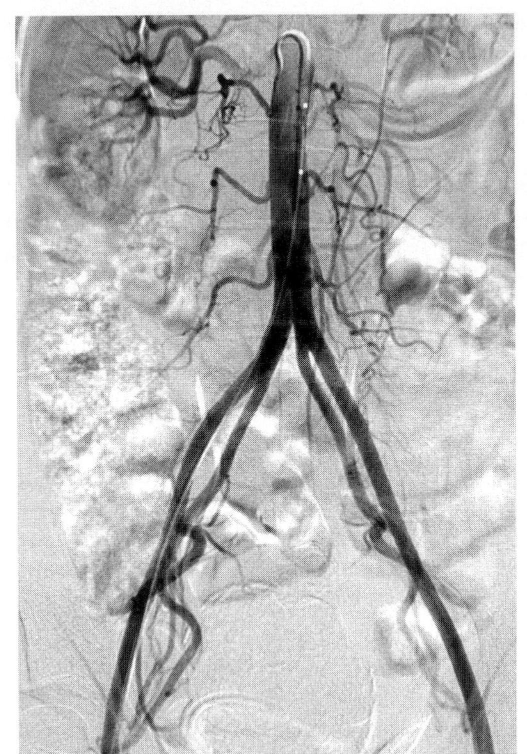

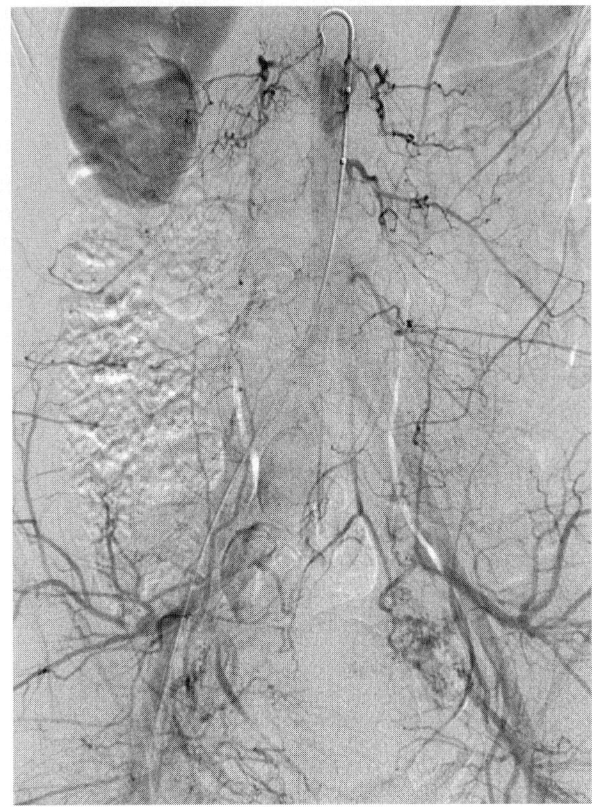

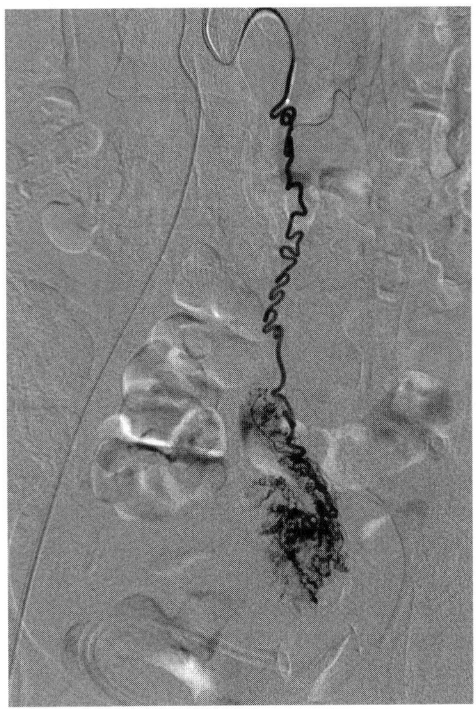

Fig. 5.6 (A,B) Two views from an abdominal aortogram after bilateral uterine artery embolization demonstrating significant flow in the left ovarian artery that is associated with an angiographic blush within the uterus. **(C)** A selective angiogram of the left ovarian artery confirming the role that this vessel plays in supplying arterial blood to the fibroid. This vessel was embolized using 500 to 700 micron Embosphere Microspheres (Biosphere Medical Corp, Rockland, MA) after this angiogram.

ine artery was agreed upon because it was the endpoint used for most embolization procedures at the time and was the most reliable endpoint to achieve with the use of particulate PVA. However, there are known shortcomings to particulate PVA that prompted investigation into optimizing the agent used during this, and other embolization procedures. These shortcomings include the inherent size variability in particle preparations, the known difficulty of injecting particulate PVA through a microcatheter, and the clumping of particles that makes the effective size of PVA larger than the actual size, leading to an embolic occlusion that is more proximal than intended.[63–66]

Once trisacryl gelatin microspheres (Embosphere Microspheres, Biosphere Medical Corp., Rockland, MA) were introduced as an alternative embolic agent to particulate PVA, embolic agent selection has been a point of controversy among interventional radiologists. This agent has been associated with significant clinical success when used for UFE (**Fig. 5.7**).[67–71] The spherical configuration of this agent was perceived as being advantageous because it addressed many of the above-listed shortcomings of particulate PVA. For example, Chua et al[72] reported that the tris-acryl gelatin microspheres measuring 700 to 900 microns in diameter penetrated deeper into the circulation of fibroids when compared with particulate PVA measuring 355 to 500 microns in diameter, implying less proximal aggregation associated with the gelatin-based microspheres. Although Spies et al failed to show any substantive differences in outcomes between the use of tris-acryl gelatin microspheres and particulate PVA, Smeets et al did demonstrate a slightly increased improvement in patient satisfaction when the gelatin-based microspheres were used.[73,74]

The clinical success of trisacryl gelatin microspheres prompted others to develop spherical agents for this procedure. PVA-based microspheres (including Contour SE Microspheres, Boston Scientific Corp., Natick, MA, and Bead Block, Terumo Corp., Somerset, NJ), were felt to have potential for this procedure because of their spherical configuration and the comfort and familiarity that interventional radiologists have had through the years with PVA. As experience with these new PVA-based microspheres increased, sentiment grew within the IR community that these products were not appropriate for UAE.[75,76] This was based on decreased clinical efficacy of these products in addition to a failure to achieve fibroid infarction to the same degree that is seen with trisacryl gelatin microspheres.[77–82] Therefore, at the present time, trisacryl gelatin microspheres are considered to be the embolic agent of choice for UFE given its success at achieving improvement in presenting symptoms, reduction of uterine and dominant fibroid volume, and infarction of the fibroids within the uterus at the time of treatment.

■ Postprocedure Recovery

One consistent feature of UFE, and one that is often the focus of patients considering this procedure and physicians discussing this procedure, is the experience of patients during the immediate postprocedure recovery period. Through the years, it has been well established that solid-organ embolization is associated with a constellation of symptoms known as the postembolization syndrome. Uterine fibroid embolization is no exception. Following UFE, patients typically experience symptoms including pelvic pain or cramping, nausea and vomiting, low-grade fever, fatigue, and generalized malaise. These symptoms last a variable amount of time across different patients, but one can generally expect the symptoms to last anywhere from 3 to 7 days. In most patients, pain generally increases over the first 2 hours after the procedure is completed and then plateaus for several hours. It then decreases fairly rapidly to a much lower level, typically following the first 8 to 10 hours after the procedure.[83] It has been shown that the severity of pain experienced after UFE cannot be predicted based on baseline uterine or fibroid volume and that the severity of pain experienced cannot be used to predict the clinical outcome from this procedure.[84] Spies et al and Ryu et al have shown that the amount of pain ex-

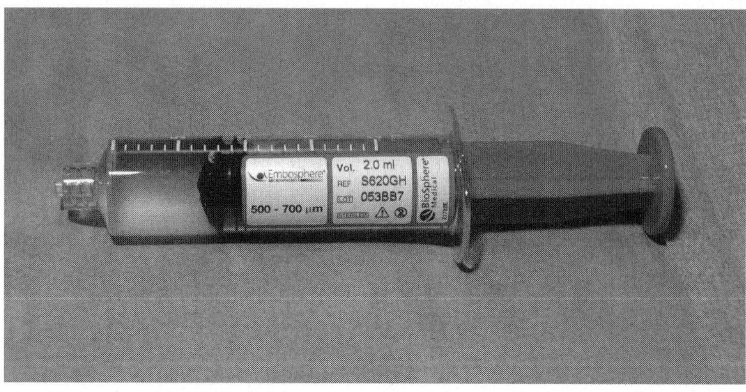

Fig. 5.7 One syringe of 500 to 700 micron trisacryl gelatin microspheres (Embosphere Microspheres, Biosphere Medical Corp., Rockland, MA).

perienced after UFE does not appear to be different when particulate PVA or trisacryl gelatin microspheres are used for the procedure.[85,86] However, Hovsepian et al[87] demonstrated that patients embolized with trisacryl gelatin microspheres experienced more pain than those embolized with PVA-based microspheres. Volkers et al,[88] reporting data from the EMMY trial, revealed that there was a relationship between the amount of embolic agent used and the risk for severe pain, postprocedural fever, and major complications.

Although the medications chosen by interventional radiologists to address these symptoms differ among the different centers offering the procedures, the concepts behind medication selection remain the same. Most centers agree that both narcotic pain medication and nonsteroidal, antiinflammatory medications are needed to address the pain associated with UFE; either used alone tends to be inadequate for relief of these symptoms. In particular, when given in combination with narcotic pain medication, ketorolac tromethamine (Abbott Laboratories, Chicago, IL) reduces postoperative pain and lessens postprocedure opioid requirements.[89–92] Medication to address nausea is important to include in a discharge medication regimen as well, because this symptom, attributed to both fibroid infarction and the effects of the narcotic pain medication, can be quite bothersome to patients as they recover from this procedure. Novel strategies for addressing postprocedure pain after embolization are being investigated presently. These include an intraarterial infusion of dilute lidocaine into the uterine artery,[93] the use of a superior hypogastric nerve block,[94] and loading embolic agents with ibuprofen for sustained release within the uterine arterial vasculature.[95]

There is some debate as to whether or not overnight observation in the inpatient setting should be a standard part of the UFE experience. Although postprocedure pain is something that most patients experience after the procedure, the degree of pain is markedly variable when comparing one patient to another. Therefore, it is certainly appropriate to have some patients initially recover as an inpatient and to then recover at home as an outpatient. The safety of outpatient UFE has been established.[89,96] In fact, there has been increasing interest in performing UFE as an outpatient procedure as more interventional radiologists are transitioning from hospital-based practices into ones based within freestanding centers. At the present time, however, overnight inpatient observation is considered typical for most patients undergoing UFE.

Hehenkamp et al[97] evaluated data from the EMMY trial concerning pain and return to daily activities after UFE. They found that patients undergoing UFE experienced significantly less pain during the first 24 hours after treatment when compared with patients undergoing a hysterectomy. In addition, UFE patients returned to daily activities significantly sooner than hysterectomy patients. Pron et al[98] reported data from the multicenter Ontario UFE trial concerning the postprocedure recovery period. In this trial, pain protocols included antiinflammatory medications and narcotics and a planned overnight hospital admission. The majority of patients had a 1-night length of stay in the hospital after UFE and recovered within 2 weeks. Worthington-Kirsch et al,[99] reporting data from the FIBROID Registry, found that the most common adverse event after discharge was inadequate pain relief requiring additional hospital treatment (2.4% of patients). Based on these data, it is fair to tell patients that they can expect the first 24 hours after UFE to be difficult, with significant pain and nausea that can be addressed with oral and/or intravenous medication. These symptoms then gradually improve over a period of several days with most patients fully recovered within 2 weeks.

■ Results

Clinical Results

To date, a large number of studies describing the clinical success associated with UFE have been published in the radiology and obstetrics and gynecology literature. The initial data published regarding UFE consisted of retrospective case series describing the success of UFE at improving clinical symptoms and reducing the volume of the uterus and dominant fibroids. White and Spies[100] have recently summarized the results of these early studies.[60–62,101–108] These 11 articles reported on 2126 patients with a mean duration of follow-up of 14.9 months. Eighty-eight percent of patients reported an improvement in menorrhagia, while 71% of patients reported improvement in bulk-related symptoms. Only eight patients underwent subsequent hysterectomy (0.3%) for complications of UFE. In these studies, the mean dominant fibroid volume decreased between 20 to 60%.

In 1999, an attempt was made to evaluate the outcomes after UFE with more uniform measures in the context of a multicenter registry sponsored by the Society of Interventional Radiology Foundation. Prior to data collection, a questionnaire called the Uterine Fibroid Symptoms and Quality of Life (UFS-QOL) questionnaire, which was specific for evaluating fibroid-related symptoms and health-related quality of life, was developed and validated.[109] Following this, prospective data concerning the technical aspects during UFE and the clinical outcomes after UFE was collected on more than 3,000 patients from 72 sites.[110] Spies et al[111] investigated the changes in symptom severity and health-related quality of life at 12 months in patients enrolled in the registry. Of 2112 eligible patients, follow-up data were obtained on 1,701 patients (80.5%) at 12 months. Based on the UFS-QOL, there were significant improvements in both symptom severity and health-related quality of life. Predictors of a greater symptom change score include smaller fibroid size, submucosal location, and presenting symptom of heavy menstrual bleeding. Of note, 5.5% of patients did not experience symptomatic improvement and 5.0% of patients did not experience improvements in health-related quality of life. In the first year after embolization, hysterectomy was performed in 2.9% of patients.

In 2004, Joffre et al[112] reported the results from a French multicenter registry evaluating the safety and efficacy of UFE performed with trisacryl gelatin microspheres. This study evaluated 85 patients with symptomatic fibroids. Complete resolution of menorrhagia was achieved in 84% of women at 24 months and significant uterine and fibroid volume reductions were noted after 6 months (37% and 73%, respectively).

As additional data has been reported regarding UFE, it is possible to begin making statements regarding the long-term outcomes after UFE and the outcomes after UFE in comparison to other gynecologic procedures. There are two studies available at the present time with 5-year follow-up after UFE. Spies et al reported on the long-term follow-up of the cohort of patients initially reported on in 2001.[28,103] In this population, there was a 93% rate of symptomatic improvement 3 months after UFE. Five years after UFE, 73% of patients reported continued control of their presenting symptoms. Subsequent interventions, including hysterectomy, myomectomy, or repeat UFE were reported in 20% of patients. Katsumori et al[113] reported 5-year follow-up data on 96 patients. In this study, the rate of symptom control after 1 year was 96.9%, which decreased to 89.5% at 5 years. The treatment failure rate in this study was 4.2% at 1 year and 12.7% at 5 years. The results of other recent studies with long-term follow-up on their patients are summarized in **Table 5.1**.[28,68,113–117] One generalization that can be made is that recurrence and hysterectomy rates tend to increase as the follow-up intervals increase.[100]

In addition to studies with long-term follow-up, studies are now available that compare UFE to standard gynecologic treatments for uterine fibroids. The EMMY trial was a randomized controlled trial comparing the effects of UFE with hysterectomy.[118] Twenty-eight Dutch hospitals participated; in this trial, 88 patients were randomized to UFE and 89 patients were randomized to hysterectomy. Two years after treatment, 23.5% of UFE patients had undergone a hysterectomy. There were no significant differences in improvement of pain and bulk-related symptoms when compared with baseline. Uterine and dominant fibroid volume reduction in UFE patients were 48.2% and 60.5%, respectively. This data allowed the investigators to consider UFE as an alternative treatment for uterine fibroids. However, given the rate of secondary procedures seen in this study, hysterectomy was also considered to be a more definitive choice for patients seeking control of abnormal bleeding.

Edwards et al[119] reported on the results of the REST trial (Randomized Trial of Embolization versus Surgical Treatment for Fibroids). This was a randomized, multicenter trial comparing UFE with abdominal surgery in women with symptomatic uterine fibroids. Patients were randomly assigned to undergo UFE (n = 106) or surgery (n = 43 hysterectomies; n = 8 myomectomies). In this study, there were no significant differences in the quality-of-life scores between the two groups at 1 year, although symptom scores were better in the surgical group at the time of follow-up. During the first year of follow-up, there were 13 major adverse events in the embolization group (12%) and 10 in the surgical group (20%), which was not statistically significant. As compared with the surgical group, the embolization group had the advantages of a significantly shorter hospital stay and a more rapid resumption of normal activities. However, 10 patients in the embolization group (9%) required a repeat UFE or hysterectomy for inadequate symptom control.

Spies et al[67] performed a multicenter, prospective study comparing UFE and hysterectomy in 152 patients (102 patients were treated with UFE and 50 were treated with hysterectomy). After 12 months of follow-up, patients in both groups experienced significant improvement in presenting symptoms and quality of life. A larger proportion

Table 5.1 Long-Term Outcomes after Uterine Fibroid Embolization

Author	No. of Patients	Follow-up	Symptom Control	Follow-up Major Intervention	% Fibroid Volume Reduction	% Uterine Volume Reduction
Broder et al, 2002[114]	59	86% at 46 mo	61%	29%		
Marret et al, 2003[115]	85	30 mo (Mean)	83.5%		60.3% (12 mo)	53.8% (12 mo)
Spies et al, 2005[111]	200	95% at 12 mo	87%	6.3%	57.8% (12 mo)	39.4% (12 mo)
		91% at 60 mo	73%	19.8%		
Katsumori et al, 2006[113]	96	100% at 36 mo	89.5%	7.3%		
Huang et al, 2006[116]	233	13 mo (Mean)	90.6%	9.4%	39.7% (6 mo)	28.4% (6 mo)
Spies et al, 2007[68]	96	72% at 36 mo	88.4%	8.3%		

of the patients who had undergone hysterectomy experienced improvements in pelvic pain. Of note, complications were more frequent in patients who underwent hysterectomy when compared with patients who had undergone UFE (50% versus 27%).

Two retrospective studies are available that compare the results after UFE with the results seen after myomectomy. Broder et al[114] reported that patients undergoing UFE were more likely to require further therapy than those patients treated with myomectomy (29% versus 3%). In this study, the overall rates of symptomatic improvement in patients not requiring subsequent intervention were similar between the two groups. In addition, patients undergoing UFE had a significantly greater degree of satisfaction after the procedure than did patients undergoing myomectomy (94% versus 79%). Razavi et al[120] reported that UFE patients had a significantly greater rate of improvement in menorrhagia (92% versus 64%), but a lower rate of improvement in bulk-related symptoms (76% versus 91%) when compared with myomectomy patients. In addition, myomectomy patients had a longer interval before resuming normal activities compared with UFE patients.

Goodwin et al[121] prospectively evaluated the differences in outcome after UFE performed with particulate PVA and myomectomy with a multicenter cohort-controlled study. There were no significant differences in bleeding improvement, quality of life improvement, and uterine volume reduction when comparing the two groups. UFE patients did have a shorter mean duration of hospital stay (<1 day versus 2.5 days) and a fewer number of days before returning to normal activity (14.6 days versus 44.4 days). Similar findings were noted by Siskin et al[122] who reported the third arm of the above study, which consisted of patients undergoing UFE with PVA microspheres. Patients undergoing UFE with this embolic agent experienced a similar degree of symptomatic improvement and improvement in health-related quality of life compared with the patients undergoing a myomectomy or embolization with particulate PVA.

Pathological Results

Following UFE, most fibroids undergo a similar pattern of degenerative change. Fibroids most commonly undergo hyaline-type necrosis,[123] but others may undergo coagulative or suppurative necrosis.[124–127] McCluggage and colleagues[128] described the findings in 10 fibroids that had previously been treated with UFE. In this report, intravascular foreign material (presumably the PVA used for embolization) was identified, which resulted in thrombosis and a histiocytic and foreign body giant cell reaction. Colgan et al[125] also reported the presence of a foreign body giant-cell reaction that was seen within 1 week of UFE and persisted for up to 14 months. When trisacryl gelatin microspheres are used for UFE, a granulomatous foreign body reaction in the vicinity of particles can be seen, which may be eventually followed by localized dissolution of the vessel wall and extravascular deposition of the embolic material.[126,129,130] Ultimately, this can lead to calcification in the periphery of the infarcted fibroid.[131]

These pathologic reports have also described embolic material found outside the confines of the treated fibroids. McCluggage et al[128] described "intravascular foreign material within the myometrium, the cervix, or paraovarian region, sometimes resulting in foci of inflammation, myometrial necrosis and microabscess formation beyond the confines of the fibroids." However, the degree of myometrial ischemia or necrosis occurring in association with UFE has not been felt to be significant.[132] Colgan et al[125] described PVA particles within the cervix, the adnexa, and the myometrium, sometimes resulting in necrotizing endomyometritis. Similar findings have been associated with the use of trisacryl gelatin microspheres.[126,129]

Imaging Findings

The early case series and the long-term and comparative studies that have been reported more recently all share the desire to report changes seen on imaging studies that have occurred as a result of the UFE procedure. Initially, the primary measure of success that was reported on postprocedure imaging studies was the degree to which the volume of the uterus and the volume of the dominant fibroid decreased after embolization. These volume measurements were obtained by using the formula for volume of a prorated ellipse.[3,58,133] This required that three linear measurements were obtained for the uterus and for each fibroid measured. Given the fact that there is still a desire to report the degree of uterine and fibroid volume reduction in association with this procedure, it is important to note the work of Joe et al.[134] They demonstrated that stereologic volume measurements made from high-resolution T2-weighted images in two planes (axial and sagittal) provided high interobserver reliability for uterine and fibroid volume measurements and was more reliable than the ellipsoid method described above.[134] The degree of uterine and fibroid volume reduction achieved with UFE is important because patient satisfaction with UFE appears to be related to the amount of volume reduction achieved.[28]

In recent years, it has been found that postprocedure-imaging studies, particularly contrast-enhanced MRI of the pelvis, have the capability of providing more information than just the degree of uterine and fibroid volume reduction. It appears that the presence or absence of fibroid infarction is one measure that is potentially predictive of long-term success after UFE.[135,136] Pelage et al[136] studied the long-term MRI outcomes in patients undergoing UFE. The data suggested that although incomplete fibroid infarction may not affect outcome immediately, regrowth of uninfarcted fibroid tissue may ultimately result in symptom recurrence. Dorenberg et al[137] similarly found that clinical improvement was more significant in patients who had evidence of complete infarction on postprocedure, contrast-enhanced MRI. This work has been far-reaching, prompting most interventionalists to evaluate their patients with contrast-enhanced MRI to determine if the treated fibroids have undergone infarction after embolization. Based on these data, fibroids that have been successfully infarcted after embolization (as evidenced by lack of enhancement on postcontrast MRI) are considered to have been treated definitively and will likely not recur whereas fibroids that have not been completely infarcted after embolization are at risk for regrowth and symptomatic recurrence (**Fig. 5.8** and **Fig. 5.9**). Yousefi et al[138] evaluated patients undergoing repeat UFE based on recurrent symptoms and found that the most common finding on MRI was a lack of tumor infarction (or persistent fibroid enhancement).

The use of contrast-enhanced MRI after UFE has also permitted studies to be performed evaluating the efficacy of the different embolic agents available for use. In large part, these imaging studies have encouraged and discouraged the use of certain agents for UFE. Spies et al performed a prospective randomized study comparing outcomes after UFE performed with PVA microspheres (Contour SE Microspheres) and trisacryl gelatin microspheres.[77] In this study, there was a high rate of failed tumor infarction (as evidenced by enhancement on postcontrast MRI) associated with a lower rate of improvement in quality of life when PVA microspheres were used for UFE. In response to this finding, a protocol recommending larger PVA microspheres (Contour SE Microspheres) for use during UFE was developed that improved the rate of fibroid infarction after UFE performed with this agent.[139] However, Siskin et al performed an additional prospective randomized study comparing trisacryl gelatin microspheres and PVA microspheres (Contour SE Microspheres) using this new protocol. The findings were similar to those reported by Spies et al: the use of PVA microspheres was associated with persistent fibroid enhancement in a significant number of patients receiving PVA microspheres during UFE.[140] Similar findings have been reported in association with the use of Bead Block, another PVA-based microsphere.[82] Therefore, contrast-enhanced MRI allows for an objective determination of procedural success that has been helpful in optimizing the technique used during UFE and for predicting long-term success for patients after UFE.

■ Complications

The complications seen after UFE have been reported in virtually every study evaluating UFE as a procedure to treat patients with fibroids. There have been case reports and small retrospective series highlighting one or more complications associated with this procedure. The larger studies and trials, however, have been helpful in understanding how often complications occur and the safety of the UFE procedure when compared with other gynecologic procedures such as hysterectomy and myomectomy.

Worthington-Kirsch et al[99] studied the short-term (30 days) efficacy of UFE from the registry data. Major in-hospital complications occurred in 0.66% of patients, and major events after discharge occurred in 4.8% of patients within the first 30 days after UFE. The most common adverse event after discharge was inadequate pain relief requiring additional hospital treatment (2.4%). Three patients (0.1%) required a hysterectomy within 30 days of treatment. There were no deaths in this period of time. Spies et al[111] reported the midterm results from the registry data. In this study, the hysterectomy rate within the first 12 months after UFE was 2.9%. In data reported from the EMMY trial, Volkers et al[88] reported that the overall complication rate (including major and minor complications) were comparable between UFE and hysterectomy. However, minor complications were more common after UFE than hysterectomy and major complications (such as pulmonary embolism, sepsis, pneumonia, etc.) were rare, but more commonly seen after hysterectomy (2.9% versus 2.7%). When comparing UFE and myomectomy, Razavi et al[120] reported that the complication rates were 11% for UFE patients and 25% for myomectomy patients.

What is clear in reviewing these studies is that complications happen in association with UFE. Most of the complications that have been reported are rare and treatable. Yet, most cannot necessarily be predicted or avoided. Therefore, it is important for anybody performing this procedure to understand the potential risks and to discuss them with every patient before moving ahead with UFE.

Premature Amenorrhea

The occurrence of premature amenorrhea after UFE is a known complication of this procedure.[141] Chrisman et al[142] studied the incidence of ovarian failure after UFE and retrospectively compared the rate of this complication in patients <age 45 with that seen in patients 45 years or older. Sixty-six premenopausal patients were included in this analysis. During follow-up, nine patients (14%) were found to have ovarian failure and presumed menopause. When divided into age groups, 9 of 21 (43%) women older than 45 years had ovarian failure after UFE. This complication was not seen in any of the women younger than age 45. They concluded that loss of menses induced by UFE is significantly more likely to occur in women older than 45 years. This finding was confirmed by Tropeano et al[143] and Ahmad et al[144] in their studies evaluating the effects of UFE on ovarian function in younger patients. Spies et al,[145] who evaluated serial basal follicle stimulating hormone (FSH)

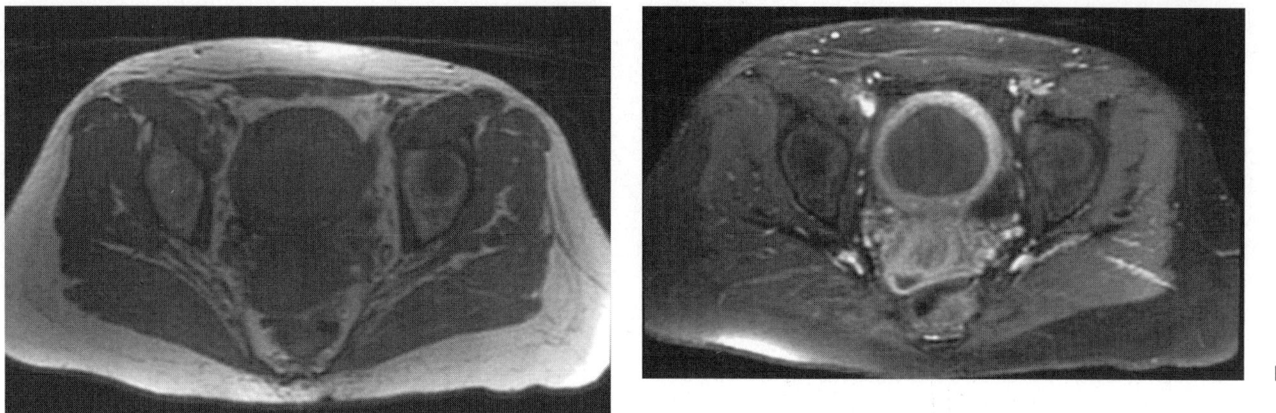

Fig. 5.8 T1-weighted axial magnetic resonance images **(A)** before and **(B)** after the administration of gadolinium demonstrating an anterior intramural fibroid that has been completely infarcted after uterine artery embolization.

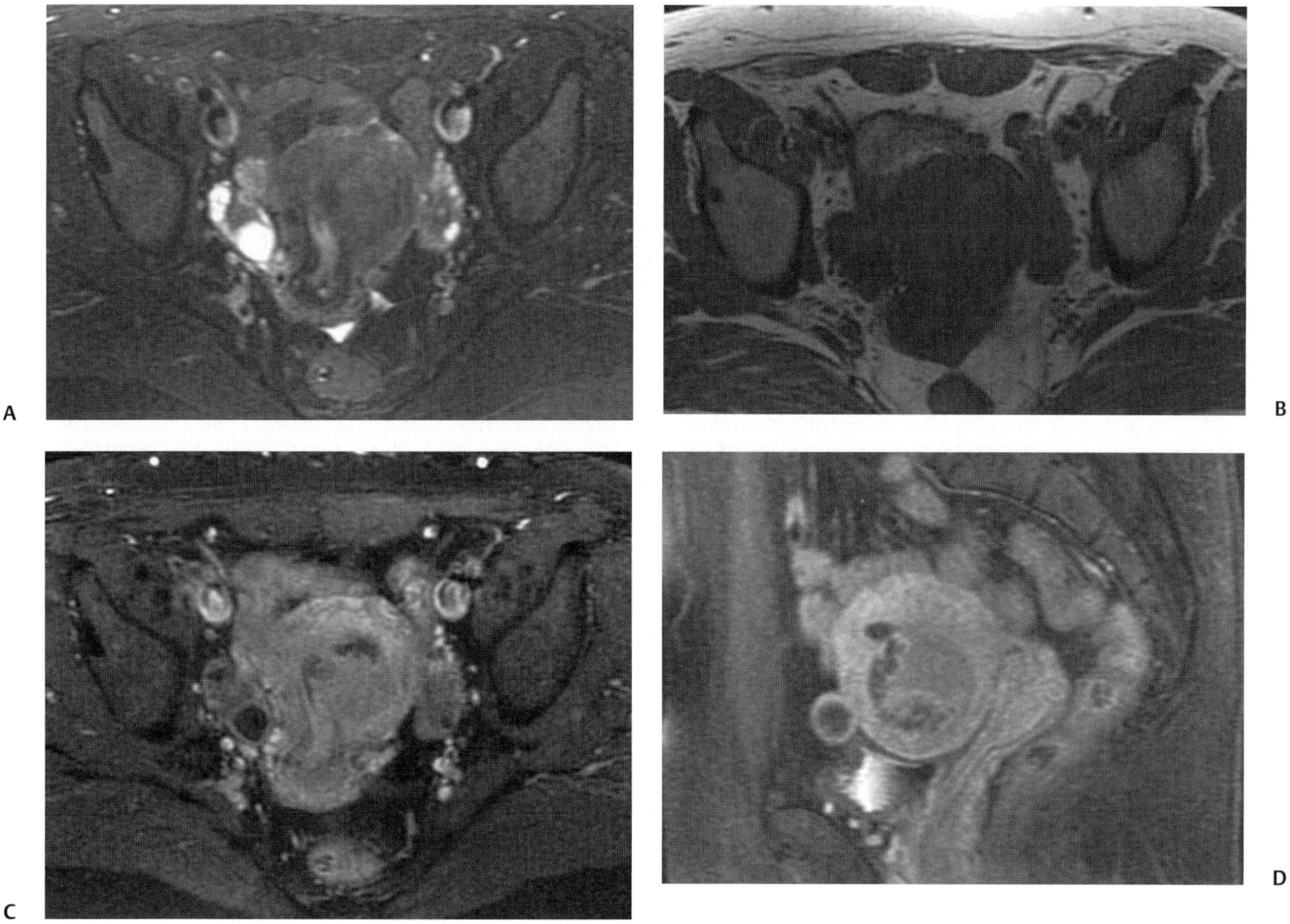

Fig. 5.9 T2- and T1-weighted axial magnetic resonance images (MRIs) **(A,B)** before the administration of contrast and T1-weighted axial and sagittal MRIs **(C,D)** after the administration of contrast demonstrating a left-sided intramural fibroid with a submucosal component, which enhances with contrast. This implies continued viability of this fibroid after embolization.

levels before and after UFE, also confirmed this finding. They found a statistically significant difference in change in basal FSH levels when comparing different age groups. A greater change was identified in patients >45 years of age and it was concluded that patients 45 years or older have a 15% chance of an increase in basal FSH into the perimenopausal range after UFE. Spies et al[111] also reported the 12-month data from the FIBROID registry. In this study, amenorrhea occurred in 7.3% of patients (86% of these patients were aged 45 years or older).

The explanation for this complication is considered to lie in the inadvertent embolization of the ovarian arterial bed that may occur secondary to the presence of anastomoses between the uterine and ovarian arterial beds. Kim et al[146] found that anastomoses between the uterine artery and ovarian artery could angiographically be demonstrated in 40.3% of patients undergoing UFE. As a result, they found that when these anastomoses can be seen angiographically, there is an increased risk of embolic particles making their way into the circulation of the fallopian tubes and adnexa and a significant increase in basal FSH levels.[147,148] Payne et al[149] also found evidence of embolic particles within the ovarian arterial vasculature after UFE. Despite the fact that adnexal tissues containing particles have been shown to be histologically viable without evidence of ischemic change or infarction, this can potentially lead to decreased ovarian arterial perfusion, increased ovarian vascular impedance, and diminished function.[150] As a result of these findings, one strategy that has been described when utero-ovarian anastomoses are visualized on angiography is to embolize the visible anastomosis with coils prior to delivery of the embolic agent.[151,152] It is important to remember that ovarian failure after UFE can be transient[153,154] and that amenorrhea after UFE can also be due to endometrial atrophy without ovarian failure.[155] Despite all of this, it has been shown that the impact on ovarian function does not differ when comparing patients who have undergone UFE, hysterectomy, or myomectomy.[156,157]

Infection

The possibility of an infection related to UFE was reported early in the experience with this procedure by Goodwin et al[3] and has since been the subject of additional case reports.[158–162] Two cases of a fatal infection related to performance of UFE have been reported.[162,163] Despite the fact that Rajan et al identified no specific risk factors for intrauterine infection following UFE, it has been suggested that fibroids at risk for transcervical expulsion (including submucosal fibroids and intramural fibroids with a submucosal component) may be at increased risk for infection, especially if the process of transcervical expulsion becomes arrested.[164] Endometritis is an infection of the endometrium that has been estimated to occur after 0.5% of UFE procedures.[165] It was originally reported in conjunction with the use of gold-colored gelatin microspheres but can occur sporadically as well.[166] Most patients will respond well to antibiotics, but if untreated, it can lead to fever, pelvic pain, and sepsis. Finally, a case of pyosalpinx after UFE has been reported in conjunction with a preexisting hydrosalpinx.[29] In this case, there was superinfection of the previously existing, simple fluid collection, which ultimately required hysterectomy and oophorectomy. As discussed earlier in this chapter, it is unclear whether or not the administration of prophylactic antibiotics has a role in preventing these rare infections after UFE.

Venous Thromboembolic Complications

Deep venous thrombosis (DVT) and pulmonary embolism have both been reported after UFE. The incidence of thromboembolic complications after UFE has been estimated at 0.4%.[167] DVT can occur due to inflammation of the major pelvic veins, especially when a patient is immobile after UFE.[165] Occurrence of pulmonary embolic disease is an equally rare phenomenon after UFE, but is potentially fatal.[168] It seems most likely that venous thromboembolic complications after UFE can be attributed to the immobility that patients experience while recovering from the procedure. However, Nikolic et al[169] demonstrated that surrogate markers of hypercoagulability increase after UFE, suggesting that a prothrombotic state may result after the procedure. Presently, early ambulation is recommended as one way to prevent DVT after UFE, but no other definitive recommendations regarding anticoagulation or lower extremity compression have been formulated for this purpose.

Transcervical Fibroid Expulsion

Transcervical expulsion of fibroid fragments or entire fibroids has been reported after UFE.[170–172] Fibroids in contact with the endometrial surface, including submucosal fibroids or intramural fibroids with a submucosal component, are at increased risk for transcervical expulsion.[173] In most cases, transcervical expulsion results in no symptoms and no significant complications, although hysteroscopy might be required for complete removal of the fibroid.[174,175] Hysteroscopy should be reserved for cases in which the patient is symptomatic or when the fibroid is partially infarcted and still attached to the wall of the endometrial cavity.[165] Patients who have arrested passage of fibroid material, however, may present with abdominal pain and signs of sepsis.[164]

Other Complications

Because UFE is an angiographic procedure performed using a percutaneous technique, there is always the risk of complications relating to arterial catheterization.[170] This includes a hematoma, pseudoaneurysm or arteriovenous fistula formation, arterial thrombosis and distal embolization, arterial dissection, vessel perforation, vasospasm, and catheterization-site infection. Similarly, reactions to the use of iodinated contrast material, including anaphylaxis and contrast nephropathy are possible as well.[170] Nontarget embolization is a possible risk of UFE as well and may have resulted in adverse events such as vesicouterine fistula formation,[176,177] labial necrosis,[178] and buttock necrosis[179] after UFE. This can potentially be avoided with the use of state-of-the-art fluoroscopic equipment and meticulous technique. In some cases, however, it may not be angiographically apparent that branches arising from the uterine artery are supplying "nontarget" tissue: in these cases, nontarget embolization may be impossible to prevent.

Other complications that have been reported include diffuse uterine necrosis,[180,181] prolapse of a cervical myoma,[182] and a small bowel volvulus requiring bowel resection due to adherence of bowel to uterine adhesions.[183] Fistula formation between the endometrial cavity and necrotic myoma has been reported as well after UFE.[184] This can potentially lead to a prolonged vaginal discharge after this procedure.

■ Conclusions

Uterine fibroid embolization (UFE) has proven itself to be a valuable addition to the treatment options now available for patients with symptomatic uterine leiomyomata. What started as an innovative use of an established procedure has grown to the point that it is now a procedure that has been formally recognized by the American College of Obstetricians and Gynecologists as an option with evidence supporting its safety and efficacy for this patient population. Future research will no doubt focus on optimizing patient selection criteria, technical modifications including the development of new embolic agents, and determining the best way to image and follow patients after UFE.

References

1. Ravina JH, Herbreteau D, Ciraru-Vigneron N, et al. Arterial embolization to treat uterine myomata. Lancet 1995;346:671–672
2. Ravina JH, Bouret JM, Ciraru-Vigneron N, et al. Recourse to particular arterial embolization in the treatment of some uterine leiomyomas. Bull Acad Natl Med 1997;181:233–243
3. Goodwin SC, Vedantham S, McLucas B, Forno AE, Perrella R. Preliminary experience with uterine artery embolization for uterine fibroids. J Vasc Interv Radiol 1997;8:517–526
4. Society of Obstetricians and Gynaecologists of Canada. SOGC Clinical Practice Guidelines. Uterine fibroid embolization (UFE). Number 150, October 2004. Int J Gynaecol Obstet 2005;89:305–318
5. Committee on Gynecolgic Practice, American College of Obstetricians and Gynecologists. ACOG Committee Opinion. Uterine artery embolization. Obstet Gynecol 2004;103:403–404
6. Jacobson GF, Shaber RE, Armstrong MA, Hung YY. Changes in rates of hysterectomy and uterine conserving procedures for treatment of uterine leiomyomas. Am J Obstet Gynecol 2007;196:e1–e6
7. Kim HS, Tsai J, Paxton BE. Safety and utility of uterine artery embolization with CO2 and a gadolinium-based contrast medium. J Vasc Interv Radiol 2007;18:1021–1027
8. Englander MJ, Siskin GP, Dowling K, Quarfordt S. Uterine fibroid embolization without the use of iodinated contrast material. J Vasc Interv Radiol 2002;13:427–429
9. Andrews RT, Spies JB, Sacks D, et al. Patient care and uterine artery embolization for leiomyomata. J Vasc Interv Radiol 2004;15:115–120
10. Ravina JH, Aymard A, Cirau-Vigneron N, et al. Embolisation arterielle particulaire: un nouveau traitement des haemorragies des leiomyomes uterins. Presse Med 1998;27:299–303
11. Braude P, Reidy J, Nott V, Taylor A, Forman R. Embolization of uterine leiomyomata: current concepts in management. Hum Reprod Update 2000;6:603–608
12. Katsumori T, Kentarou A, Mihara T. Uterine artery embolization for pedunculated subserosal fibroids. AJR Am J Roentgenol 2005;184:399–402
13. Walker WJ, Pelage JP, Sutton C. Fibroid embolization. Clin Radiol 2002;57:325–331
14. Margau R, Simons M, Rajan DK, et al. Outcomes after uterine artery embolization for pedunculated subserosal leiomyomas. J Vasc Interv Radiol 2008;19:657–661
15. Verma SK, Bergin D, Gonsalves CF, et al. Submucosal fibroids becoming endocavitary following uterine artery embolization: risk assessment by MRI. AJR 2008;190:1220–1226
16. Levgur M. Therapeutic options for adenomyosis: a review. Arch Gynecol Obstet 2007;276:1–15
17. Goodwin SC, McLucas B, Lee M, et al. Uterine artery embolization for the treatment of uterine leiomyomata: midterm results. J Vasc Interv Radiol 1999;10:1159–1165
18. Smith SJ, Smith SJ, Sewall LE, Handelsman A. A clinical failure of uterine fibroid embolization due to adenomyosis. J Vasc Interv Radiol 1999;10:1171–1174
19. Siskin GP, Tublin ME, Stainken BF, Dowling K, Dolen EG. Uterine artery embolization for the treatment of adenomyosis: clinical response and evaluation with MR imaging. AJR Am J Roentgenol 2001;177:297–302
20. Kim MD, Won JW, Lee DY, Ahn CS. Uterine artery embolization for adenomyosis without fibroids. Clin Radiol 2004;59:520–526
21. Jha RC, Takahama J, Imaoka I, et al. Adenomyosis: MRI of the uterus treated with uterine artery embolization. AJR Am J Roentgenol 2003;181:851–856
22. Chen CL, Liu P, Zeng BL, Ma B, Zhang H. Intermediate and long term clinical effects of uterine arterial embolization in treatment of adenomyosis. Zhonghua Fu Chan Ke Za Zhi 2006;41:660–663
23. Lohle PN, De Vries J, Klazen CA, et al. Uterine artery embolization for symptomatic adenomyosis with or without uterine leiomyomas with the use of calibrated tris-acryl gelatin microspheres: midterm clinical and MR imaging follow-up. J Vasc Interv Radiol 2007;18:835–841
24. Kim MD, Kim S, Kim NK, et al. Long-term results of uterine artery embolization for symptomatic adenomyosis. AJR Am J Roentgenol 2007;188:176–181
25. Pelage JP, Jacob D, Fazel A, et al. Midterm results of uterine artery embolization for symptomatic adenomyosis: initial experience. Radiology 2005;234:948–953
26. Goldberg J. Uterine artery embolization for adenomyosis: looking at the glass half full. Radiology 2005;236:1111–1112
27. Prollius A, de Vries C, Loggenberg E, du Plessis A, Nel M, Wessels PH. Uterine artery embolization for symptomatic fibroids: the effect of the large uterus on outcome. BJOG 2004;111:239–242

28. Spies JB, Bruno J, Czeyda-Pommersheim F, et al. Long-term outcome of uterine artery embolization of leiomyomas. Obstet Gynecol 2005;106:933–939
29. Nikolic B, Nguyen K, Martin LG, Redd DC, Best I, Silverstein MI. Pyosalpinx developing from a preexisting hydrosalpinx after uterine artery embolization. J Vasc Interv Radiol 2004;15:297–301
30. Siskin GP, Bagla S, Sansivero GE, Mitchell NL. The interventional radiology clinic: key ingredients for success. J Vasc Interv Radiol 2004;15:681–688
31. Chrisman HB, Minocha J, Ryu RK, Vogelzang RL, Nikolaidis P, Omary RA. Uterine artery embolization: a treatment option for symptomatic fibroids in postmenopausal women. J Vasc Interv Radiol 2007;18:451–454
32. Dueholm M, Lundorf E, Hansen ES, et al. Magnetic resonance imaging, transvaginal sonography, hysterosonographic examination and diagnostic hysteroscopy in evaluation of the uterine cavity. Fertil Steril 2001;76:350–357
33. Woodward PJ, Sohaey R, Mezzetti TP Jr. Endometriosis: radiologic-pathologic correlation. Radiographics 2001;21:193–216
34. Ascher SM, Arnold LL, Patt RH, et al. Adenomyosis: prospective comparison of MR imaging and transvaginal sonography. Radiology 1994;190:803–806
35. Spielmann AL, Keogh C, Forster BB, Martin ML, Machan LS. Comparison of MRI and sonography in the preliminary evaluation for fibroid embolization. AJR Am J Roentgenol 2006;187:1499–1504
36. Cura M, Cura A, Bugone A. Role of magnetic resonance imaging in patient selection for uterine artery embolization. Acta Radiol 2006;47:1105–1114
37. Kroncke TJ, Hamm B. Role of magnetic resonance imaging (MRI) in establishing the indication for, planning, and following up uterine artery embolization (UAE) for treating symptomatic leiomyomas of the uterus. Radiologe 2003;43:624–633
38. Omary RA, Vasireddy S, Chrisman HB, et al. The effect of pelvic MR imaging on the diagnosis and treatment of women with presumed symptomatic uterine fibroids. J Vasc Interv Radiol 2002;13:1149–1153
39. Nikolaidis P, Siddiqi AJ, Carr JC, et al. Incidence of nonviable leiomyomas on contrast material-enhanced pelvic MR imaging in patients referred for uterine artery embolization. J Vasc Interv Radiol 2005;16:1465–1471
40. Harman M, Zeteroglu S, Arslan H, Sengul M, Etlik O. Predictive value of magnetic resonance imaging signal and contrast enhancement characteristics on post-embolization volume reduction of uterine fibroids. Acta Radiol 2006;47:427–435
41. Burn PR, McCall JM, Chinn RJ, Vashisht A, Smith JR, Healy JC. Uterine fibroleiomyoma: MR imaging appearances before and after embolization of uterine fibroids. Radiology 2000;214:729–734
42. Jha RC, Ascher SM, Imaoka I, Spies JB. Symptomatic fibroleiomyomata: MR imaging of the uterus before and after uterine arterial embolization. Radiology 2000;217:228–235
43. Ryan JM, Ryan BM, Smith TP. Antibiotic prophylaxis in interventional radiology. J Vasc Interv Radiol 2004;15:547–556
44. Pelage JP, Cazejust J, Pluot E, et al. Uterine fibroid vascularization and clinical relevance to uterine fibroid embolization. Radiographics 2005;25(Suppl 1):S99–S117
45. Worthington-Kirsch RL, Andrews RT, Siskin GP, et al. Uterine fibroid embolization: technical aspects. Tech Vasc Interv Radiol 2002;5:17–34
46. Lai AC, Goodwin SC, Bonilla SM, et al. Sexual dysfunction after uterine artery embolization. J Vasc Interv Radiol 2000;11:755–758
47. Waltman AC, Courey W, Athanasoulis C, Baum S. Technique for left gastric artery catheterization. Radiology 1973;109:732–734
48. Nicholson T. Outcome in patients undergoing unilateral uterine artery embolization for symptomatic fibroids. Clin Radiol 2004;59:186–191
49. Gabriel-Cox K, Jacobson GF, Armstrong MA, Hung YY, Learman LA. Predictors of hysterectomy after uterine artery embolization for leiomyoma. Am J Obstet Gynecol 2007;196:e1–e6
50. Binkert CA, Andrews RT, Kaufman JA. Utility of nonselective abdominal aortography in demonstrating ovarian artery collaterals in patients undergoing uterine artery embolization for fibroids. J Vasc Interv Radiol 2001;12:841–845
51. Saraiya PV, Chang TC, Pelage JP, Spies JB. Uterine artery replacement by the round ligament artery: an anatomic variant discovered during uterine artery embolization for leiomyomata. J Vasc Interv Radiol 2002;13(9 Pt 1):939–941
52. White AM, Banovac F, Yousefi S, Slack RS, Spies JB. Uterine fibroid embolization: the utility of aortography in detecting ovarian artery collateral supply. Radiology 2007;244:291–298
53. White AM, Banovac F, Spies JB. Patient radiation exposure during uterine fibroid embolization and the dose attributable to aortography. J Vasc Interv Radiol 2007;18:573–576
54. Kroencke TJ, Scheurig C, Kluner C, Taupitz M, Schnorr J, Hamm B. Uterine fibroids: contrast-enhanced MR angiography to predict ovarian artery supply – initial experience. Radiology 2006;241:181–189
55. Abbara S, Nikolic B, Pelage JP, Banovac F, Spies JB. Frequency and extent of uterine perfusion via ovarian arteries observed during uterine artery embolization for leiomyomas. AJR Am J Roentgenol 2007;188:1558–1563
56. Andrews RT, Bromley PJ, Pfister ME. Successful embolization of collaterals from the ovarian artery during uterine artery embolization for fibroids: a case report. J Vasc Interv Radiol 2000;11:607–610
57. Razavi MK, Wolanske KA, Hwang GL, Sze DY, Kee ST, Dake MD. Angiographic classification of ovarian artery-to-uterine artery anastomoses: initial observations in uterine fibroid embolization. Radiology 2002;224:707–712
58. Spies JB, Scialli AR, Jha RC, et al. Initial results from uterine fibroid embolization for symptomatic leiomyomata. J Vasc Interv Radiol 1999;10:1149–1157
59. Worthington-Kirsch RL, Popky GL, Hutchins FL. Uterine arterial embolization for the management of leiomyomas: quality of life assessment and clinical response. Radiology 1998;208:625–629
60. Pron G, Bennett J, Common A, et al. The Ontario uterine fibroid embolization trial: part 2. Uterine fibroid reduction and symptoms relief after uterine artery embolization for fibroids. Fertil Steril 2003;79:120–127
61. Walker WJ, Pelage J. Uterine artery embolization for symptomatic fibroids: clinical results in 400 women with imaging follow-up. BJOG 2002;109:1262–1272
62. Brunereau L, Herbreteau D, Gallas S, et al. Uterine artery embolization in the primary treatment of uterine leiomyomas: technical features and prospective follow-up with clinical and sonographic examination in 58 patients. AJR Am J Roentgenol 2000;175:1267–1272
63. Laurent A, Beaujeux R, Wassef M, et al. Trisacryl gelatin microspheres for therapeutic embolization: I. Development and in-vitro evaluation. AJNR Am J Neuroradiol 1996;17:533–540
64. Derdeyn CP, Graves VG, Salamant MS, et al. Collagen-coated acrylic microspheres for embolotherapy: in vivo and in vitro characteristics. AJNR Am J Neuroradiol 1997;18:647–653
65. Choe DH, Moon HH, Gyeong HK, et al. An experimental study of embolic effect according to infusion rate and concentration of suspension in transarterial particulate embolization. Invest Radiol 1997;32:260–267
66. Siskin GP, Englander M, Stainken BF, et al. Embolic agents used for uterine fibroid embolization. AJR Am J Roentgenol 2000;175:767–773
67. Spies JB, Cooper JM, Worthington-Kirsch R, et al. Outcome of uterine artery embolization and hysterectomy for leiomyomas: results of a multicenter study. Am J Obstet Gynecol 2004;191:22–31
68. Spies JB, Cornell C, Worthington-Kirsch R, Lipman JC, Benenati JF. Long-term outcome from uterine fibroid embolization with tris-acryl gelatin microspheres: results of a multicenter study. J Vasc Interv Radiol 2007;18:203–207
69. Pelage JP, LeDref O, Beregi J, et al. Limited uterine embolization with tris-acryl gelatin microspheres for uterine fibroids. J Vasc Interv Radiol 2003;14:15–20
70. Spies JB, Benenati J, Worthington-Kirsch R, et al. Initial US experience using tris-acryl gelatin microspheres for uterine artery embolization for leiomyomata. J Vasc Interv Radiol 2001;12:1059–1061

71. Lohle PN, Boekkooi FP, Smeets AJ, et al. Limited uterine artery embolization for leiomyomas with tris-acryl gelatin microspheres. 1 year follow-up. J Vasc Interv Radiol 2006;17:283–287
72. Chua GC, Wilsher M, Young MP, Manyonda I, Morgan R, Belli AM. Comparison of particle penetration with non-spherical polyvinyl alcohol versus trisacryl gelatin microspheres in women undergoing premyomectomy uterine artery embolization. Clin Radiol 2005;60:116–122
73. Smeets AJ, Lohle PN, Vervest HA, Boekkooi PF, Lampmann LE. Midterm clinical results and patient satisfaction after uterine artery embolization in women with symptomatic uterine fibroids. Cardiovasc Intervent Radiol 2006;29:188–191
74. Spies JB, Allison S, Flick P, et al. Polyvinyl alcohol particles and tris-acryl gelatin microspheres for uterine artery embolization for leiomyomas: results of a randomized comparative study. J Vasc Interv Radiol 2004;15:793–800
75. Ryu RK. Uterine artery embolization: current implications of embolic agent choice. J Vasc Interv Radiol 2005;16:1419–1422
76. Golzarian J, Lang E, Hovsepian D, et al. Higher rate of partial devascularization and clinical failure after uterine artery embolization for fibroids with spherical polyvinyl alcohol. Cardiovasc Intervent Radiol 2006;29:1–3
77. Spies JB, Allison S, Flick P, et al. Spherical polyvinyl alcohol versus tris-acryl gelatin microspheres for uterine artery embolization for leiomyomas: results of a limited randomized comparative study. J Vasc Interv Radiol 2005;16:1431–1437
78. Golzarian J, Sabri S, Small S, Stolpen A, Vibhakar J, Sun S. High rate of partial devascularization demonstrated by MR after uterine artery embolization for fibroids with spherical PVA. Abstract presented at: Annual Meeting and Postgraduate Course of the Cardiovascular and Interventional Radiological Society of Europe; September 10–14, 2005; Nice, France
79. Shlansky-Goldberg RD, Levin DA, Rosen M, et al. PVA boulders or spheres for UFE: Is there a difference? Abstract presented at: 30th Annual Meeting of the Society of Interventional Radiology, April 2, 2005; New Orleans, LA
80. Kroencke TJ, Lampmann L, Boekkooi F, et al. Initial experience with use of PVA microspheres for UFE: results of a prospective two-center registry. [abstract] J Vasc Interv Radiol 2005;15:S79
81. Mjoomdar A, Rafat Zand R, Torres CI, et al. Initial experience with spherical PVA in comparison with irregular PVA in UFE. [abstract] J Vasc Interv Radiol 2005;16:S65
82. Dhand S, Rajeswaran HB, Chrisman AA, et al. Evaluation of the embolic agent Bead Block in the treatment of uterine fibroids with uterine artery embolization. Abstract presented at: 32nd Annual Meeting of the Society of Interventional Radiology; March 2, 2007; Seattle, WA
83. Worthington-Kirsch RL, Koller NE. Time course of pain after uterine artery embolization for fibroid disease. Medscape Womens Health 2002;7:4
84. Roth AR, Spies JB, Walsh SM, Wood BJ, Gomez-Jorge J, Levy FB. Pain after uterine artery embolization for leiomyomata: can its severity be predicted and does severity predict outcome? J Vasc Interv Radiol 2000;11:1047–1052
85. Spies JB, Allison S, Flick P, et al. Polyvinyl alcohol particles and tris-acryl gelatin microspheres for uterine artery embolization for leiomyomas: results of a randomized comparative study. J Vasc Interv Radiol 2004;15:793–800
86. Ryu RK, Omary RA, Sichlau MJ, et al. Comparison of pain after uterine artery embolization using tris-acryl gelatin microspheres versus polyvinyl alcohol particles. Cardiovasc Intervent Radiol 2003;26:375–378
87. Hovsepian DM, Mandava A, Pilgram TK, et al. Comparison of adjunctive use of rofecoxib versus ibuprofen in the management of postoperative pain after uterine artery embolization. J Vasc Interv Radiol 2006;17:665–670
88. Volkers NA, Hehenkamp WJ, Birnie E, et al. Uterine artery embolization in the treatment of symptomatic uterine fibroid tumors (EMMY trial): periprocedural results and complications. J Vasc Interv Radiol 2006;17:471–480
89. Siskin GP, Stainken BF, Dowling K, Meo P, Ahn J, Dolen EG. Outpatient uterine artery embolization for symptomatic uterine fibroids: experience in 49 patients. J Vasc Interv Radiol 2000;11:305–311
90. Prados W, Blaylock S. The effect of ketorolac on the postoperative narcotic requirements of gynecologic surgery outpatients. [abstract] Anesthesiology 1991;75:A6
91. Parker RK, Holtmann B, Smith I, White PF. Use of ketorolac after lower abdominal surgery. Anesthesiology 1994;80:6–12
92. Liu J, Ding Y, White PF, et al. Effects of ketorolac on postoperative analgesia and ventilatory function after laparoscopic cholecystectomy. Anesth Analg 1993;76:1061–1066
93. Zhan S, Li Y, Wang G, Han H, Yang Z. Effectiveness of intra-arterial anesthesia for uterine fibroid embolization using dilute lidocaine. Eur Radiol 2005;15:1752–1756
94. Rasuli P, Jolly EE, Hammond I, et al. Superior hypogastric nerve block for pain control in outpatient uterine artery embolization. J Vasc Interv Radiol 2004;15:1423–1429
95. Borovac T, Pelage JP, Kasselouri A, Prognon P, Guiffant G, Laurent A. Release of ibuprofen from beads for embolization: in vitro and in vivo studies. J Control Release 2006;115:266–274
96. Klein A, Schwartz ML. Uterine artery embolization for the treatment of uterine fibroids: an outpatient procedure. Am J Obstet Gynecol 2001;184:1556–1560
97. Hehenkamp WJ, Volkers NA, Birnie E, Reekers JA, Ankum WM. Pain and return to daily activities after uterine artery embolization and hysterectomy in the treatment of symptomatic uterine fibroids: results from the randomized EMMY trial. Cardiovasc Intervent Radiol 2006;29:179–187
98. Pron G, Mocarski E, Bennett J, et al. Tolerance, hospital stay, and recovery after uterine artery embolization for fibroids: the Ontario Uterine Fibroid Embolization Trial. J Vasc Interv Radiol 2003;14:1243–1250
99. Worthington-Kirsch R, Spies JB, Myers ER, et al. The Fibroid Registry for Outcomes Data (FIBROID) for Uterine Embolization: short-term outcomes. Obstet Gynecol 2005;106:52–59
100. White AM, Spies JB. Uterine fibroid embolization. Tech Vasc Interv Radiol 2006;9:2–6
101. Hutchins FL Jr, Worthington-Kirsch R, Berkowitz R. Selective uterine artery embolization as primary treatment for symptomatic leiomyomata uteri. J Am Assoc Gynecol Laparosc 1999;6:279–284
102. Katsumori T, Nakajima K, Mihara T, et al. Uterine artery embolization using gelatin sponge particles alone for symptomatic uterine fibroids: midterm results. AJR Am J Roentgenol 2002;178:135–139
103. Spies JB, Ascher SA, Roth AR, et al. Uterine artery embolization for leiomyomata. Obstet Gynecol 2001;98:29–34
104. Andersen PE, Lund N, Justesen P, et al. Uterine artery embolization for symptomatic uterine fibroids: initial success and short-term results. Acta Radiol 2001;42:234–238
105. Goodwin SC, McLucas B, Lee M, et al. Uterine artery embolization for the treatment of uterine leiomyomata: midterm results. J Vasc Interv Radiol 1999;10:1159–1165
106. McLucas B, Adler L, Perella R. Uterine fibroid embolization: nonsurgical treatment for symptomatic fibroids. J Am Coll Surg 2001;192:95–105
107. Pelage JP, LeDref O, Soyer P, et al. Fibroid-related menorrhagia: treatment with superselective embolization of the uterine arteries and mid-term follow-up. Radiology 2000;215:428–431
108. Ravina J, Ciraru-Vigneron N, Aymard A, et al. Uterine artery embolization for fibroid disease: results of a 6 year study. Minim Invasive Ther Allied Technol 1999;8:441–447
109. Spies JB, Coyne K, Guaou Guaou N, et al. The UFS-QOL, a new disease-specific symptom and health-related quality of life questionnaire for leiomyomata. Obstet Gynecol 2002;99:290–300
110. Myers ER, Goodwin S, Landow W, et al. Prospective data collection of a new procedure by a specialty society: the FIBROID registry. Obstet Gynecol 2005;106:44–51
111. Spies JB, Myers ER, Worthington-Kirsch R, et al. The FIBROID registry: symptom and quality of life status 1 year after therapy. Obstet Gynecol 2005;106:1309–1318

112. Joffre F, Tubiana JM, Pelage JP, et al. FEMIC (Fibromes Embolises aux MICrospheres calibrees): uterine fibroid embolization using tris-acryl microspheres. A French multicenter study. Cardiovasc Intervent Radiol 2004;27:600–606
113. Katsumori T, Kashara T, Akazawa K. Long-term outcomes of uterine artery embolization using gelatin sponge particles alone for symptomatic fibroids. AJR Am J Roentgenol 2006;186:848–853
114. Broder MS, Goodwin S, Chen G, et al. Comparison of long-term outcomes of myomectomy and uterine artery embolization. Obstet Gynecol 2002;100(Pt 1):864–868
115. Marret H, Alonso AM, Cottier JP, et al. Leiomyoma recurrence after uterine artery embolization. J Vasc Interv Radiol 2003;14:1395–1399
116. Huang JY, Kafy S, Dugas A, et al. Failure of uterine artery embolization. Fertil Steril 2006;85:30–35
117. Radeleff BA, Satzl S, Eiers M, et al. Clinical 3-year follow-up of uterine fibroid embolization. Rofo 2007;179:593–600
118. Volkers NA, Hehenkamp WJ, Birnie E, Ankum WM, Reekers JA. Uterine artery embolization versus hysterectomy in the treatment of symptomatic uterine fibroids: 2 years' outcome from the randomized EMMY trial. Am J Obstet Gynecol 2007;196:e1–e11
119. Edwards RD, Moss JG, Lumsden MA, et al. Uterine artery embolization versus surgery for symptomatic uterine fibroids. N Engl J Med 2007;356:360–370
120. Razavi MK, Hwang G, Jahed A, et al. Abdominal myomectomy vs. uterine fibroid embolization in the treatment of symptomatic uterine leiomyomas. AJR Am J Roentgenol 2003;180:1571–1575
121. Goodwin SC, Bradley LD, Lipman JC, et al. Uterine artery embolization versus myomectomy: a multicenter comparative study. Fertil Steril 2006;85:14–21
122. Siskin GP, Shlansky-Goldberg RD, Goodwin SC, et al. A prospective multicenter comparative study between myomectomy and uterine artery embolization with polyvinyl alcohol microspheres: long-term clinical outcomes in patients with symptomatic uterine fibroids. J Vasc Interv Radiol 2006;17:1287–1295
123. Siskin GP, Eaton LA, Stainken BF, Dowling K, Herr A, Schwartz J. Pathologic findings in a uterine leiomyoma after bilateral uterine artery embolization. J Vasc Interv Radiol 1999;10:891–894
124. Dundr P, Mara M, Maskova J, Fucikova Z, Povysil C, Tvrdik D. Pathological findings of uterine leiomyomas and adenomyosis following uterine artery embolization. Pathol Res Pract 2006;202:721–729
125. Colgan TJ, Pron G, Mocarski EJ, Bennett JD, Asch MR, Common A. Pathologic features of uteri and leiomyomas following uterine artery embolization for leiomyomas. Am J Surg Pathol 2003;27:167–177
126. Weichert W, Denkert C, Gauruder-Burmester A, et al. Uterine arterial embolization with tris-acryl gelatin microspheres: a histopathologic evaluation. Am J Surg Pathol 2005;29:955–961
127. Katsumori T, Bamba M, Kobayashi TK, et al. Uterine leiomyoma after embolization by means of gelatin sponge particles alone: report of a case with histopathologic features. Ann Diagn Pathol 2002;6:307–311
128. McCluggage WG, Ellis PK, McClure N, Walker WJ, Jackson PA, Manek S. Pathologic features of uterine leiomyomas following uterine artery embolization. Int J Gynecol Pathol 2000;19:342–347
129. Chiesa AG, Hart WR. Uterine artery embolization of leiomyomas with trisacryl gelatin microspheres (TGM): pathologic features and comparison with polyvinyl alcohol emboli. Int J Gynecol Pathol 2004;23(4):386–392
130. Siskin GP, Dowling K, Virmani R, Jones R, Todd D. Pathologic evaluation of a spherical polyvinyl alcohol embolic agent in a porcine renal model. J Vasc Interv Radiol 2003;14:89–98
131. Nicholson TA, Pelage JP, Ettles DF. Fibroid calcification after uterine artery embolization: ultrasonographic appearance and pathology. J Vasc Interv Radiol 2001;12:443–446
132. Banu NS, Gaze DC, Bruce H, Collinson PO, Belli AM, Manyonda IT. Markers of muscle ischemia, necrosis, and inflammation following uterine artery embolization in the treatment of symptomatic uterine fibroids. Am J Obstet Gynecol 2007;196:e1–e5
133. Orsini LF, Salardi S, Pilu G, Bovicelli L, Cacciari E. Pelvic organs in premenarcheal girls: real-time ultrasonography. Radiology 1984;153:113–116
134. Joe BN, Suh J, Hildebolt CF, Hovsepian DM, Johnston B, Bae KT. MR volumetric measurements of the myomatous uterus: improved reliability of stereology over linear measurements. Acad Radiol 2007;14:455–462
135. Banovac F, Ascher S, Jones D, et al. MR imaging outcome after uterine artery embolization for leiomyomata using tris-acryl gelatin microspheres. J Vasc Interv Radiol 2002;13:681–687
136. Pelage JP, Guaou Guaou N, Jha R, et al. Long-term imaging outcome after embolization for uterine fibroid tumors. Radiology 2004;230:803–809
137. Dorenberg EJ, Novakovic Z, Smith HJ, Hafsahl G, Jakobsen JA. Uterine fibroid embolization can still be improved: observations on post-procedure magnetic resonance imaging. Acta Radiol 2005;46:547–553
138. Yousefi S, Czeyda-Pommersheim F, White AM, Banovac F, Hahn WY, Spies JB. Repeat uterine artery embolization: indications and technical findings. J Vasc Interv Radiol 2006;17:1923–1929
139. Pelage JP. Technical optimization of uterine fibroid embolization using polyvinyl alcohol microspheres. [abstract] J Vasc Interv Radiol 2005; 16(suppl):568
140. Siskin GP, Beck A, Schuster M, et al Leiomyoma infarction after uterine artery embolization: a prospective randomized study comparing tris-acryl gelatin microspheres versus polyvinyl alcohol microspheres. J Vasc Interv Radiol 2008;19:58–65
141. Stringer NH, Grant T, Park J, Oldham L. Ovarian failure after uterine artery embolization for treatment of myomas. J Am Assoc Gynecol Laparosc 2000;7:395–400
142. Chrisman HB, Saker MB, Ryu RK, et al. The impact of uterine fibroid embolization on resumption of menses and ovarian function. J Vasc Interv Radiol 2000;11:699–703
143. Tropeano G, Di Stasi C, Litwicka K, Romano D, Draisci G, Mancuso S. Uterine artery embolization for fibroids does not have adverse effects on ovarian reserve in regularly cycling women younger than 40 years. Fertil Steril 2004;81:1055–1061
144. Ahmad A, Qadan L, Hassan N, Najarian K. Uterine artery embolization treatment of uterine fibroids: effect on ovarian function in younger women. J Vasc Interv Radiol 2002;13:1017–1020
145. Spies JB, Roth AR, Gonsalves SM, Murphy-Skrzyniarz KM. Ovarian function after uterine artery embolization for leiomyomata: assessment with use of serum follicle stimulating hormone assay. J Vasc Interv Radiol 2001;12:437–442
146. Kim HS, Tsai J, Patra A, Lee JM, Griffith JG, Wallach EE. Effects of utero-ovarian anastomoses on clinical outcomes and repeat intervention rates after uterine artery embolization. J Vasc Interv Radiol 2006;17:783–789
147. Kim HS, Tsai J, Lee JM, Vang R, Griffith JG, Wallach EE. Effects of utero-ovarian anastomoses on basal follicle-stimulating hormone level change after uterine artery embolization with tris-acryl gelatin microspheres. J Vasc Interv Radiol 2006;17:965–971
148. Kim HS, Thonse VR, Judson K, Vang R. Utero-ovarian anastomosis: histopathologic correlation after uterine artery embolization with or without ovarian artery embolization. J Vasc Interv Radiol 2007;18(1 Pt 1):31–39
149. Payne JF, Robboy SJ, Haney AF. Embolic microspheres within ovarian arterial vasculature after uterine artery embolization. Obstet Gynecol 2002;100(5 Pt 1):883–886
150. Ryu RK, Chrisman HB, Omary RA, et al. The vascular impact of uterine artery embolization: prospective sonographic assessment of ovarian arterial circulation. J Vasc Interv Radiol 2001;12:1071–1074
151. Wolanske KA, Gordon RL, Wilson MW, Kerlan RK, LaBerge JM, Jacoby AF. Coil embolization of a tuboovarian anastomosis before uterine artery embolization to prevent nontarget particle embolization of the ovary. J Vasc Interv Radiol 2003;14:1333–1338

152. Marx M, Wack JP, Baker EL, Stevens SK, Barakos JA. Ovarian protection by occlusion of uteroovarian collateral vessels before uterine fibroid embolization. J Vasc Interv Radiol 2003;14:1329–1332
153. Amato P, Roberts AC. Transient ovarian failure: a complication of uterine artery embolization. Fertil Steril 2001;75:438–439
154. Hascalik S, Celik O, Sarac K, Hascalik M. Transient ovarian failure: a rare complication of uterine fibroid embolization. Acta Obstet Gynecol Scand 2004;83:682–685
155. Tropeano G, Litwicka K, Di Stasi C, Romano D, Mancuso S. Permanent amenorrhea associated with endometrial atrophy after uterine artery embolization for symptomatic uterine fibroids. Fertil Steril 2003;79:132–135
156. Healey S, Buzaglo K, Seti L, Valenti D, Tulandi T. Ovarian function after uterine artery embolization and hysterectomy. J Am Assoc Gynecol Laparosc 2004;11:348–352
157. Hovsepian DM, Ratts VS, Rodriguez M, Huang JS, Aubuchon MG, Pilgram TK. A prospective comparison of the impact of uterine artery embolization, myomectomy, and hysterectomy on ovarian function. J Vasc Interv Radiol 2006;17:1111–1115
158. Aungst M, Wilson M, Vournas K, McCarthy S. Necrotic leiomyomas and gram-negative sepsis eight weeks after uterine artery embolization. Obstet Gynecol 2004;104(5 Pt 2):1161–1164
159. Robson S, Wilson K, Munday D, Sebben R. Pelvic sepsis complicating embolization of a uterine fibroid. Aust N Z J Obstet Gynaecol 1999;39:516–517
160. Payne JF, Haney AF. Serious complications of uterine artery embolization for conservative treatment of fibroids. Fertil Steril 2003;79:128–131
161. Rajan DK, Beecroft JR, Clark TW, et al. Risk of intrauterine infectious complications after uterine artery embolization. J Vasc Interv Radiol 2004;15:1415–1421
162. Vashisht A, Studd J, Carey A, Burn P. Fatal septicaemia after fibroid embolization. Lancet 1999;354:307–308
163. de Blok S, de Vries C, Prinssen HM, Blaauwgeers HL, Jorna-Meijer LB. Fatal sepsis after uterine artery embolization with microspheres. J Vasc Interv Radiol 2003;14:779–783
164. Messina ML, Bozzini N, Baracat EC. Necrotic fibroid expulsion with intrauterine infection after uterine fibroid embolization. Int J Gynaecol Obstet 2007;97:158–159
165. Kitamura Y, Ascher SM, Cooper C, et al. Imaging manifestations of complications associated with uterine artery embolization. Radiographics 2005;25(Suppl 1):S119–S132
166. Richard HM, Siskin GP, Stainken BF. Endometritis after uterine artery embolization with gold-colored gelatin microspheres. J Vasc Interv Radiol 2004;15:406–407
167. Czeyda-Pommersheim F, Magee ST, Cooper C, Hahn WY, Spies JB. Venous thromboembolism after uterine fibroid embolization. Cardiovasc Intervent Radiol 2006;29:1136–1140
168. Lanocita R. A fatal complication of percutaneous transcatheter embolization for treatment of uterine fibroids. Paper presented at: 11th Annual Scientific Meeting of SMIT/CIMIT; September 16–18, 1999; Boston, MA
169. Nikolic B, Kessler CM, Jacobs HM, et al. Changes in blood coagulation markers associated with uterine artery embolization for leiomyomata. J Vasc Interv Radiol 2003;14(9 Pt 1):1147–1153
170. Sterling KM, Vogelzang RL, Chrisman HB, et al. V. Uterine fibroid embolization: management of complications. Tech Vasc Interv Radiol 2002;5:56–66
171. Berkowitz RP, Hutchins FL, Worthington-Kirsch RL. Vaginal expulsion of submucosal fibroids after uterine artery embolization. A report of three cases. J Reprod Med 1999;44:373–376
172. Abbara S, Spies JB, Scialli AR, et al. Transcervical expulsion of a fibroid as a result of uterine artery embolization for leiomyomata. J Vasc Interv Radiol 1999;10:409–411
173. Spies JB, Spector A, Roth AR, Baker CM, Mauro L, Murphy-Skrynarz K. Complications after uterine artery embolization for leiomyomas. Obstet Gynecol 2002;100:873–880
174. Park HR, Kim MD, Kim NK, et al. Uterine restoration after repeated sloughing of fibroids or vaginal expulsion following uterine artery embolization. Eur Radiol 2005;15:1850–1854
175. Kroencke TJ, Gauruder-Burmester A, Enzweiler CN, Taupitz M, Hamm B. Disintegration and stepwise expulsion of a large uterine leiomyoma with restoration of the uterine architecture after successful uterine fibroid embolization: case report. Hum Reprod 2003;18:863–865
176. Sultana CJ, Goldberg J, Aizenman L, Chon JK. Vesicouterine fistula after uterine artery embolization: a case report. Am J Obstet Gynecol 2002;187:1726–1727
177. Price N, Golding S, Slack RA, Jackson SR. Delayed presentation of vesicouterine fistula 12 months after uterine artery embolization for uterine fibroids. J Obstet Gynaecol 2007;27:205–207
178. Yeagley TJ, Goldberg J, Klein TA, Bonn J. Labial necrosis after uterine artery embolization for leiomyomata. Obstet Gynecol 2002;100(5 Pt 1):881–882
179. Dietz DM, Stahlfeld KR, Bansal SK, Christopherson WA. Buttock necrosis after uterine artery embolization. Obstet Gynecol 2004;104(5 Pt 2):1159–1161
180. Godfrey CD, Zbella EA. Uterine necrosis after uterine artery embolization for leiomyomas. Obstet Gynecol 2001;98(5 Pt 2):950–952
181. Torigian DA, Siegelman ES, Terhune KP, Butts SF, Blasco L, Shlasky-Goldberg RD. MRI of uterine necrosis after uterine artery embolization for treatment of uterine leiomyomata. AJR Am J Roentgenol 2005;184:555–559
182. Pollard RR, Goldberg JM. Prolapsed cervical myoma after uterine artery embolization. A case report. J Reprod Med 2001;46:499–500
183. Gavrilescu T, Sherer DM, Temkin S, Zinn H, Abulafia O. Small bowel volvulus after uterine artery embolization requiring bowel resection: a case report. J Reprod Med 2006;51:739–741
184. Ogliari KS, Mohallem SV, Barrozo P, Viscomi F. A uterine cavity-myoma communication after uterine artery embolization: two case reports. Fertil Steril 2005;83:220–222

6 New Treatments for Uterine Fibroids

Gary P. Siskin, Suzanne D. LeBlang, and Kristof Chwalisz

For decades, there was very little innovation in the treatment of uterine fibroids.[1] During that time, the standard treatment for fibroids had been hysterectomy or myomectomy, primarily because they are effective and offer a solution to the problem. There have been significant advances in surgical technique to avoid the morbidity associated with laparotomy,[2] including laparoscopic and hysteroscopic resection of subserosal and submucosal fibroids, respectively. However, these approaches are often not appropriate for many patients and this has prompted the search for novel treatment options for these patients.[1] With the success of uterine artery embolization (UAE) as an alternative to surgery, it now appears that a multitude of different approaches to treat these patients has been introduced into both the literature and into current medical practice. The purpose of this article is to review the different approaches to fibroid therapy and the data supporting their use.

■ Lesion-based Treatment

The fundamental concept behind lesion-based treatment options for uterine fibroids is that fibroids represent a focal problem within the uterus that can potentially be treated by directing therapy toward one lesion at a time. The most invasive form of this therapy is myomectomy because conceptually, this procedure involves removing specific lesions and leaving the remaining portions of the uterus intact. It is clear, however, that less invasive forms of management have become a popular alternative to traditional surgical resection. If a less invasive approach is desired, then nonsurgical lesion-based therapy will require accurate imaging guidance to be certain that therapy is being directed at abnormal tissue with the intention of sparing as much normal uterine tissue as possible. This concept is one that is familiar to most interventional radiologists who are involved with using ablation techniques (e.g., radiofrequency ablation [RFA], cryoablation, microwave ablation) to treat hepatic, renal, and pulmonary malignancies. In fact, many of these interventions have been applied in limited fashion toward the treatment of uterine fibroids and the clinical results will be reviewed in this section.

Thermal Ablation

A variety of thermal ablation techniques has been applied to the treatment of uterine fibroids. This includes RFA, cryoablation, laser ablation, and MR-guided focused ultrasound (MRgFUS). The use of RFA to achieve local control of a wide variety of tumors in many locations has become more accepted in recent years. It has been theorized that RFA treats fibroids by inducing coagulative necrosis and depressing the expression of estrogen and progesterone receptors.[3]

Bergamini et al[4] were the first to report the use of laparoscopic RFA to treat symptomatic uterine fibroids. In this study, 18 patients, all of whom were older than age 40 and premenopausal with fewer than three fibroids were treated with RFA. All of the procedures were performed under general anesthesia using the system manufactured by Rita Medical Systems (part of Angiodynamics, Queensbury, NY) under laparoscopic guidance. The operative time ranged from 20 to 40 minutes and there were no intraoperative or postoperative complications reported. Only two patients complained of mild abdominal pain, both of whom did not require postprocedure pain medication. All patients were observed overnight and discharged on the following day. Nine patients were available for 12-month imaging follow-up, which demonstrated a mean fibroid volume reduction of 85%. Significant improvements in both symptom severity and health-related quality of life were observed based on pre- and postprocedure administration of the Uterine Fibroids Symptom and Quality of Life (UFS-QOL) questionnaire. Ghezzi et al[5] later reported the results of laparoscopic RFA on 25 patients with at least one-year follow-up, including the 18 patients reported by Bergamini et al.[4] The median baseline diameter and volume of the dominant fibroid were 5.3 cm (range 3.0 to 8.6 cm) and 76.8 cm^3 (range 14.8 to 332.8 cm^3). In these patients, the median reduction in fibroid volume was 68.8% and 77.9% at 6 and 12 months, respectively. No intraoperative or postoperative complications were reported in this study. One patient required a hysterectomy for symptom recurrence at one year. All other patients had significant improvement in symptom severity and health-related quality of life.

Milic et al[6] have also reported their experience with laparoscopic RFA. They treated four patients with fibroids <6 cm in diameter with the LeVeen Needle Electrode system (Boston Scientific Corp., Natick, MA). These patients were observed for 6 hours and discharged home the same day. The procedure was technically successful in 3 of 4 patients: one patient had a firm, mobile, posterior fibroid that could not be treated. Symptomatic relief was achieved in two of the three treated patients: the one patient with persistent postprocedure pain was later found to have adenomyosis in addition to fibroids. Magnetic resonance imaging (MRI) performed at 3 months in the three treated patients, revealed lack of fibroid enhancement in all three patients. However, at 7 months, a focal area of enhancement within a treated fibroid was seen in one patient and this particular patient experienced recurrence of pain and bleeding within 9 months of the procedure. Kim et al[7] also evaluated the use of percutaneous RFA for uterine fibroids, but did so in patients with large fibroids (>5 cm) who had been treated with UAE. Thirty-five patients were included in this study and were treated with moderate sedation. Significant improvements were seen in both symptom severity and health-related quality of life after the procedures were performed. In addition, the mean fibroid volume reduction was 56.5%. There were no immediate percutaneous RFA-related complications. However, one patient did have delayed drainage via the transabdominal tract, which was ultimately self-limiting. Kim et al[7] theorized that percutaneous RFA may improve the clinical results of UAE by providing targeted treatments to areas of residual fibroid enhancement after UAE. Despite the small number of studies and the limited numbers of patients reported, the conclusions from the groups authoring the above articles are that RFA may offer a realistic alternative to surgery for symptomatic uterine fibroids.

Laser myolysis was first described in 1990 by Donnez et al[8] using hysteroscopic technique and by Nisolle et al[9] in 1993 using laparoscopic technique. By placing laser fibers directly within the target fibroid, laser energy can be converted to heat. An attempt is made to coagulate the entire fibroid by placing laser fibers at multiple sites within the fibroid.[10] As the temperature increases within the fibroid to ~56°C, protein denaturation develops, which causes coagulative necrosis within the fibroid.[11] When initially reported in the mid-1990s, this laparoscopic procedure resulted in uterine volume decreases of 83% and fibroid volume decreases of 50 to 70% 3 to 6 months after the procedure.[12,13] One problem associated with this technique was the significant incidence of pelvic adhesions in these patients. These adhesions appear to be secondary to the use of multiple fibroid punctures and thermal damage to the serosal surface.[9]

In 1999, Law et al reported on the use of MR-guided percutaneous laser ablation of uterine fibroids.[14,15] The benefits of this approach were felt to be the real-time imaging guidance for needle placement and monitoring of the thermal ablation.[16] The monitoring is important because a maximum ablation can be achieving before damaging the serosal and adjacent structures, which can potentially lead to adhesion formation.[17] Law et al studied 12 patients who were awaiting hysterectomy and underwent laser myolysis. Technically, four MR-compatible 18 g needles were placed within the fibroid under MR guidance while the patient received intravenous (IV) sedation. Laser fibers were then advanced into the needles and the needles were withdrawn to expose the tip of the laser fiber. Laser light at a wavelength of 810 nm was then delivered to the fibroid tissue via each laser fiber. The mean ablation time was 15 minutes (range 10 to 25 minutes). Eleven of the 12 patients went home on the same day: one patient chose to remain in the hospital overnight. Of the 12 treated patients, 4 underwent hysterectomy with well-defined areas of coagulative necrosis seen within the excised fibroids. The remaining eight patients declined surgery after laser ablation and were found to have a fibroid volume reduction of 37.5% on MRI performed 3 months after the procedure. Law et al[11] subsequently reported their experience with their first 30 patients. Treatment in 29 of 30 patients was considered technically successful; one patient terminated the procedure after 12 minutes due to abdominal pain. All but one patient was discharged on the day of the procedure. Of the 30 patients treated, 26 patients declined their planned surgery with all of these women reporting significant symptomatic improvement. After 3 months, the mean fibroid volume reduction was 37.5% (range 25 to 49%). As this pilot study continued, Hindley et al[17] reported on 66 patients. MRI at 3 and 12 months revealed a fibroid volume reduction of 31% and 41%, respectively. All patients were noted to have a decrease in mean menstrual blood loss after treatment. In addition, the Menorrhagia Outcomes Questionnaire (MOQ), which was used to assess clinical outcomes, revealed that outcomes were not as good as those seen after hysterectomy in a historical control group, but that there were no significant differences in quality of life and satisfaction between the two groups of patients.

Cryoablation appears to be the lesion-based approach that has the most literature supporting its use in patients with symptomatic uterine fibroids. It is thought that cooling the target tissue to -20°C with cryoablation destroys tissues by intracellular freezing and extracellular crystallization of interstitial water leading to cellular dehydration, thrombosis of small blood vessels, and mechanical damage to cellular integrity by expansion of large ice crystals within the interstitial space.[18–22] Olive et al were the first to report the use of cryoablation to treat uterine fibroids.[23] In this early report, cryoablation was performed using laparoscopic guidance on 14 patients; the authors subsequently reported a 10% fibroid volume reduction on follow-up imaging. Since then, other studies have been performed evaluating the use of laparoscopic cryoablation. Ciavattini et al[25] treated 76 fibroids in 61 patients under general anesthesia with procedure times ranging from 20 to 60 minutes.[24–28] After the procedure, 8.3% of patients complained of pain and 5% had a postoperative fever. Most patients (83.6%) reported symptomatic relief after the procedure and the mean fibroid volume reduction was 60.3% and 69.8% at 12 and 24 months, respectively. Zupi et al[26] subsequently treated 20 patients using this technique. All procedures were performed with general anesthesia and all patients were discharged within 24 hours. No postprocedure analgesia was required and no procedural complications were reported. During follow-up, 95% of patients reported elimination or improvement of their symptoms; the mean fibroid volume reduction was 24.9% and 60% at 1 and 12 months, respectively.[27] The ultrasound findings were further evaluated in 10 of these patients by Exacoustos et al, who found decreased blood flow in all treated fibroids, even when peripheral surrounding vessels remained intact.[28] This was seen 1 month after treatment and remained unchanged 3 to 6 months after treatment. In addition, a hyperechoic avascular central zone was seen in 80% of treated fibroids that persisted (although reduced in size) 6 months after treatment.

There is limited data on pregnancy outcomes after laparoscopic cryomyolysis. Ciavattini et al[29] reported their experience with nine pregnancies in nine patients who underwent this procedure to treat symptomatic uterine fibroids. Two of these patients had an early miscarriage while seven pregnant patients had a regular, uncomplicated course with three patients delivering by cesarean section and four patients delivering vaginally. Therefore, it was concluded that this procedure does not compromise a good pregnancy outcome and vaginal delivery.

In 2001, reports regarding the percutaneous performance of cryoablation using MRI guidance became available. The first report was by Sewell et al[30] who treated two patients with large symptomatic fibroids. A 10F access sheath was placed transabdominally into the target fibroid and a 6F cryoablation probe was then advanced through the sheath into the fibroid. Cryoablation was performed until the "ice ball," which was well seen on MRI, encompassed the fibroid with minimal overlap into the surrounding myometrium. Once the cryoprobe was removed, the access sheath was filled with SurgiSeal (Confluent Surgical, Inc., Waltham, MA) for hemostasis. After 2 and 3 months, MRI revealed fibroid volume reductions of 65% and 53%, respectively. Cowan et al[31] later reported a similar mean fibroid volume reduction of 65% when nine patients were treated using a similar technique. In this series, complications were reported including nausea requiring an overnight admission, mild foot drop due to a peroneal nerve defect that resolved after 4 months, and laceration of a vessel coursing over the serosal surface of a fibroid that led to bleeding requiring laparotomy and myomectomy. Sakuhara et al[32] also reported on their experience with six patients undergoing MR-guided cryoablation. All of these patients experienced a fever after treatment with one patient requiring surgical drainage of an abscess in the probe channel. The mean fibroid volume reduction rate in these patients in these patients was 79.4% at 9 to 12 months.

Dohi et al were the first to report the use of cryoablation from a transvaginal approach to treat eight patients with symptomatic fibroids.[18] Cryoprobes were introduced utilizing MRI guidance under epidural and local anesthesia into the targeted fibroids using a transvaginal approach. Lower abdominal pain occurred after the procedure in 3 patients, which was addressed with analgesic medication. All patients were discharged on the day following the procedure. Clinically, the menstrual score improved in 75% of the patients with pain and anemia successfully addressed in all patients with these symptoms. At 6 to 7 weeks after the procedure, the mean fibroid volume reduction was 59%; at 9 to 12 months, it was 67.7% (in five patients). Interestingly, Dohi et al suggested that the optimal size of the ice ball formed during cryoablation may not need to be larger than the fibroid to cause alleviation of symptoms in these patients.

When evaluating the data for lesion-based therapy (irrespective of the actual technique used) and the imaging modality used for guidance (laparoscopy or MRI), it appears that the short-term data are promising in terms of the ability of these procedures to improve symptoms and reduce fibroid volume. An additional benefit of these procedures is the clear absence of significant postprocedure pain, a finding that differentiates these procedures from UAE and other more invasive therapies. This may be due to the fact that these targeted therapies are successful in limiting treatment to the fibroids, reducing the effect of treatment on normal myometrium. This may therefore represent an advantage for this type of therapy when compared with a more organ-based treatment such as UAE.

However, a lesion-based approach also has limitations. Because each fibroid requires individually targeted therapy, there are restrictions to the number of fibroids that can be present before this would be considered an unreasonable approach. If multiple procedures are required to treat multiple fibroids, then the overall risk of utilizing this approach would be increased as well. In addition, if small fibroids are left untreated, then symptom recurrence may become a potential long-term issue. Multiple fibroids were therefore a limitation that was mentioned in many of the above-quoted studies and was often used as selection criteria for deciding which patients would be eligible for participation. Given the fact that many patients present with multiple fibroids, these ablative techniques may not be appropriate for many of the patients who present with symptomatic fibroids. An additional limitation is that at this time, all of the patients described above were not evaluated with contrast-enhanced MRI. The global experience with UAE has emphasized the importance of utilizing contrast-enhanced MRI as the imaging modality of choice after UAE to confirm that fibroid infarction has been induced by the procedure.[33] Without this information, it is not possible to know if these targeted ablation techniques result in tissue infarction. Although this may open up the possibility of future recurrence, it also may help explain why these patients experienced less postprocedure pain than typically seen after UAE. Therefore, additional studies with contrast-enhanced MRI as the follow-up imaging modality would be required to better characterize the tissue changes induced by these procedures.

Magnetic Resonance–guided Focused Ultrasound Surgery

The use of MR-guided focused ultrasound surgery (MRgFUS) to treat patients with symptomatic uterine fibroids is an exciting step forward in lesion-based therapy because it truly defines noninvasive medicine. Although MRgFUS has been studied for over six decades,[34,35] it was only approved by the United States Food and Drug Administration (FDA) for the treatment of uterine fibroids in October, 2004. By definition, noninvasive surgery means that the skin remains intact with no incisions, catheters, or laparoscopic portholes. Despite the fact that this technology has been evaluated for a long time, improvements in MRI, MR thermometry images, and the ability to combine the software components of the MRI machine with the focused ultrasound transducer has propelled it into clinical use.

This procedure delivers high-energy ultrasound waves into the fibroid under direct MRI guidance. The patient lies in the prone position with the pelvis overlying the phased array ultrasound transducer, which is encased in a degassed water tank within the MRI table (**Fig. 6.1**). This table is able to dock with a 1.5 or 3.0 Tesla MRI scanner. Similar to how a magnifying glass focuses light energy, the ultrasound waves are focused into a small region of tissue inside the fibroid called the focal spot;[35] this can range in size from a small jellybean to a large coffee bean. The MRI T2-weighted planning images in three planes are utilized to determine the focal spot location. The ultrasound beam

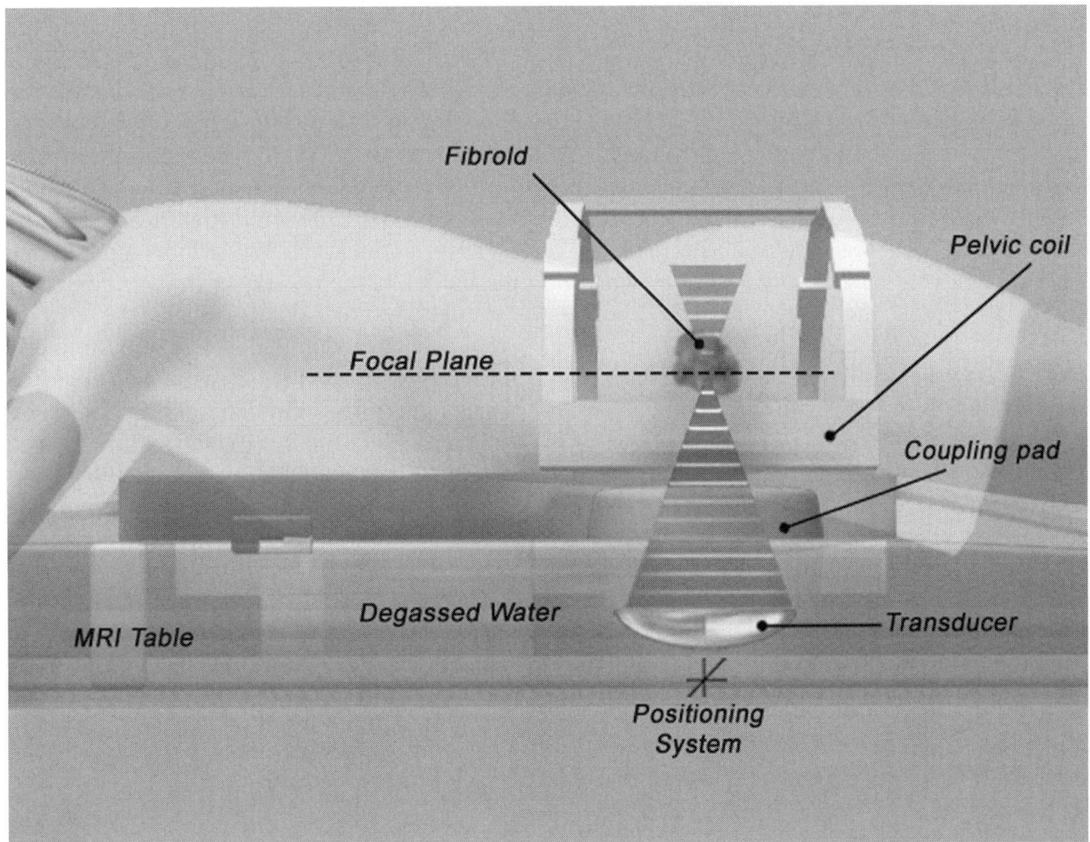

Fig. 6.1 Diagrammatic representation of a patient in the prone position receiving magnetic resonance-guided focused ultrasound (MRgFUS) to treat a uterine fibroid.

path is depicted overlying these anatomic images to ensure a safe passageway into the fibroid. The transducer can be tilted ~15 to 20 degrees in all directions to avoid scars or nearby loops of bowel. During the 20- to 30-second sonications when the ultrasound waves are focused into the fibroid, heat is generated in the focal spot resulting in thermal ablation. Studies have shown that if the temperature remains above 57°C for >1 second, then coagulative necrosis occurs leading to irreversible cell death.[36,37] Every 3 seconds during the sonications, MR thermometry images are obtained that follow the temperature within the focal spot during the sonciation to ensure that the temperature is high enough to induce cell death and tissue ablation. Various parameters can be altered during the procedure to reach critical temperatures such as the amount of energy in the ultrasound beam, the frequency of the ultrasound beam, the size of the focal spot, and the duration of the sonications.

Patient selection is important to ensure a safe and effective outcome after MRgFUS. The published clinical trials limited inclusion to premenopausal women with no plans for future childbearing with a uterus <24 weeks in size. The timing of the procedure relative to the phase of the menstrual cycle has not been shown to be important.[38] A screening MRI of the pelvis with and without contrast is necessary prior to the procedure to determine candidacy and several parameters should be noted carefully. Perhaps the most important reason to screen these patients is to ensure that the patient does have fibroids and not other pathology that can mimic a fibroid on the ultrasound images (e.g., endometrial cancer, sarcoma, or a focal adenomyoma). Patients with more than five fibroids are usually not good candidates because the time to ablate these fibroids can be prohibitively long. In addition, the signal characteristics of the fibroid should be assessed because low-signal lesions on T2-weighted images tend to respond better to MRgFUS than high-signal lesions.[39] Postcontrast images should demonstrate diffuse enhancement of the fibroid ensuring that it is not already necrotic or hemorrhagic as there would be no viable tissue to ablate in such cases. Scrutiny of the images for bowel loops interposed between the anterior abdominal wall and the uterus is critical to note as the air inside these bowel loops could deflect the ultrasound beam and heat other surrounding tissues. Abdominal scar tissue, including that seen after abdominal liposuction, represents a contraindication to this procedure as well, if the scar tissue would be in the path of the ultrasound beam. In our practice, 73% of patients screened with MRI are found to be good candidates for MRgFUS (LeBlang). Findings that have excluded patients include malignancy (including endometrial cancer and uterine leiomyosarcoma), adenomyosis, nonenhancing fibroids, large number of fibroids, endometrial polyps, fibroids of inappropriate size (too large and too small), highly vascularized fibroids, clips along the beam path, or fibroids that are inaccessible to the beam path.

Prior to the procedure, patients are instructed to shave the area from the umbilicus to the pubic symphysis because hair increases the risk of thermal injury to the skin.[40] No oils or creams can be placed on the skin of the lower abdominal wall before treatment. A Foley catheter is placed to keep the bladder empty because a distending bladder can cause changes in the uterine position compared with the T2-weighted planning images, resulting in misplacement of the focal spot.[40] The Foley catheter is also needed to maintain the bladder filled at a constant level when used to push intervening bowel loops out of the beam path. These bowel loops can be displaced laterally and superiorly by filling the bladder immediately prior to the procedure. Conscious sedation is typically used to minimize patient motion and minimize any discomfort during the procedure.

Once this technology was shown to effectively reduce uterine fibroid tumor size in a nude mouse model,[41] trials began in humans. The initial feasibility data obtained on patients with symptomatic uterine fibroids was reported by Tempany et al.[42] In this study, nine patients were treated with MRgFUS prior to a planned hysterectomy. Six of these nine patients received the entire planned thermal dose to their target fibroid. Two of the patients did not complete the treatment due to pain on the anterior abdominal wall during the sonications or because the MR thermometry images did not detect the temperature changes. The other treatment was not performed as there were bowel loops in the beam path on the day of treatment. During the procedure, seven patients received intravenous conscious sedation and two utilized oral sedation and all patients were discharged home the day of the procedure. Two patients experienced minor skin burns after the procedures (one of whom had an abdominal scar). MRI performed after treatment revealed discrete areas of decreased contrast enhancement in the treated fibroids, which were confirmed to represent tissue devascularization and necrosis after hysterectomy (**Fig. 6.2**).

Stewart et al[43] then reported on an initial multicenter experience treating 55 patients with clinically significant uterine fibroids. For each of these patients, one myoma was targeted for treatment. The goal of treatment was to induce coagulative necrosis within an operator-defined portion of the targeted tumor and not to cause necrosis within the entire fibroid. The median treatment time was 1 hour 45 minutes; the mean total time in the scanner was equal to 3 hours. Most patients reported only limited pain and discomfort after the procedure and all were treated as outpatients. Interestingly, posttreatment MRI scans revealed areas of nonperfusion within the treated fibroids, which was noted to often be larger than expected based on treatment volumes and confirmed at hysterectomy.

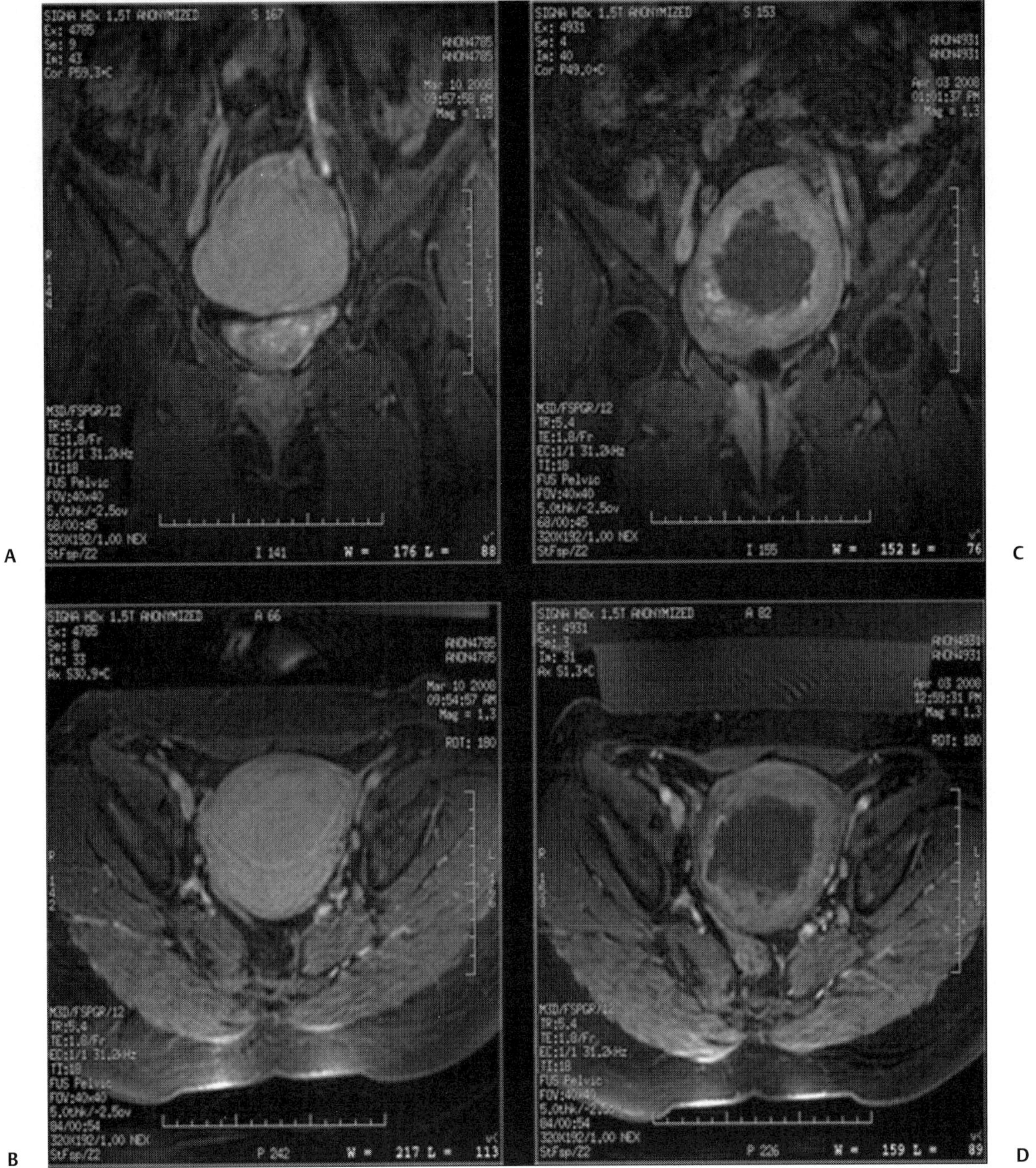

Fig. 6.2 T1-weighted magnetic resonance images (MRIs) obtained before **(A,B)** and after **(C,D)** treatment with MR-guided focused ultrasound (MRgFUS). This is a 55-year-old patient with an 8 cm fibroid causing urinary frequency, pelvic pressure, and menorrhagia. She received 81 sonications over a 3-hour period. The images obtained after treatment demonstrate the nonperfused volume caused by this therapy.

Hindley et al and Stewart et al have all reported on the results from the phase III clinical trial to evaluate the MR-guided focused ultrasound therapy system known as the ExAblate 2000 (Insightec, Haifa Tel Aviv, Israel).[44–46] In this study, 176 patients were enrolled and screened and 62% (n = 109) of these women underwent treatment at seven sites, based on the initial inclusion criteria. The FDA limited the amount of tissue that could be treated to a maximum of 100 cm^3 per myoma or 150 cm^3 per treatment.[45] In addition, the target regions must have been >1.5 cm from the serosal and endometrial surface and 0.5 cm from the fibroid capsule.[45] The treatment time was limited to 2 hours. Overall, 10 to 11% of the fibroid volume was treated using this protocol by the FDA.[46] Eighty-two percent of patients reported pain during the procedure, although only 16% described the pain as severe. After the procedure, only 1% reported severe pain and 7% reported moderate pain. During follow-up, one patient complained of leg and buttock pain, which was attributed to sciatic nerve palsy secondary to exposure of the sciatic nerve to the high frequency ultrasound beam; this complication resolved by the time of her 12-month follow-up visit. In response to this complication, the FDA recommended that the target region be >4 cm from the spine along the beam path as bone absorbs more heat than soft tissues and could secondarily heat the adjacent nerves. At 6 months, 70.6% of patients experienced a significant decrease in symptom severity (defined as 10-point improvement in the symptom severity score of the UFS-QOL). This decreased to 51.2% of patients after 12 months of follow-up. At 6 months, the mean fibroid volume reduction was 13.5% with a mean nonperfused volume of ~25% (which was greater than the volume targeted for treatment). One explanation why the prescribed treatment volume was smaller than the actual treated volume may be due to a vascular effect. As small regions of cells die, there is probably ischemia to the adjacent cells as the small capillaries are no longer needed to supply the region. From pelvic angiographic studies, we know that the surrounding normal uterine tissue is supplied by different, more proximal vessels and thus, the tissue outside the fibroid capsule is not compromised by the UAE effect of those small capillaries inside the fibroid during ablation.[47] Within 12 months of follow-up, 28% of the patients treated underwent alternative treatment.

When the above data was analyzed, it was felt that patients did quite well after MRgFUS, especially considering the significant limitations placed on the amount of fibroid that could be treated. After April 30, 2004, the FDA modified these limitations, enabling a greater percentage of the fibroid tissue to be treated over a longer period.[48,49] Allowed treatment volumes were increased from 33% of all fibroids to 50% for all fibroids except submucosal ones, and maximal treatment volume was increased to 150 cm^3, regardless of the number of fibroids. The treatment time was increased from 120 to 180 minutes and the restriction of treatment borders of 1.5 cm from the endometrium and 0.5 cm from the fibroid capsule were eliminated. Finally, two treatment sessions were allowed if performed within a 14-day period. Fennessy et al[48] reported on this change in the protocol by evaluating 96 patients treated using the original treatment guidelines and 64 patients treated with the modified guidelines. This study demonstrated that use of the modified protocol resulted in a larger nonperfused volume than the original protocol (25.8% versus 16.7%). This correlated with the observation that the change in the symptom severity score was greater in the modified group than the original group and that this difference continued to be seen 12 months after treatment. In addition, fewer adverse events were seen in the modified group compared with the original group.

Stewart et al[49] then reported data on 2-year outcomes after MRgFUS. This study evaluated 359 patients treated with MRgFUS who had been enrolled in previous clinical trials and had completed 24 months of follow-up. Because the guidelines for treatment changed as patients were recruited into clinical trials, this review evaluated outcomes against nonperfused volume. This study demonstrated that there was an improvement in symptom severity for patients with >20% and <20% nonperfused volume 3 months after treatment with the higher nonperfused group experiencing more significant improvement. At both 12 and 24 months after treatment, significantly fewer patients in the higher nonperfused group required additional treatment for their fibroids. Given the fact that the adverse event rates are low with the modified protocol, it certainly appears based on these studies that long-term symptom control can be achieved with MRgFUS and that the results are improved as more tissue is treated. Based on this data, the authors predicted that with a negative predictive value (NPV) >60%, there would be only a 3% chance of needing an alternative treatment at 12 months and a 10% chance at 24 months. These numbers compare favorably with other uterine-sparing procedures such as laparoscopic myomectomy and uterine artery embolization.[50,51]

MR-guided focused ultrasound surgery represents an idealized form of lesion-based therapy. To be able to specially ablate tissue and treat it in a completely noninvasive manner while sparing a maximum amount of surrounding normal tissue should be the goal of any form of lesion-based therapy.[52] However, as a form, albeit advanced form of lesion-based therapy, many of the same limitations that were described previously in the context of RFA, laser ablation, and cryoablation, can be applied to this procedure as well. The ability of this treatment to address patients with multiple fibroids may represent a significant limitation to widespread applicability. Although multiple treatments are certainly possible, especially given the noninvasive nature of this therapy, the reported procedure times may be seen as a limitation, both from a patient perspective and an economic perspective when one focuses on throughput on an expensive piece of capital equipment. A second important limitation concerns the restrictions on this technology by the FDA. At the present time, it is not permitted to treat the fibroids in their entirety and time required to do so may again be seen as prohibitive. A recent report suggests that pretreatment with Lupron (TAP Pharmaceutical Products, Inc., Lake Forest, IL) for 3 months enhances the efficacy of MRgFUS by initially shrinking the fibroid (so there is less tissue to treat) and by improving the thermoablative effect resulting in a more complete treatment with higher NPVs.[53] However, until fibroids are treated in their entirety, the data obtained in the context of

UAE indicates that these patients may be at risk for fibroid regrowth and symptom recurrence. That said, if nonperfused volume on MRI continues to exceed treated volume, then treating entire fibroids may not be necessary and we do also know that inducing fibroid infarction is not always necessary to achieve symptomatic relief in these patients. Despite all of this, there is no doubt that the results seen after MRgFUS are extremely promising, especially given the completely noninvasive nature of this treatment. Future studies should continue the effort to answer these questions.

■ Organ-based Treatment

The concept behind organ-based treatment options for uterine fibroids is that fibroids represent a diffuse problem within the uterus that can potentially be treated by directing therapy toward the entire uterus. This concept forms the basis for hysterectomy, which can be seen as the ultimate form of organ-based therapy: remove the organ and the problem is solved. This concept also forms the basis for UAE because embolizing both uterine arteries creates an ischemic environment within the uterus that ultimately leads to fibroid infarction and symptomatic relief. Utilizing this philosophy has led to alternative methods of reducing blood flow within the uterus arteries to induce an effect similar to UAE. In some way, this has validated the methodology that interventional radiologists have long perceived as being an effective way to treat uterine fibroids and other tumors throughout the body. Besides UAE (which has been reviewed in previous chapters), the procedures in this section include laparoscopic occlusion of the uterine arteries, laparoscopic bipolar coagulation of the uterine arteries, and transvaginal clamping of the uterine arteries.

Laparoscopic occlusion of the uterine arteries is a procedure during which the uterine arteries are identified and clipped at a level near their origin from the internal iliac artery. Once this is completed, the visible collaterals between the ovaries and the uterus are coagulated with bipolar forceps. Hald et al[54] studied this technique by evaluating 46 patients undergoing either UAE ($n = 24$) or laparoscopic closure of the uterine arteries ($n = 22$) to treat their fibroids. This study was not randomized; patients were assigned to laparoscopic occlusion when the size of the fibroid did not exceed the umbilicus and patients were assigned to UAE independently of the size of the fibroid. Postoperative pain was found to be more severe in the UAE group. Six months after therapy, patients undergoing laparoscopic uterine artery occlusion experienced mean uterine and fibroid volume reductions of 36.7% and 36.2%, respectively, while the mean uterine and fibroid volume reductions in the UAE group were 40.1% and 45.1%, respectively. Of the 16 patients available for follow-up in the laparoscopy group, 14 experienced a reduction in bleeding and were satisfied with their clinical outcome. Of note, three patients undergoing laparoscopic uterine artery occlusion complained of skin sensation abnormalities and reduction of leg adduction due to the procedure affecting the obturator nerve, which was ultimately self-limited in all patients. Hald et al[55] followed that study up with a prospective randomized comparison of laparoscopic uterine artery occlusion and UAE. In this study, 66 patients were randomized to the two groups, but only 58 patients were treated (29 patients in each group). Twenty-eight patients in each group completed 6-month follow-up, at which time 21% of patients undergoing laparoscopic uterine artery occlusion complained of heavy bleeding compared with 4% of the patients undergoing UAE. However, in patients reporting improvement, the degree of improvement was similar in both groups. In the uterine artery occlusion group, complications included pulmonary embolism in one patient, temporary adductor muscle weakness in two patients, and buttock claudication due to internal iliac artery occlusion in one patient.

Laparoscopic bipolar coagulation of the uterine arteries is another potential treatment option for patients with uterine fibroids. In this procedure, the uterine artery is directly visualized and desiccated using bipolar forceps once it is separated from the ureter and other surrounding structures. The anastomotic sites of the uterine and ovarian arteries are coagulated as well. The uterine nerve can be ablated at the same time, which may help to decrease postoperative ischemic pain and improve the dysmenorrhea associated with uterine fibroids.[56] Liu et al[57] reported on their experience with treating 87 patients with symptomatic uterine fibroids using this technique. In these patients, laparoscopy was performed under general anesthesia. The procedure was technically successful in 97.7%. Following the procedure, 27.6% of patients experienced lower abdominal pain that persisted for ~2 weeks and were treated with nonsteroidal antiinflammatory medications. Symptomatic improvement was found in most patients: 93.1% of patients with menorrhagia reported improvement, 87% of patients with bladder compressive symptoms reported improvement, and 81.1% of patients with dysmenorrhea reported improvement. Using ultrasound for imaging follow-up, it was found that the mean fibroid volume reduction was 76%, with greater decreases seen in fibroids >5 cm in diameter compared with fibroids <5 cm in diameter. Simsek et al[58] have found similar findings in their study of 21 patients undergoing this procedure. Successful pregnancies have been reported after this procedure, but there has been a relatively high rate (41.2%) of early miscarriages observed in these pregnancies.[59,60]

One of the newer methods that has been recently described to treat uterine fibroids is the use of a transvaginal clamp to occlude the uterine arteries.[61,62] The Flostat system (Vascular Control Systems, San Juan Capistrano, CA) consists of a guiding cervical tenaculum, a transvaginal vascular clamp with integrated Doppler ultrasound, and a small transceiver that generates audible Doppler sound. With the patient in the lithotomy position, a guiding cervical tenaculum is placed in the cervix and the vascular clamp is attached to this tenaculum. The clamp is then slid along the tenaculum to the level of the lateral vaginal fornices. At this point, Doppler signals from the uterine arteries are detected. The clamp is advanced along the tenaculum, displacing the arteries superiorly. At this point, the clamp is closed, which occludes the uterine arteries by squeezing them along the lateral borders of the uterus. The clamp remains in place for 6 hours and is then released, with immediate return of Doppler signal from each uterine artery. The 6-hour duration was derived from a previous study of laparoscopic bilateral uterine artery occlusion that indicated that the myometrium was reperfused within 6 hours in ~80% of women.[63] This procedure has been performed with a paracervical block and an epidural. Istre et al[61] and Vilos et al[62] have both described case reports using this technique. Both cases resulted in improvement in abnormal bleeding and significant reductions of both uterine and dominant fibroid volume.

Each of these procedures, in addition to UAE, demonstrates the potential role that arterial occlusive therapy and subsequent tissue ischemia can potentially play in the treatment of patients with symptomatic uterine fibroids. However, from the perspective of an interventional radiologist, these alternative procedures are troubling in that they appear to disregard what is perceived as a fundamental understanding of tissue perfusion and ischemia induction that has been gained through more than three decades of experience with transcatheter embolization procedures. The premise is that when the level of occlusion produced during an embolization procedure within the vasculature of a target organ is distal, the potential for true tissue infarction is higher than when the level of occlusion is proximal, primarily because proximal occlusions tend to leave open the possibility of collateral flow bypassing the occlusion induced by the embolization procedure. UAE is based on this through its use of flow-directed particles that presumably occlude the uterine vasculature beyond the point where significant collaterals can become an issue. All of the procedures described produce a proximal uterine artery occlusion, and therefore leave open the possibility of collateral flow and continued perfusion. Therefore, although each of these alternative therapies presents promising data, the absence of follow-up imaging using contrast-enhanced MRI is a limitation because there is no documentation that any of these procedures resulted in true fibroid infarction. It is known that fibroid ischemia, even in the absence of tissue infarction, can lead to symptomatic improvement and even uterine and fibroid volume reduction after UAE. However, it has been demonstrated that the lack of tissue infarction can predispose patients to incomplete treatment and symptomatic recurrence.[33] Therefore, MRI will be needed to demonstrate tissue infarction to support the premise that a proximal uterine artery occlusion will lead to permanent changes within the treated fibroids.

■ Pharmacologic Treatment

Interventional radiologists, gynecologists, and any other physicians performing procedures to treat uterine fibroids should be aware of the fact that medical management of the symptoms caused by uterine fibroids is an impending reality.[2,53,64] Today, oral contraceptives are often used to treat abnormal uterine bleeding, but this effect is usually temporary and they do not reduce fibroid and uterine volume. Leuprolide acetate, which is a gonadotropin-releasing hormone agonist, is used as a preoperative treatment of fibroids associated with anemia and is effective at reducing both abnormal bleeding and uterine and fibroid volume prior to surgery. In addition, early results from Europe suggest that Lupron can be used to increase the efficacy of MRgFUS by shrinking the fibroid so that there is less tissue to treat and making the tissue more sensitive to the heating caused by this procedure.[53] However, associated symptoms such as vaginal dryness, bone loss, headache, and hot flushes limit its potential use as long-term, stand-alone therapy. The use of add-back therapy while on leuprolide acetate may counteract some of these hypoestrogenic effects. The progestin norethindrone acetate is FDA-approved as an add-back therapy for Lupron Depo for the treatment of endometriosis. However, it is not approved for the treatment of uterine fibroids. Initial studies with Lupron and norethindrone acetate add-back therapy in women with uterine fibroids showed that norethindrone acetate decreased the efficacy of Lupron on fibroid volume reduction, which is most likely due to proliferative effects of a progestin on uterine fibroid tissue. Tibolone (Organon, West Orange, NJ), which is not approved for use in the United States, is a synthetic compound that has intrinsic estrogenic, progestogenic, and androgenic properties. It has been shown to reduce bone mineral density loss and vasomotor symptoms without affecting fibroid shrinkage in patients receiving GnRH agonist treatment for fibroids.[65]

It has been established that the development of fibroids is dependent on ovarian steroid hormones, including both estrogen and progesterone.[66] Observations such as the growth of fibroids during reproductive years (especially during pregnancy) and in the setting of postmenopausal hormone therapy, and the decrease in size seen within fibroids after menopause support their dependence on hormones. Traditionally, estrogen has been felt to be the dominant fibroid involved in the pathogenesis of fibroids. However, the role of progesterone and progesterone receptors has been recently studied.[67] This has led to biochemical, histological, clinical, and pharmacologic evidence that supports an important role for progesterone in the pathogenesis of fibroids.[66,68–71]

This focus on the role of progesterone in this condition essentially began with the discovery of mifepristone (RU-486), a progesterone receptor modulator with primarily antagonistic properties.[72–74] Discovered in 1981 as a new glucocorticoid receptor antagonist, its possible role as a progesterone antagonist quickly became realized.[75] The double-blind, placebo controlled study performed by Fiscella et al showed that treatment with mifepristone 5 mg daily for 6 months significantly improved quality of life, reduced uterine bleeding, and reduced uterine and fibroid volume.[74] These effects have been shown to be accompanied by a reduction in uterine blood flow, suggesting that progesterone plays an important role in the regulation of uterine perfusion.[75,76] At higher doses (>10 mg/day), unopposed estrogenic effects including a high rate of endometrial hyperplasia have been reported in association with the use of mifepristone.[77–79] There have also been reports in ~10% of patients that hepatic enzymes become elevated with mifepristone treatment, but these normalize once therapy is stopped.[79,80] Although this drug has antiglucocorticoid properties, elevated cortisol levels have been noted with the use of daily, low-dose mifepristone.[80] Interestingly, regrowth of the fibroids has been shown to occur slowly following cessation of the medication.[73] Although this medication did address the symptoms of uterine fibroids to some degree, these concerns directed research toward finding compounds with increased progesterone antagonistic potency along with reduced antiglucocorticoid activity.[81] CDB-2914 is another pure progesterone antagonist that appears to have less antiglucocorticoid activity, which is a potential advantage for long-term use. In a small, randomized study, Levens et al have demonstrated that CDB-2914 significantly reduces fibroid volume without antiglucocorticoid effects after 90 days of treatment.[82] This agent continues to be studied for the treatment of fibroids.

The next class of compounds to be evaluated as a medical treatment for fibroids was the selective progesterone receptor modulators (SPRMs). These compounds exert selective progesterone agonist, antagonist, or mixed agonist and antagonist effects on various progesterone target tissues depending on the biological action studied.[75,77] These J compounds, which are characterized structurally by 11 β-benzaldoxime substitutions, demonstrate less agonist activity than progesterone and less antagonist activity then mifepristone; therefore, their effects differ from these other compounds.[83]

Specifically, these compounds can maintain estrogen secretion, decrease or not change progesterone secretion, and cause amenorrhea via a direct effect on the endometrium.[77] Importantly, they tend to have low antiglucocorticoid effects as well.[81,84]

Asoprisnil is a selective progesterone receptor modulator and is the first SPRM to reach an advanced stage of clinical development for the treatment of uterine fibroids.[85] This agent has been shown to inhibit the expression of growth factors and growth factor-induced proliferation of uterine leiomyomata.[86] In a phase 1 study on healthy volunteers having regular menstrual cycles, asoprisnil suppressed menstruation in a dose-dependent manner.[66,87] The dose-dependent induction of amenorrhea by asoprisnil was then confirmed in a phase 2 study in patients with uterine fibroids.[88] In 2007, Chwalisz et al reported the findings of a prospective, randomized, double-blind, placebo-controlled study of 129 patients with fibroids receiving a placebo or asoprisnil (5, 10, or 25 mg) for 12 weeks.[89] This study demonstrated that asoprisnil was effective at controlling abnormal bleeding, reducing uterine and fibroid volume, and improving bulk-related symptoms, especially at higher doses. These effects occurred with minimal symptoms of estrogen deprivation and no significant bone resorption. This mechanism for uterine bleeding suppression is still unknown, but may involve an interaction between asoprisnil, perivascular cells, and spiral vessels based on full-thickness endometrial samples obtained during hysterectomy in patients receiving asoprisnil prior to surgery.[90] This interaction likely alters the responsiveness of the spiral arteries to modulations by ovarian steroids.[77] Of note, Chwalisz et al reported that there was a small increase in the frequency of breast pain and in the incidence of functional, asymptomatic ovarian cysts >4 cm in diameter in patients receiving asoprisnil.[89] Mutter et al[91] have raised an additional safety concern by noting that chronic use of progesterone antagonists and SPRMs is associated with endometrial changes. These agents continue to be studied and new administration regimens are being developed to address these safety concerns.

Varelas et al[92] have evaluated the potential role of anastrazole as a medical treatment option for fibroids. Anastrazole is a nonsteroidal aromatase inhibitor used to treat advanced breast cancer in menopausal patients. It may have a role in the treatment of fibroids because aromatase, which catalyzes the conversion of androstenedione and testosterone to estrone and estradiol, has been shown to be present in fibroid tissue.[93] If the aromatase in fibroids leads to the production of in-situ estrogen, then that could promote cell proliferation and growth.[94] Varelas et al[92] studied the effects of a 3-month cycle of anastrazole on patients with fibroids and found that this medication reduces the size of uterine fibroids, improves symptoms, and is well tolerated. Similar findings were also demonstrated by Hilario et al.[95] However, in premenopausal women, aromatase inhibitors have been associated with the formation of ovarian cysts, which may limit their use.[96] This compound continues to be tested as a treatment for fibroids.

There has also been some interest in exploring gene therapy approaches to the treatment of uterine fibroids.[97] Al-Hendy and Salama[97] have theorized that uterine fibroids may be an attractive target for gene therapy because they are well-circumscribed lesions and easily differentiated from surrounding normal tissue. This may make it possible to deliver viral vectors by direct injection or by intraarterial injection as with UFE, both of which might limit systemic toxicity and immunologic reactions. In addition, complete resolution is not necessarily needed to achieve some degree of symptomatic improvement. Preliminary work by Niu et al demonstrated that nonviral mediated transfer of a suicide gene for thymidine kinase can result in leiomyoma cell death.[98] In addition, dominant-negative estrogen receptor gene therapy proposed by Al-Hendy et al can also work by intercepting the estrogen signaling pathway.[99] This early work demonstrating the potential of gene therapy continues to be explored.

■ Conclusions

In conclusion, the introduction of UAE as a treatment option for patients with symptomatic fibroids has changed the landscape of fibroid therapy. It was not very long ago that articles were being written and lectures were being delivered to encourage patients and physicians to consider UAE as an alternative to surgery for uterine fibroids. With the success of UAE, others have now been seeking additional, nonsurgical options for these patients. The innovative attempts that have been reported during the past decade have given an unprecedented amount of attention to this condition and these patients. Now, with UAE as an accepted treatment option for uterine fibroids, all of the procedures described in this article are "alternatives" to UAE. Because of the potential for success demonstrated by many of these techniques, it is important that any interventional radiologist offering UAE be familiar with these other less invasive and noninvasive procedures, not only for his or her own education and practice, but also to facilitate appropriate discussions with patients regarding the best available treatment options.

References

1. Walker CL, Stewart EA. Uterine fibroids: the elephant in the room. Science 2005;308:1589–1592
2. Munro MG. Management of leiomyomas: is there a panacea in Pandora's box? Fertil Steril 2006;85:40–43
3. Luo X, Shen Y, Song WX, Chen PW, Xie XM, Want XY. Pathologic evaluation of uterine leiomyoma treated with radiofrequency ablation. Int J Gynaecol Obstet 2007;99:9–13
4. Bergamini V, Ghezzi F, Cromi A, et al. Laparoscopic radiofrequency thermal ablation: a new approach to symptomatic uterine myomas. Am J Obstet Gynecol 2005;192:768–773
5. Ghezzi F, Cromi A, Bergamini V, et al. Midterm outcome of radiofrequency thermal ablation for symptomatic uterine myomas. Surg Endosc 2007;21:2081–2085
6. Milic A, Asch MR, Hawrylyshyn PA, et al. Laparoscopic ultrasound-guided radiofrequency ablation of uterine fibroids. Cardiovasc Intervent Radiol 2006;29:694–698
7. Kim HS, Tsai J, Jacobs MA, Kamel IR. Percutaneous image-guided radiofrequency thermal ablation for large symptomatic uterine leiomyomata after uterine artery embolization: a feasibility and safety study. J Vasc Interv Radiol 2007;18:41–48
8. Donnez J, Gillerot S, Bourgonjon D, et al. Neodymium: YAG laser hysteroscopy in large submucous fibroids. Fertil Steril 1990;54:999–1003
9. Nisolle M, Smets M, Malvaux V, et al. Laparoscopic myolysis with the neodymium-ytrium aluminum garnet laser. Int J Gynaecol Surg 1993;9:95–99
10. Zupi E, Sbracia M, Marconi D, Munro MG. Myolysis of uterine fibroids: is there a role? Clin Obstet Gynecol 2006;49:821–833
11. Law P, Gedroyc WMW, Regan L. Magnetic-resonance guided percutaneous laser ablation of uterine fibroids. Lancet 1999;354:2049–2050
12. Phillips DR, Nathanson HG, Milim SJ, Haselkorn JS. Laparoscopic leiomyomas coagulation. J Am Assoc Gynecol Laparosc 1996; 3(4, Suppl)S39
13. Goldfarb HA. Laparoscopic coagulation of myoma (myolysis). Obstet Gynecol Clin North Am 1995;22:807–819
14. Law P, Gedroyc WMW, Regan L. Magnetic resonance-guided percutaneous laser ablation of uterine fibroids. J Magn Reson Imaging 2000;12:565–570
15. Parker DL, Smith V, Sheldon P, et al. Temperature distribution measurements in two dimensional NMR imaging. Med Phys 1983;10:321–325
16. Law P, Regan L. Interstitial thermo-ablation under MRI guidance for the treatment of fibroids. Curr Opin Obstet Gynecol 2000;12:277–282
17. Hindley JT, Law PA, Hickey M, et al. Clinical outcomes following percutaneous magnetic resonance image guided laser ablation of symptomatic uterine fibroids. Hum Reprod 2002;17:2737–2741
18. Dohi M, Harada J, Mogami T, et al. MR-guided transvaginal cryotherapy of uterine fibroids with a horizontal open MRI system: initial experience. Radiat Med 2004;22:391–397
19. Tacke J, Adam G, Haage P, et al. MR-guided percutaneous cryotherapy of the liver: in-vivo evaluation with histologic correlation in an animal model. J Magn Reson Imaging 2001;13:50–56
20. Rubinsky B, Lee CY, Bastacky J, et al. The process of freezing and the mechanism of damage during hepatic cryosurgery. Cryobiology 1990;27:85–97
21. Bischof J, Fahssi WM, Smith D, et al. A parametric study of freezing injury in ELT-3 uterine leiomyoma tumour cells. Hum Reprod 2001;16:340–348
22. Rupp CC, Nagel TC, Swanlund DK, et al. Cryothermic and hyperthermic treatments of human leiomyoma and adjacent myometrium and their implications for laparoscopic surgery. J Am Assoc Gynecol Laparosc 2003;10:90–98
23. Olive DL, Rutherford T, Zreik T, et al. Cryomyolysis in the conservative treatment of uterine fibroids. J Am Assoc Gynecol Laparosc 1996; 3(4, Suppl)S36
24. Zreik TG, Rutherford TJ, Palter SF, et al. Cryomyolysis, a new procedure for the conservative treatment of uterine fibroids. J Am Assoc Gynecol Laparosc 1998;5:33–38
25. Ciavattini A, Tsiroglou D, Piccioni M, et al. Laparoscopic cryomyolysis. An alternative to myomectomy in patients with symptomatic fibroids. Surg Endosc 2004;18:1785–1788
26. Zupi E, Piredda A, Marconi D, et al. Directed laparoscopic cryomyolysis: a possible alterantive to myomectomy and/or hysterectomy for symptomatic leiomyomas. Am J Obstet Gynecol 2004;190:639–643

27. Zupi E, Marconi D, Sbracia M, et al. Directed laparoscopic cryomyolysis for symptomatic leiomyomata: one-year follow-up. J Minim Invasive Gynecol 2005;12:343–346
28. Exacoustos C, Zupi E, Marconi D, et al. Ultrasound-assisted, laparoscopic cryomyolysis: two- and three-dimensional findings before, during and after treatment. Ultrasound Obstet Gynecol 2005;25:393–400
29. Ciavattini A, Tsiroglou D, Litta P, Vichi M, Tranquilli AL. Pregnancy outcome after laparoscopic cryomyolysis of uterine myomas: report of nine cases. J Minim Invasive Gynecol 2006;13:141–144
30. Sewell PE, Arriola RM, Robinette L, et al. Real-time I-MR-guided cryoablation of uterine fibroids. J Vasc Interv Radiol 2001;12:891–893
31. Cowan BD, Sewell PE, Howard JC, et al. Interventional magnetic resonance imaging cryotherapy of uterine fibroid tumors: preliminary observation. Am J Obstet Gynecol 2002;186:1183–1187
32. Sakuhara Y, Shimizu T, Kodama Y, et al. Magnetic resonance-guided percutaneous cryoablation of uterine fibroids: early clinical experiences. Cardiovasc Intervent Radiol 2006;29:552–558
33. Pelage JP, Guaou NG, Jha RC, et al. Uterine fibroid tumors: long-term MR imaging outcome after embolization. Radiology 2004;230:803–809
34. Chapman A, ter Haar G. Thermal ablation of uterine fibroids using MR-guided focused ultrasound – a truly non-invasive treatment modality. Eur Radiol 2007;17:2505–2511
35. Lynn JG, Zwemer RL, Chick AJ, et al. A new method for the generation and use of focused ultrasound in experimental biology. J Gen Physiol 1942;26:179–183
36. Kennedy JE, Haar GR, Cranston D. High intensity focused ultrasound: surgery of the future? Br J Radiol 2003;76:590–599
37. Fennessy FM, Tempany CM. A review of magnetic resonance imaging-guided focused ultrasound surgery of uterine fibroids. Top Magn Reson Imaging 2006;17:173–179
38. So MJ, Fennessy FM, Zou KH, et al. Does the phase of menstrual cycle affect MR-guided focused ultrasound surgery of uterine leiomyomas? Eur J Radiol 2006;59:203–207
39. Funaki K, Fukunishi H, Funaki T, et al. Mid-term outcome of magnetic resonance-guided focused ultrasound surgery for uterine myomas: from six to twelve months after volume reduction. J Minim Invasive Gynecol 2007;14:616–621
40. Hudson SBA, Stewart EA. Magnetic resonance-guided focused ultrasound surgery. Clin Obstet Gynecol 2008;51:159–166
41. Vaezy S, Fujimoto VY, Walker C, et al. Treatment of uterine fibroid tumors in a nude mouse model using high-intensity focused ultrasound. Am J Obstet Gynecol 2000;183:6–11
42. Tempany CMC, Stewart EA, McDannold N, et al. MR-imaging-guided focused ultrasound surgery of uterine leiomyomas: a feasibility study. Radiology 2003;226:897–905
43. Stewart EA, Gedroyc WMW, Tempany CMC, et al. Focused ultrasound treatment of uterine fibroid tumors: safety and feasibility of a noninvasive thermoablative technique. Am J Obstet Gynecol 2003;189:48–54
44. Hindley J, Gedroyc WMW, Regan L, et al. MRI guidance of focused ultrasound therapy of uterine fibroids: early results. AJR Am J Roentgenol 2004;183:1713–1719
45. Stewart EA, Rabinovici J, Tempany CMC, et al. Clinical outcomes of focused ultrasound surgery for the treatment of uterine fibroids. Fertil Steril 2006;85:22–29
46. Stewart EA, Rabinovici J, Tempany CMC, et al. Clinical outcomes of focused ultrasound surgery for the treatment of uterine fibroids. Fertil Steril 2006;85:22–29
47. McDannold N, Tempany CM, Fennessy FM, et al. Uterine leiomyomas: MR imaging-based thermometry and thermal dosimetry during focused ultrasound thermal ablation. Radiology 2006;240:263–272
48. Fennessy FM, Tempany CM, McDannold NJ, et al. Uterine leiomyomas: MR imaging-guided focused ultrasound surgery – results of different treatment protocols. Radiology 2007;243:885–893
49. Stewart EA, Gostout B, Rabinovici J, et al. Sustained relief of leiomyoma symptoms by using focused ultrasound surgery. Obstet Gynecol 2007;110:279–287
50. Stewart EA, Faur AV, Wise LA, Reilly RJ, Harlow BL. Predictors of subsequent surgery for uterine leiomyomata development after abdominal myomectomy. Obstet Gynecol 2002;99:426–432
51. Marret H, Cottier JP, Alonso AM, et al. Predictive factors for fibroid recurrence after uterine artery embolization. BJOG 2005;112:461–465
52. Siskin G. New treatments for uterine fibroids. Tech Vasc Interv Radiol 2006;9:12–18
53. Smart OC, Hindley JT, Regan L, Gedroyc WG. Gonadotropin-releasing hormone and magnetic resonance guided ultrasound surgery for uterine leiomyomata. Obstet Gynecol 2006;108:49–54
54. Hald K, Langebrekke A, Klow NE, et al. Laparoscopic occlusion of uterine vessels for the treatment of symptomatic uterine fibroids: initial experience and comparison to uterine artery embolization. Am J Obstet Gynecol 2004;190:37–43
55. Hald K, Klow NE, Qvigstad E, Istre O. Laparoscopic occlusion compared with embolization of uterine vessels. A randomized controlled trial. Obstet Gynecol 2007;109:20–27
56. Yen YK, Liu WM, Yuan CC, Ng HT. Addition of laparoscopic uterine nerve ablation to laparoscopic bipolar coagulation of uterine vessels for women with uterine myomas and dysmenorrhea. J Am Assoc Gynecol Laparosc 2001;8:573–578
57. Liu WM, Ng HT, Wu YC, et al. Laparoscopic bipolar coagulation of uterine vessels: a new method for treating symptomatic uterine fibroids. Fertil Steril 2001;75:417–422
58. Simsek M, Sadik S, Taskin O, et al. Role of laparoscopic uterine artery coagulation in management of symptomatic myomas: a prospective study using ultrasound and magnetic resonance imaging. J Minim Invasive Gynecol 2006;13:315–319
59. Chen YJ, Wang PH, Yuan CC, et al. Successful pregnancy in a woman with symptomatic fibroids who underwent laparoscopic bipolar coagulation of uterine vessels. Fertil Steril 2002;77:838–840
60. Chen YJ, Wang PH, Yuan CC, et al. Pregnancy following treatment of symptomatic myomas with laparoscopic bipolar coagulation of uterine vessels. Hum Reprod 2003;18:1077–1081
61. Istre O, Hald K, Qvigstad E. Multiple myomas treated with a temporary, noninvasive Doppler-directed transvaginal uterine artery clamp. J Am Assoc Gynecol Laparosc 2004;11:273–276
62. Vilos GA, Vilos EC, Romano W, Abu-Rafea B. Temporary uterine artery occlusion for treatment of menorrhagia and uterine fibroids using an incisionless Doppler-guided transvaginal clamp: case report. Hum Reprod 2006;21:269–271
63. Lichtinger M, Burbank F, Hallson L, et al. The time course of myometrial ischemia and reperfusion after laparoscopic uterine artery occlusion. Theoretical implications. J Am Assoc Gynecol Laparosc 2003;10:553–556
64. Young SL, Al-Hendy A, Copland JA, et al. Potential nonhormonal therapeutics for medical treatment of leiomyoma. Semin Reprod Med 2004;22:121–130
65. Morris EP, Rymer J, Robinson J, Fogelman I. Efficacy of tibolone as "add-back therapy" in conjunction with a gonadotropins-releasing hormone analogue in the treatment of uterine fibroids. Fertil Steril 2008;89:421–428
66. Chwalisz K, DeManno D, Garg R, et al. Therapeutic potential for the selective progesterone receptor modulator asoprisnil in the treatment of leiomyomata. Semin Reprod Med 2004;22:113–119
67. Rein MS, Barbieri RL, Friedman AJ. Progesterone: a critical role in the pathogenesis of uterine myomas. Am J Obstet Gynecol 1995;172:14–18
68. Brandon DD, Bethea CL, Strawn EY, et al. Progesterone receptor messenger ribonucleic acid and protein are overexpressed in human uterine leiomyomas. Am J Obstet Gynecol 1993;169:78–85
69. Harrison-Woolrych ML, Charnock-Jones DS, Smith SK. Quantification of messenger ribonucleic acid for epidermal growth factor in human myometrium and leiomyomata using reverse transcriptase polymerase chain reaction. J Clin Endocrinol Metab 1994;78:1179–1184
70. Maruo T, Matsuo H, Samoto T, et al. Effects of progesterone on uterine leiomyoma growth and apoptosis. Steroids 2000;65:585–592

71. Maruo T, Matsuo H, Shimomura Y, et al. Effects of progesterone on growth factor expression in human uterine leiomyoma. Steroids 2003;68:817–824
72. Murphy AA, Kettel LM, Morales AJ, et al. Regression of uterine leiomyomata in response to the antiprogesterone RU 486. J Clin Endocrinol Metab 1993;76:513–517
73. Eisinger SH, Bonfiglio T, Fiscella K, et al. Twelve month safety and efficacy of low-dose mifepristone for uterine myomas. J Minim Invasive Gynecol 2005;12:227–233
74. Fiscella K, Eisinger SH, Meldrum S, et al. Effect of mifepristone for symptomatic leiomyomata on quality of life and uterine size: a randomized controlled trial. Obstet Gynecol 2006;108:1381–1387
75. Spitz IM. Progesterone receptor antagonists and selective progesterone receptor modulators (SPRMs). Semin Reprod Med 2005;23:3–7
76. Reinsch RC, Murphy AA, Morales AJ, et al. The effects of RU 486 and leuprolide acetate on uterine artery blood flow in the fibroid uterus: a prospective, randomized study. Am J Obstet Gynecol 1994;170:1623–1628
77. Chwalisz K, Perez MC, DeManno D, et al. Selective progesterone receptor modulator development and use in the treatment of leiomyomata and endometriosis. Endocr Rev 2005;26:423–438
78. Murphy AA, Kettel LM, Morales AJ, et al. Endometrial effects of long-term low-dose administration of RU-486. Fertil Steril 1995;63:761–766
79. Eisinger SH, Meldrum S, Fiscella K, et al. Low-dose mifepristone for uterine leiomyomata. Obstet Gynecol 2003;101:243–250
80. Steinauer J, Pritts EA, Jackson R, Jacoby AF. Systemic review of mifepristone for the treatment of uterine leiomyomata. Obstet Gynecol 2004;103:1331–1336
81. Schubert G, Elger W, Kaufmann G, et al. Discovery, chemistry, and reproductive pharmacology of asoprisnil and related 11B-benzaldoxime substituted selective progesterone receptor modulators (SPRMs). Semin Reprod Med 2005;23:58–73
82. Levens ED, Potlog-Nahari C, Armstrong AY, et al. CDB-2914 for uterine leiomyomata treatment. Obstet Gynecol 2008;111:1129–1136
83. Elger W, Bartley J, Schneider B, et al. Endocrine pharmacological characterization of progesterone antagonists and progesterone receptor modulators with respect to PR-agonistic and antagonistic activity. Steroids 2000;65:713–723
84. DeManno D, Elger W, Garg R, et al. Asoprisnil (J867): a selective progesterone receptor modulator for gynecological therapy. Steroids 2003;68:1019–1032
85. Bachmann G. Expanding treatment options for women with symptomatic uterine leiomyomas: timely medical breakthroughs. Fertil Steril 2006;85:46–47
86. Wang J, Ohara N, Wang Z, et al. A novel selective progesterone receptor modulator asoprisnil (J867) downregulates the expression of EGF, IGF-I, TGFbeta3, and their receptors in cultured uterine leiomyoma cells. Hum Reprod 2006;21:1869–1877
87. Chwalisz K, Elger W, McCrary K, et al. Reversible suppression of menstruation in normal women irrespective of the effect on ovulation with the noval selective progesterone receptor modulator (SPRM) J867. J Soc Gynecol Investig 2002;9:82A
88. Chwalisz K, Parker L, Williamson S. Treatment of uterine leiomyomas with the novel selective progesterone receptor modulator (SPRM). J Soc Gynecol Investig 2003;10:301A
89. Chwalisz K, Larsen L, Mattia-Goldberg C, et al. A randomized, controlled trial of asoprisnil, a novel selective progesterone receptor modulator, in women with uterine leiomyomata. Fertil Steril 2007;87:1399–1412
90. Williams ARW, Critchley HOD, Osei J, et al. The effects of the selective progesterone receptor modulator asoprisnil on the morphology of uterine tissues after 3 months treatment in patients with symptomatic uterine leiomyomata. Hum Reprod 2007;22:1696–1704
91. Mutter GL, Bergeron C, Deligdisch L, et al. The spectrum of endometrial pathology induced by progesterone receptor modulators. Mod Pathol 2008;21:591–598
92. Varelas FK, Papanicolaou AN, Vavatsi-Christaki N, Makedos G, Vlassis GD. The effect of anastrazole on symptomatic uterine leiomyomata. Obstet Gynecol 2007;110:643–649
93. Shozu M, Murakami K, Inoue M. Aromatase and leiomyoma of the uterus. Semin Reprod Med 2004;22:51–60
94. Sumitani H, Shozu M, Segawa T, et al. In situ estrogen synthesized by aromatase P450 in uterine leiomyoma cells promotes cell growth probably via an autocrine/intracrine mechanism. Endocrinology 2000; 141:3852–3861
95. Hilario SG, Bozzini N, Borsari R, Baracat EC. Action of aromatase inhibitor for treatment of uterine leiomyoma in perimenopausal patients. Fertil Steril 2009;91(1):240–243
96. Attar E, Bulun SE. Aromatase inhibitors: the next generation of therapeutics for endometriosis? Fertil Steril 2006;85:1307–1318
97. Al-Hendy A, Salama S. Gene therapy and uterine leiomyoma: a review. Hum Reprod Update 2006;12:385–400
98. Niu H, Simari RD, Zimmermann EM, Christman GM. Nonviral vector-mediated thymidine kinase gene transfer and ganciclovir treatment in leiomyoma cells. Obstet Gynecol 1998;91:735–740
99. Al-Hendy A, Lee EJ, Wang HQ, Copland JA. Gene therapy of uterine leiomyomas: adenovirus-mediated expression of dominant negative estrogen receptor inhibits tumor growth in nude mice. Am J Obstet Gynecol 2004;191:1621–1631

7 Uterine Fibroid Embolization and Infertility

Gary P. Siskin

Since the first reports of utilizing uterine fibroid embolization (UFE) as a treatment for symptomatic uterine fibroids surfaced in the early 1990s, this procedure has gained both acceptance and popularity as a nonsurgical alternative used to manage this condition. As the success of UFE in addressing fibroid-related symptoms has been established, more women have been asking their gynecologist, primary-care physician, and interventional radiologist about UFE and its potential role in their care. This includes patients who express a desire to preserve future fertility options. Therefore, most interventionalists with active UFE practices are facing decisions regarding the appropriate management of a patient with fibroids who has stated her desire to either definitely or possibly have a child in the future.

To provide guidance for the interventionalists facing this dilemma in everyday practice, it is important to recognize that these patients typically fall into three very different categories characterized by the objectives of the patients. The first category includes patients who have fibroids and wish to preserve their fertility options, but do not have definite plans to have a child in the immediate future. The second category includes patients with fibroids who have definite plans for childbearing in the immediate future. Finally, the third category includes patients with fibroids who have been experiencing difficulties in becoming pregnant or carrying a pregnancy to term. The purpose of this chapter is to provide recommendations regarding the role that UFE may play in the care of all of these patients based on a current review of the literature regarding fertility issues in patients with fibroids and fertility preservation after procedures used to treat symptomatic uterine fibroids.[1]

■ Infertility and Uterine Fibroids

Infertility is a problem affecting many women and many couples in today's world. Based on the 2002 National Survey of Family Growth, 7.4% of married women (~2.1 million women) were infertile and 12% of women aged 15 to 44 (~7.3 million women) had difficulty getting pregnant or carrying a baby to term.[2] Classically, infertility has been defined as a failure to conceive after one year of failed intercourse. With this definition in mind, however, only a minority of patients are considered to have true infertility because they can only conceive and successfully carry a pregnancy with medical assistance. These patients may have conditions such as occluded fallopian tubes, an absent uterus, absent ovarian follicles, or male partners with an inability to produce sperm. The remaining patients can be considered subfertile because there is a chance that conception could happen without medical intervention. However, fertility treatment is often recommended for these patients if it is felt that treatment can improve their situation and increase the odds of conception.

There is no consensus about the impact of uterine fibroids on female subfertility.[3] It is known that fibroids are present in 5 to 10% of infertility patients and may be the sole factor identified in 1 to 2.5% of patients. However, the exact role that fibroids play in recurrent pregnancy loss and infertility is uncertain. This is because it has been historically difficult to assess the direct impact of fibroids on fertility due to the following: the incidence of fibroids increases with age, fertility declines with age, and many women with fibroids conceive spontaneously. That said, there are anatomic and physiologic factors attributed to the presence of uterine fibroids over the years, which may contribute to subfertility in this patient population.[4–8] As a space-occupying lesion, fibroids can be responsible for anatomic changes that can lead to subfertility, including distortion of the endometrial cavity, obstruction of the tubal ostia or cervical canal, and displacement of the cervix within the vagina. Physiologically, fibroids also have the potential to impair uterine contractility and impair implantation due to endometrial vascular disturbances resulting in inflammation, ulceration, thinning, and atrophy.

The problem that is considered by most to be responsible for fibroid-related subfertility is the distortion of the endometrial cavity because it can create an abnormal site for placental implantation which, in turn, can lead to increases in the rate of both spontaneous abortion and premature labor. This is why fibroid location and size are often the most important factors in determining the impact of fibroids.[3] Because of this, few dispute the fact that submucosal fibroids or intramural fibroids, which have a submucosal component, influence pregnancy rates. Even this, however, is controversial in the obstetrics-gynecology literature. When looking at this issue in the context of assisted reproductive technologies (such as in-vitro fertilization, intracytoplasmic sperm injection, etc.), some investigators have found that intramural and/or subserosal fibroids do not affect the outcome of these procedures.[9–11]

Others, however, have found that even small intramural fibroids that do not distort the endometrial cavity have a significant effect on pregnancy, implantation, and ongoing pregnancy rates.[11–14] This debate has led to differences regarding which patients should undergo treatment for fibroids, such as myomectomy, prior to attempts with assisted reproductive techniques.[15,16]

Given the importance of fibroid-related distortion of the endometrial cavity, one of the first steps that an interventional radiologist can take when evaluating a patient with fibroids and fertility concerns is to participate in the imaging evaluation of these patients and render an opinion as to whether or not the fibroids may be contributing to subfertility. Therefore, patients who have had fertility problems or wish to preserve fertility options after treating their fibroids should undergo an imaging evaluation of their endometrial cavity to determine the anatomic relationship between the fibroids and the cavity. There are many imaging tests that can potentially answer this question, including transvaginal ultrasound, sonohysterography, hysterosalpingogram, and hysteroscopy.[17–19] In addition, pelvic MRI, which is growing in importance as the imaging modality of choice before and after UFE, can provide this information as well.[20,21] At the very least, MRI will provide the information necessary to determine if the fibroids are distorting the endometrial cavity and if any other conditions are present that may explain infertility. MRI can also help determine if a patient is a candidate for myomectomy based on the size, number, and position of their fibroids.

■ Review of the Literature on Uterine Fibroid Treatment and Future Fertility

Once the fertility status of a patient is known and her childbearing plans have been discussed, an interventional radiologist can utilize the available imaging data and confer on the patient's treatment options. At the present time, a review of available literature supports the position that myomectomy is the preferred treatment option for a patient with symptomatic uterine fibroids and a desire to preserve fertility options. In 1998, Vercellini et al[22] performed a comprehensive review of the literature that estimated the effect of abdominal myomectomy on infertility. Twenty-three studies were reviewed, all of which were noncomparative. The pregnancy rate after myomectomy, based on 138 patients, was 57%; the conception rate ranged from 58 to 65% in patients with intramural and/or subserosal fibroids. This rate was similar to that found by Campo et al,[23] who evaluated 41 patients with intramural or subserosal patients and found a conception rate of 61%; Marchionni et al[24] in their evaluation of 72 patients with intramural or subserosal fibroids found a conception rate of 70%. Importantly, Campo et al found that myomectomy was associated with a decrease in the rate of miscarriage from 57.1% to 13.9%, which was similar to the decrease in miscarriages from 69% to 25% found by Marchionni et al.[23,24] Vercellini also found a conception rate ranging from 53 to 70% in patients with only submucosal fibroids.[22] This was similar to that reported by Shokeir et al[25] who found a 72.4% pregnancy rate after a hysteroscopic myomectomy was performed on 29 patients with submucosal fibroids. Similarly, they found that the miscarriage rate had dropped from 62% to 26% after myomectomy.

Despite the fact that there are a reasonably large number of studies available that have reported increases in conception and pregnancy rates and decreases in miscarriage rates, there remain differences of opinion regarding the role that myomectomy should play in patients with fibroids and a desire for fertility preservation. For example, in her 2001 review of fibroids and infertility, Pritts[4] stated that the only analysis of myomectomy outcomes stratified by location was for women with submucosal fibroids, with results supporting the use of myomectomy for these patients. However, given the lack of data suggesting a cause and effect relationship between intramural and subserosal fibroids and infertility, and given the potential complications of myomectomy, she felt that the use of myomectomy for these patients may be unjustified.[4] This differs from the data of Campo et al, who found that performing a myomectomy in patients with subserosal and/or intramural fibroids does help to improve pregnancy rates.[24] Therefore, although there certainly does seem to be data supporting the use of myomectomy in patients with symptomatic fibroids desiring future childbearing, this data certainly seems to leave room for questions and differences of opinion. It may also open the door for a possible role for UFE in the care of these patients.

As more interventional radiologists are performing UFE procedures on patients with symptomatic fibroids who desire future fertility, the number of reports and studies commenting on the successes and failure of this approach has increased. There are, at the present time, several case reports[26–35] and clinical studies[36–42] that support the observation that patients can become pregnant and carry a pregnancy to term after UFE. The outcomes of these clinical studies are summarized in **Table 7.1**. These reports all enable an interventional radiologist to say that patients can successfully conceive and deliver a healthy baby after UFE is performed. Although not exactly a quantitative statement, this is meaningful given the definitive early warnings against UFE in this patient population that were issued by the American College of Obsetetrics and Gynecology in 2000[43] and the inclusion of "desire to maintain childbearing potential" on the list of relative contraindica-

Table 7.1 Summary of Outcomes Concerning Pregnancy after Uterine Artery Embolization to Treat Symptomatic Uterine Fibroids

Author	No. of Patients	No. of Pregnancies	No. of Live Births	% Preterm Delivery	% C-section Delivery
Ravina et al[36]	9	12	7	43	57
McLucas et al[37]	14	17	10		
Carpenter & Walker[38]	24	29	16	25	88
Pron et al[39]	21	24	18	22	50
Kim et al[40]	7	8	7	14	29
Dutton et al[41]	27	37	19		79
Walker & McDowell[42]	33	56	33	18	73

tions to UFE by the Society of Interventional Radiology in their Quality Improvement Guidelines prepared in 2004.[44] However, despite the optimism generated by these case studies and limited reports, an interventional radiologist may not tell an infertile patient with fibroids that UFE can improve her chances to conceive and carry a pregnancy to term. The type of data that was presented earlier in support of myomectomy in this patient population is not yet available for patients undergoing UFE to treat symptomatic fibroids who have the hope of preserving or improving their chances for future childbearing. This is why myomectomy still remains the treatment of choice for patients with symptomatic uterine fibroids desiring both treatment and the possibility of fertility preservation.

To understand the issues surrounding UFE and future fertility more fully, it is important to review the work of Goldberg et al.[29] In 2002, Goldberg et al[29] reviewed 50 published cases of pregnancies after UFE. They found that several complications arose in these reported cases including cesarean delivery (58%), premature delivery (28%), malpresentation (17%), postpartum hemorrhage (13%); 7% of the infants born were small for gestational age. As a result, concerns were raised regarding the appropriateness of performing UFE in this patient population. In 2004, Goldberg et al[29] performed an additional literature-based comparison of pregnancies reported after UFE (n = 53) and after laparoscopic myomectomy (n = 139) and found a significantly higher rate of preterm delivery and malpresentation after UFE when compared with myomectomy. However, it is generally known that the rates of these complications are higher in all patients with uterine fibroids and therefore may not be a direct result of a UFE procedure. Still, the questions raised by Goldberg et al and others,[45] are largely responsible for the hesitation that presently exists when recommending UFE to patients desiring fertility preservation.

On the more positive side, it is important to review some of the larger case series mentioned earlier to gain additional insight into this issue. Pron et al[39] reported on the pregnancy data obtained during the Ontario Multicenter Study. This study evaluated 555 patients undergoing UFE to treat symptomatic uterine fibroids. In this population, they found that there had been 24 pregnancies in 21 patients during the follow-up period (23 of the pregnancies were spontaneous and 1 was attributed to in-vitro fertilization). Of these 24 pregnancies, there were 18 live births, 4 spontaneous abortions, and 2 elective terminations. Further analysis of the 18 live births revealed that the average time from UFE to conception was 15 months. Fourteen of the pregnancies were fullterm and four patients delivered prematurely. Six infants had low birth weight (four of whom were the infants delivered prematurely), whereas 12 had an appropriate weight for gestational age. Of the 18 live births, three were complicated by abnormal placentation: two patients had complete placenta previa, and one had placenta accrete. When evaluating this data, Pron et al[39] commented on how difficult it can be to determine why a complication with pregnancy occurs in a patient with fibroids who has undergone UFE because one can never know if the problem was due to the UFE procedure or other factors such as the presence of fibroids, patient age, etc. Pron and colleagues however, did feel that the rate of abnormal placentation was higher than that seen in the general population, despite the fact that the incidence of this complication is known to increase with patient age (which could have potentially explained the findings in this study). They felt that this complication could be explained by UFE because this procedure could potentially lead to reductions in endometrial perfusion and endometrial abnormalities that could contribute to abnormal placentation. Therefore, they suggested the use of hysteroscopy to confirm endometrial integrity after UFE if pregnancy is being considered.

Carpenter and Walker[38] reported on the pregnancy data obtained during review of 671 patients undergoing UFE to treat symptomatic fibroids. During the follow-up period, 29 pregnancies in 24 patients were identified. With the use of a questionnaire, 27 of these pregnancies were further evaluated and the incidence rates for several complications were recorded. Specifically, the following information was obtained: C-section (52%), preterm delivery (31%), miscarriage (27%), postpartum hemorrhage (20%), placenta previa (6.6%), placental abruption (6.6%), and intrauterine growth retardation (6.6%). When evaluating this data, Carpenter and Walker focused on the incidence of preterm delivery and miscarriages after UFE. The 31% preterm delivery rate they noted, which was similar to that reported by Goldberg et al[28] and Ravina et al[36] is higher than the 8 to 15% rate seen in the general population. However, they believed that the patients they identified in their study who had a preterm delivery had other potential explanations for this occurring, including the HELLP syndrome (hemolysis, elevated liver enzyme levels, and a low platelet count), preeclampsia, chorioamnionitis, placental abruption, and spontaneous rupture of membranes. Therefore, they were hesitant to attribute the 31% preterm delivery rate to UFE, a point echoed in a later study by Walker and McDowell.[42] Similarly, they believed that the 27% miscarriage rate was anticipated for this age group (age 15 to 35) and were unwilling to definitively attribute this finding to UFE as well. This too was mentioned in the later study by Walker and McDowell, when discussing their miscarriage rate of 30.4%.[42] Despite their interpretation of this data, these studies can lend support to the belief that UFE may adversely affect the ability of the uterus to support a pregnancy, which would potentially make a patient susceptible to potential complications including spontaneous abortions, abnormal placentation, uterine rupture, malpresentation, and preterm delivery. However, this clearly needs more study in an attempt to determine if the incidence of these complications increases as a result of UFE.

When evaluating the utility of UFE in patients desiring future fertility, one cannot forget about the established complications associated with UFE that can certainly occur in patients who either are or are not interested in having children. These have been described in Chapter 5, Uterine Fibroid Embolization. It is, however, particularly important to highlight the possibility of postprocedure amenorrhea and the premature onset of menopause with any patient that has a desire for fertility preservation who is considering undergoing UFE. Several studies have reported data concerning the incidence of amenorrhea and ovarian failure after UFE.[44,46–49] Given the findings in these studies, we know that amenorrhea due to ovarian failure and/or endometrial atrophy are possible after UFE and tend to be seen more often in patients older than age 45. The available data seems to suggest that younger patients experience no change in ovarian reserve, no change in ovarian volume, and no change in follicle count after UFE. However, it must also be stressed that although the risk is low, this complication can occur in younger patients and these patients must therefore be counseled appropriately due to the impact this complication would have on childbearing potential.

■ Counseling the Patient on Treatment for Uterine Fibroids

When any patient enters the office of an interventional radiologist to be evaluated for UFE, it is incumbent upon the interventional radiologist to perform a complete evaluation of the patient. The number, size, and position of the fibroids must be documented with imaging and their correlation with any number of possible presenting symptoms must be made to determine if performing UFE will help address that patient's chief complaint. Once this has been established, and once the presence or absence of absolute and relative contraindications to UFE has been confirmed, then attention should be paid to the patient's fertility status and her desire to have or not have children in the future. With this information, a complete picture of the patient can be obtained and appropriate patient-specific recommendations can be made.[1]

Patients with fibroids, who present because they have fibroids and are experiencing difficulties in either becoming pregnant or carrying a pregnancy to term, are asking about UFE as a potential treatment option. This is because these patients are often seeking to avoid myomectomy, a procedure perceived by these patients to be significantly more invasive than UFE, potentially placing them at an increased risk for an unplanned hysterectomy. If this patient is not experiencing any of the typical fibroid-related symptoms, then in our opinion, the recommendation is fairly straightforward. UFE should not be the first procedure offered to an asymptomatic patient with fibroids and infertility. As described, data exists in support of myomectomy, demonstrating improvements in conception, miscarriage, and delivery rates. This data does not yet exist to support the use of UFE in this setting. Because it cannot yet be said that UFE will improve a patient's chance of becoming pregnant and/or carrying a pregnancy to term, then exposing the patient to the potential risks of UFE and the potential issues surrounding pregnancies after UFE should not be supported on a first-line basis. The recommendation for these patients is that they should be counseled regarding the role of myomectomy and should be referred back to their gynecologist or to a gynecologist specializing in this procedure to have this discussion. This recommendation is supported by Mara et al[50] who performed a prospective, randomized study to compare fertility after UFE and myomectomy. In this study of 121 patients, myomectomy was found to have superior reproductive outcomes compared to UFE. UFE can, however, be considered as a potential option for a patient with fibroid-related subfertility who is not a candidate for myomectomy, but only after an imaging evaluation demonstrating the possible contribution of fibroids to the patient's infertility and after careful discussion with the patient.

Other patients will present to the office of an interventional radiologist with symptomatic fibroids and definite plans for future childbearing once they recover from a procedure to address their fibroid-related symptoms. In our opinion, these patients should be treated in a similar manner to the patient-type described above. Because these patients have expressed a strong desire for future childbearing and in fact have definite plans to that effect, the emphasis during the course of making a treatment decision must be placed on doing everything possible to preserve this patient's fertility. Although most interventional radiologists would be confident in the ability of UFE to address this patient's symptoms, for the reasons listed above we cannot be entirely confident that UFE will address this patient's symptoms while preserving fertility. Therefore, these patients should be encouraged to pursue more information about myomectomy and to consider myomectomy if they are not a candidate for UFE or do not wish to undergo that procedure.

Finally, there is the patient that presents with symptomatic fibroids and a desire to preserve fertility options. These patients do not yet have definite plans for future childbearing but simply want to "preserve the option." With these patients, counseling must be performed in such a way that enables these patients to determine the priority for seeking treatment for their symptomatic fibroids. The need for these patients to feel better must be balanced with their desire to have children in the future. If their priority is to address fibroid-related symptoms with future childbearing being an appealing idea but not something they are likely to pursue, then the level of confidence in offering them UFE as first-line therapy is increased. If, after counseling, these patients determine that symptomatic relief is a priority but only if done in such a way that optimizes their potential for fertility preservation, then additional discussions with a gynecologist regarding myomectomy would be the most appropriate next step. Once again, if the patient is not a candidate for myomectomy or does not wish to undergo that procedure, then UFE should be considered.

■ Conclusions

The most important thing that an interventional radiologist can do for a patient with fibroids and a desire for fertility preservation is to make sure that they are informed of the risks and benefits of all available treatment options. It is therefore important for us to acknowledge that we do not yet know enough about UFE and future fertility to make many definitive statements (other than "women have become pregnant after UFE"). We must be cautious in our recommendations regarding UFE, keeping in mind what has been reported in the literature and what the most important goal is for each individual patient. Ultimately, patients need to make decisions that will work best for them; a consultation that is designed to inform patients about their options in a nonbiased fashion will enable most patients to do just that.

References

1. Domenico L, Siskin GP. Uterine artery embolization and infertility. Tech Vasc Interv Radiol 2006;9:7–11
2. Fertility, Family Planning, and Reproductive Health of U.S. Women: Data from the 2002 National Survey of Family Growth. Center for Disease Control: National Center for Health Statistics. Series 23, No. 25: (PHS) 2006–1977. Available at: http://www.cdc.gov/nchs/products/pubs/pubd/series/sr23/pre-1/sr23_25.htm. Accessed July 24, 2006
3. Rackow BW, Arici A. Fibroids and in-vitro fertility: which comes first? Curr Opin Obstet Gynecol 2005;17:225–231
4. Pritts EA. Fibroids and infertility: a systematic review of the evidence. Obstet Gynecol Surv 2001;56:483–491
5. Deligdish L, Lowenthal M. Endometrial changes associated with myomata of the uterus. J Clin Pathol 1970;23:676–680
6. Forssman L. Venous changes in the endometrium of the myomatous uteri as measured by locally injected 133 xenon. Acta Obstet Gynecol Scand 1976;55:101–104
7. Jacobson FJ, Enzer N. Uterine myomas and endometrium. Obstet Gynecol 1956;7:206–210
8. Iosif CS, Akerlund M. Fibromyomas and uterine activity. Acta Obstet Gynecol Scand 1983;62:165–167
9. Oliveira FG, Abdelmassih VG, Diamond MP, Dozortsev D, Melo NR, Abdelmassih R. Impact of subserosal and intramural uterine fibroids that do not distort the endometrial cavity on the outcome of in-vitro fertility-intracytoplasmic sperm injection. Fertil Steril 2004;81:582–587
10. Yarali H, Bukulmez O. The effect of intramural and subserous uterine fibroids on implantation and clinical pregnancy rates in patients having intracytoplasmic sperm injection. Arch Gynecol Obstet 2002;266:30–33
11. Healy DL. Impact of uterine fibroids on ART outcome. Environ Health Perspect 2000;108(Suppl 5):845–847
12. Khalaf Y, Ross C, El-Toukhy T, Hart R, Seed P, Braude P. The effect of small intramural uterine fibroids on the cumulative outcome of assisted conception. Hum Reprod 2006;21:2640–2644
13. Hart R, Khalaf Y, Yeong CT, Seed P, Taylor A, Braude P. A prospective controlled study of the effect of intramural uterine fibroids on the outcome of assisted conception. Hum Reprod 2001;16:2411–2417
14. Eldar-Geva T, Meagher S, Healy DL, MacLachlan V, Breheny S, Wood C. Effect of intramural, subserosal, and submucosal uterine fibroids on the outcome of assisted reproductive technology treatment. Fertil Steril 1998;70:687–691
15. Bajekal N, Li TC. Fibroids, infertility, and pregnancy wastage. Hum Reprod Update 2000;6:614–620
16. Casini ML, Rossi F, Agostini R, Unfer V. Effects of the position of fibroids on fertility. Gynecol Endocrinol 2006;22:106–109
17. Roma Dalfo A, Ubeda B, Ubeda A, et al. Diagnostic value of hysterosalpingography in the detection of intrauterine abnormalities: a comparison with hysteroscopy. AJR Am J Roentgenol 2004;183:1405–1409
18. Soares SR, Barbosa dos Reis MM, Camargos AF. Diagnostic accuracy of sonohysterography, transvaginal sonography, and hysterosalpingography in patients with uterine cavity diseases. Fertil Steril 2000;73:406–411
19. Preutthipan S, Linasmita V. A prospective comparative study between hysterosalpingography and hysteroscopy in the detection of intrauterine pathology in patients with infertility. J Obstet Gynaecol Res 2003;29:33–37
20. Nalaboff KM, Pellerito JS, Ben-Levi E. Imaging the endometrium: disease and normal variants. Radiographics 2001;21:1409–1424
21. Imaoka I, Wada A, Matsuo M, et al. MR imaging of disorders associated with female infertility: use in diagnosis, treatment, and management. Radiographics 2003;23:1401–1421

22. Vercellini P, Maddalena S, De Giorgi O, et al. Abdominal myomectomy for infertility: a comprehensive review. Hum Reprod 1998;13:873–879
23. Campo S, Campo V, Gambadauro P. Reproductive outcome before and after laparoscopic or abdominal myomectomy for subserous or intramural myomas. Eur J Obstet Gynecol Reprod Biol 2003;110:215–219
24. Marchionni M, Fambrini M, Zambelli V, et al. Reproductive performance before and after abdominal myomectomy: a retrospective analysis. Fertil Steril 2004;82:154–159
25. Shokeir TA. Hysteroscopic management in submucous fibroids to improve fertility. Arch Gynecol Obstet 2005;273:50–54
26. Vashisht A, Smith JR, Thorpe-Beeston G, et al. Pregnancy subsequent to uterine artery embolization. Fertil Steril 2001;75:1246–1248
27. Kovacs P, Stangel JJ, Santoro NF, et al. Successful pregnancy after transient ovarian failure following treatment of symptomatic leiomyomata. Fertil Steril 2002;77:1292–1295
28. Goldberg J, Pereira L, Berghella V. Pregnancy after uterine artery embolization. Obstet Gynecol 2002;100(5 Pt 1):869–872
29. Goldberg J, Pereira L, Berghella V, et al. Pregnancy outcomes after treatment for fibromyomata: uterine artery embolization versus laparoscopic myomectomy. Am J Obstet Gynecol 2004;191:18–21
30. D'Angelo A, Amso NN, Wood A. Spontaneous multiple pregnancy after uterine artery embolization for uterine fibroid: case report. Eur J Obstet Gynecol Reprod Biol 2003;110:245–246
31. Kostal M, Tosner J, Natekova J, et al. Pregnancy after uterine artery embolization in uterine myoma. Ceska Gynekol 2004;69:48–50
32. Pietura R, Jakiel G, Swatowski D, et al. Pregnancy 4 months after uterine artery embolization. Cardiovasc Intervent Radiol 2005;28:117–119
33. Ng C, Lavery S, Hemingway A, et al. Successful spontaneous pregnancy following surgical removal of a post uterine artery embolized necrotic fibroid capsule: a case report. Hum Reprod 2006;21:380–383
34. Price N, Gillmer MD, Stock A, Hurley PA. Pregnancy following uterine artery embolization. J Obstet Gynaecol 2005;25:28–31
35. Trastour C, Bongain A, Rogopoulos A, Gillet JY. Pregnancy after embolization of uterine leiomyomata. Gynecol Obstet Fertil 2003;31:243–245
36. Ravina JH, Vigneron NC, Aymard A, et al. Pregnancy after embolization of uterine myoma: report of 12 cases. Fertil Steril 2000;73:1241–1243
37. McLucas B, Goodwin S, Adler L, et al. Pregnancy following uterine fibroid embolization. Int J Obsetet Gynecol 2001;74:1–7
38. Carpenter TT, Walker WJ. Pregnancy following uterine artery embolization for symptomatic fibroids: a series of 26 completed pregnancies. BJOG 2005;112:321–325
39. Pron G, Mocarski E, Bennett J, et al. Pregnancy after uterine artery embolization for leiomyomata: the Ontario multicenter trial. Obstet Gynecol 2005;105:67–76
40. Kim MD, Kim NK, Kim HJ, Lee MH. Pregnancy following uterine artery embolization with polyvinyl alcohol particles for patients with uterine fibroids or adenomyosis. Cardiovasc Intervent Radiol 2005;28:611–615
41. Dutton S, Hirst A, McPherson K, Nicholson T, Maresh MA. UK multicentre retrospective cohort study comparing hysterectomy and uterine artery embolisation for the treatment of symptomatic fibroids (HOPEFUL study): main results on medium-term safety and efficacy. BJOG 2007;114:1340–1351
42. Walker WJ, McDowell SJ. Pregnancy after uterine artery embolization for leiomyomata: a series of 56 completed pregnancies. Am J Obstet Gynecol 2006;195:1266–1271
43. American College of Obstetricians and Gynecologists (ACOG). Surgical alternatives to hysterectomy in the management of leiomyomas. ACOG Practice Bulletin No. 16. Washington, DC: American College of Obstetricians and Gynecologists; 2000:10
44. Hovsepian DM, Siskin GP, Bonn J, et al. Quality improvement guidelines for uterine artery embolization in symptomatic leiomyomata. J Vasc Interv Radiol 2004;15:535–542
45. El-Miligy M, Gordon A, Houston G. Focal myometrial defect and partial placenta accreta in a pregnancy following bilateral uterine artery embolization. J Vasc Interv Radiol 2007;18:789–791
46. Chrisman HB, Saker MB, Ryu RK, et al. The impact of uterine fibroid embolization on resumption of menses and ovarian function. J Vasc Interv Radiol 2000;11:699–703
47. Spies JB, Roth AR, Gonsalves SM, et al. Ovarian function after uterine artery embolization for leiomyomata: assessment with use of serum follicle stimulating hormone assay. J Vasc Interv Radiol 2001;12:437–442
48. Tropeano G, Di Stasi C, Litwicka K, et al. Uterine artery embolization for fibroids does not have adverse effects on ovarian reserve in regularly cycling women younger than 40 years. Fertil Steril 2004;81:1055–1061
49. Tropeano G, Litwicka K, Di Stasi C, et al. Permanent amenorrhea associated with endometrial atrophy after uterine artery embolization for symptomatic uterine fibroids. Fertil Steril 2003;79:132–135
50. Mara M, Maskova J, Fucikova Z, et al. Midterm clinical and first reproductive results of a randomized controlled trial comparing uterine fibroid embolization and myomectomy. Cardiovasc Interven Radiol 2008;31:73–85

8 Applications of Pelvic Embolization Beyond Uterine Fibroid Embolization

Jean-Claude Veille and Gary P. Siskin

■ Postpartum Hemorrhage

Postpartum hemorrhage (PPH) is the leading cause of maternal morbidity and mortality in the world.[1] It has been reported to cause at least 17% of maternal mortality in some parts of the world, but this number has been reported as high as over 50%.[2–5] In developing countries, PPH is also the most common reason for blood transfusion after delivery.[3] Even in developed countries, where maternal morbidity has declined significantly, fatal hemorrhage can still occur when blood or blood components are not readily available or if patients refuse blood products for religious reasons.[3,6] In the United States, it has been reported that obstetric hemorrhage is responsible for 13% of maternal death with PPH being the lethal event in more than one-third of these cases.[3,5]

PPH has been defined by the World Health Organization (WHO) as postpartum blood loss >500 cc.[7,8] Other definitions using higher volumes of blood before labeling an episode as a PPH have been established based on the fact that the average volume of blood loss at delivery can approach 500 cc.[9,10] Some have defined PPH as a 10% change in hematocrit; others define it as postpartum blood loss that requires the patient to have a transfusion.[11,12] Postpartum hemorrhage can be classified as either primary PPH, when blood loss occurs during the first 24 hours after delivery, or secondary PPH, when blood loss occurs from 24 hours to 6 weeks after delivery.[3]

Postpartum hemorrhage is an urgent situation that requires immediate attention. Unfortunately, by the time a significant hemorrhage is recognized the patient is often hemodynamically compromised. Because up to one-fifth of maternal cardiac output, which is >600 mL/minute, enters the uteroplacental circulation at term, it is understandable that primary PPH can be catastrophic, capable of exsanguinating a mother within minutes. Consequences of PPH include a consumptive coagulopathy with disseminated intravascular coagulation (DIC) and multiple organ failure due to circulatory collapse and decreased end-organ perfusion.

Primary postpartum hemorrhage occurs in 4 to 6% of pregnancies.[12] The most frequent causes are listed in **Fig. 8.1** and can be remembered by applying the "Four Ts": tone (uterine atony), trauma, tissue, and thrombophilia. The main causes of primary PPH are uterine atony, retained placenta or placental fragments, abnormal attachment of the placenta to the inner uterine wall (placenta accreta), and lower genital tract trauma.[8,13,14] Uterine atony is the most common cause of PPH and may be responsible for 80% or more of cases.[12] Primary PPH due to uterine atony occurs when the relaxed myometrium fails to constrict maternal spiral arteries in the placental bed, which allows for hemorrhage to occur.

Abnormal attachment of the placenta is the second most common cause of PPH.[15,16] Placenta previa can lead to hemorrhage following removal of the placenta due to the abnormal insertion of its lower edge. When there is invasion of the placenta into the myometrium, the placenta can be difficult to remove. The degree of the abnormal invasion will cause poor hemostasis at that particular site, rendering control of bleeding more difficult. Risk factors for placenta accreta include placenta previa with or without previous uterine surgery, prior myomectomy, prior cesarean delivery, Asherman syndrome, submucosal fibroids, and maternal age older than 35 years.[17] When these risk factors are present, one must have a high degree of clinical suspicion for placenta accreta because it is possible to take measures to reduce the likelihood of a significant PPH in these patients.

Patients are at increased risk for lower genital tract trauma when there is a difficult cesarean delivery or when there is an instrumented vaginal delivery of the fetus. Hereditary and acquired defects of hemostasis are uncom-

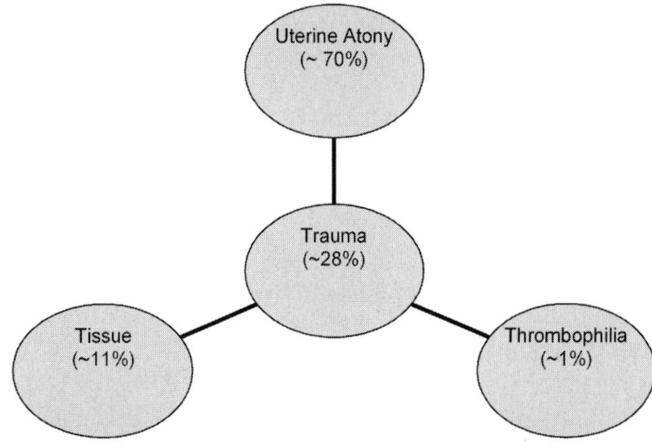

Fig. 8.1 The four Ts summarize the most common causes of postpartum hemorrhage.

Table 8.1 Potential Causes for Postpartum Hemorrhage

Uterine atony
Retained products of conception
Vaginal/cervical laceration
Placenta previa
Placenta accreta/increta/percreta
Placental abruption
Uterine fibroids

mon causes of PPH as are uterine inversion and uterine rupture.[18] Uterine rupture can occur spontaneously or at the site of a previous cesarean delivery or other surgical procedure involving the uterine wall. In addition, abnormal labor and placenta accreta can lead to rupture. Surgical repair is usually required when uterine rupture occurs.[8] Uterine inversion, in which the uterine corpus descends to and possibly through the cervix, is associated with PPH as well (**Table 8.1**).

Secondary hemorrhage occurs in ~1% of pregnancies.[8] Causes of secondary PPH include subinvolution of the placental site, retained products of conception, infection, and inherited coagulation defects.[8] Uterine atony, with or without infection, can also contribute to secondary hemorrhage, although bleeding is usually less than that seen with primary PPH. Postpartum hemorrhage may actually be the first indication for von Willebrand disease for many patients. Therefore, some have suggested testing for bleeding disorders in patients with a history of menorrhagia to prepare for this possibility.[19]

Whenever possible, some of the maternal conditions that potentially could lead to a postpartum hemorrhage should be identified. The most common predisposing conditions are listed in **Table 8.2**, including nulliparity, ma-

Table 8.2 Maternal Conditions That Increase the Risk for Postpartum Hemorrhage

Patients with a previous cesarean scar
Patients with a previous myomectomy scar
Patients at risk for uterine dehiscence/rupture
Leiomyomata uteri
Polyhydramnios
Multifetal pregnancies (twins or higher order)
Prolonged labor
Signs of chorioamnionitis
Grand multiparity
Large fetal weight
Diabetes
Retained placenta
Soft-tissue laceration
Episiotomy

ternal obesity, a large baby, prolonged third stage of labor, antepartum hemorrhage, previous postpartum hemorrhage and operative deliveries (especially emergent cesarean sections).[14] When these conditions are identified, preparation can take place, which is important for any hospital or medical center managing patients who are at increased risk for this complication. A team can be put in place (e.g., high-risk obstetrics-gynecology, obstetrical anesthesia, interventional radiology, urology, etc.) and there can be regular "drills" involving everybody potentially involved in the care of these patients to enable the team to deliver the best care if this type of event occurs. In our institution, we also have a "postpartum medicinal kit" (**Fig. 8.2**), which has a seal that can be easily broken at the bedside in the event of a hemorrhagic event. If PPH occurs,

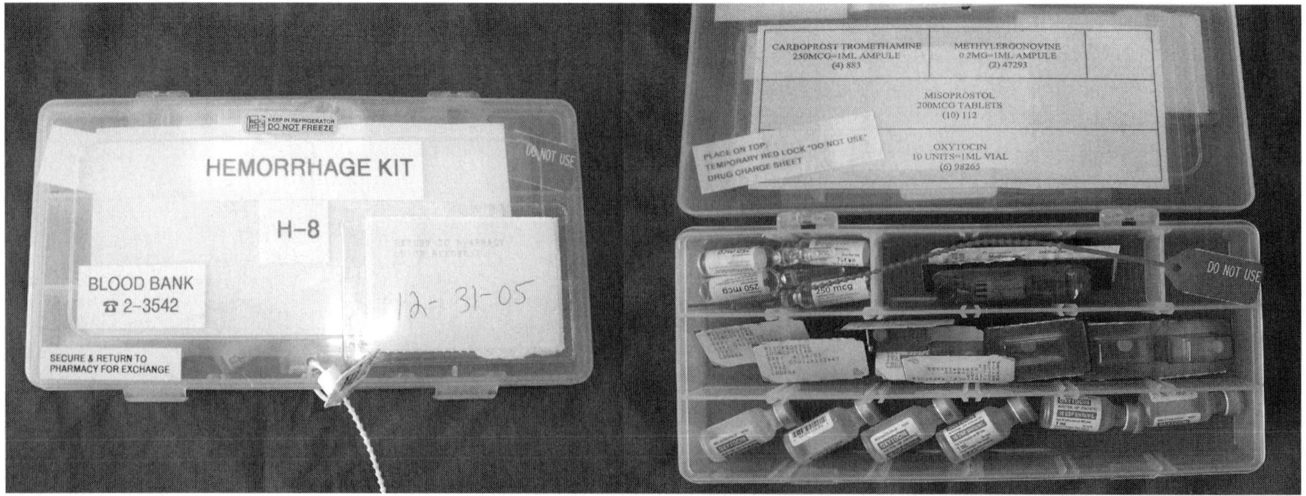

Fig. 8.2 The hemorrhagic kit available in the event of a postpartum hemorrhage.

Fig. 8.3 Contents of the hemorrhagic kit.

this kit, which contains all of the necessary medications to use in this scenario, is therefore immediately available to the care provider. In this way, a PPH is treated as any other "emergency code" in the hospital, which allows our pharmacy department to check these kits on a regular basis for accuracy and expiration. The contents of a typical PPH kit are shown in **Fig. 8.3**. All of these steps increase the probability that a potentially catastrophic event can be avoided.

Medical Treatment of Postpartum Hemorrhage

Given the possible morbidity and mortality associated with postpartum hemorrhage, an attempt to prevent this is being made with the growing use of active management during the third stage of labor.[20] Active management of the third stage of labor is felt to be the best preventive strategy for PPH, with its goal being to hasten and augment uterine contraction and retraction after delivery of the baby and placenta.[20–22] The main components of active management include administration of a prophylactic uterotonic agent (typically oxytocin) soon after the delivery of the baby, early clamping and cutting of the umbilical cord, early delivery of the placenta by controlled cord traction after the uterus has contracted, and uterine massage after delivery of the placenta.[21,23]

The International Federation of Gynecology and Obstetrics (FIGO) has recently removed early umbilical cord clamping from its guidelines for active management of the third stage of labor: delaying the clamping can increase iron stores and decrease the incidence of anemia in newborn infants.[24] The prophylactic administration of oxytocin has been shown to reduce the rate of postpartum hemorrhage by 40%; this risk reduction can also be seen if oxytocin is given after delivery of the placenta.[8,22,25] Several randomized and controlled trials have been performed comparing active with expectant management (allowing the placenta to deliver spontaneously) during the third stage of labor. These trials have found that active management is associated with reduced risks of maternal blood loss, reduced incidence of postpartum anemia, and a reduced requirement for blood transfusions.[14,26–28] This has prompted the recommendation that active management should be used routinely in women undergoing a vaginal delivery.[20]

In the setting of decreased uterine tone (based on physical examination and clinical suspicion), the administration of additional uterotonic medications is considered first-line treatment for PPH.[8] Uterotonics (including oxytocin, ergotamines, prostaglandins, and combinations of these medications) have been shown to effectively achieve hemostasis and allow most patients with PPH due to uterine atony to avoid surgery. Hence, the use of these medications has become widespread.[3] Interestingly, although a bolus and infusion of oxytocin is considered standard practice in the treatment of PPH, there is little research to support the use of this regimen.[29] Initially, 20 to 40 units of oxytocin is administered intravenously. Methergine (methylergonovine; Novartis Pharmaceuticals, Inc., Basel, Switzerland) is administered as well if the patient is not hypertensive. Injectable prostaglandins, such as prostaglandin 15-methyl prostaglandin F2-α (carboprost), can also be used, but are associated with significant gastrointestinal side effects. It is often reserved for use only when other measures fail.[20,30,31] Misoprostol (Cytotec; Pfizer, Inc., New York, NY) is a synthetic analogue of prostaglandin E1 that has been shown in many randomized, controlled trials to be an effective way to prevent PPH.[20,32–35] It is administered rectally or vaginally: the resulting uterine contractility is more potent when compared with the oral route.[3] However, recent reviews have shown that misoprostol is not as effective as conventional uterotonics; side effects such as shivering and fever make it less desirable to use.[36,37] However, its ease of use and storage relative to conventional medications and its low cost prevent misoprostol from being dismissed as a uterotonic agent.[20] Activated Factor VII

Table 8.3 Summary of Medical Treatment for Postpartum Hemorrhage

Oxytocin 40 units/L rapid IV infusion
Cytotec 400–1,000µg administered intrarectally
15-Methyl PGF2-α 0.25–1.5 mg IM or intramyometrial (up to 7 ampules)
Methylergonovine 0.2 mg IM

Abbreviations: IM, intramuscular; IV, intravenous; PGF2-α; prostaglandin F2-alpha.

has also been described as helpful for intractable PPH.[38,39] However, because it works on the extrinsic clotting pathway, it may be associated with an increased risk for future thromboembolic events.[40] Further studies evaluating the use of Factor VIIa for postpartum hemorrhage are needed to better assess its optimal dose, safety, and effectiveness.[41] A summary of the medical treatment for postpartum hemorrhage is given in **Table 8.3**.

When uterotonics fail to cause sustained uterine contractions and hemorrhage control, packing or tamponade of the uterine cavity can be considered an additional form of conservative management. First, an examination under anesthesia is generally recommended to rule out genital tract lacerations and retained placental fragments.[14] Uterine packing with gauze can address PPH, but should only be entertained once a genital tract laceration has been excluded. Packing has been shown to effectively address PPH due to uterine atony, placenta accreta, and placenta previa.[14,42] Uterine tamponade may serve to address PPH on an acute basis as well.[43] Success has been demonstrated with use of a Foley catheter, a Sengstaken–Blakemore tube, a Rusch urological catheter (which has a larger volume balloon than a Foley catheter), or an SOS Bakri Tamponade Balloon (Cook Medical Inc., Bloomington, IN).[13,43,44] The use of topical agents for hemostasis, such as FloSeal (Baxter, Deerfield, IL), has also been described in cases of PPH.[45]

Surgical Treatment of Postpartum Hemorrhage

When conservative management cannot control a postpartum hemorrhage, a surgical or interventional approach is usually the next line of treatment. The acuity of a patient's condition and the wishes of a patient to preserve her ability to have other children will help determine whether surgery or interventional treatment is selected. The surgical management of PPH has traditionally relied on hysterectomy and ligation of the internal iliac arteries.[13] Today, it is felt that hysterectomy should be reserved for when all other available measures have been exhausted, when persistent or recurrent bleeding following conservative surgical intervention occurs, and when a patient becomes coagulopathic and there is a lack of replacement blood products.[13,14]

If the uterus is not firm on examination and uterotonics have failed, then consideration can be given toward using the O'Leary technique for ligating the uterine arteries and veins.[46] This has shown success for controlling bleeding seen after cesarean sections and is quicker and easier to perform than ligation of the internal iliac arteries.[47] Success after ligation of the internal iliac arteries has been described in patients with placenta accreta.[48] A B-Lynch suture of the uterus may be attempted as well, especially if bimanual compression of the uterus works to decrease the bleeding.[13] This technique involves a pair of vertical brace sutures around the uterus to appose the anterior and posterior walls.[13,49] It works by direct application of pressure on the placental bed bleeding and by reducing blood flow to the uterus.[8,13] Cho et al[50] have also described the use of multiple square suturing to treat an uncontrolled PPH. The technique entails square suturing of the entire uterine wall, including the uterine cavity, around the bleeding area. If the bleeding persists, another square is inserted until the bleeding stops.[14] If the uterus is firm on examination, then ligation of the internal iliac or uterine arteries can be considered.[13]

The presence of a vulvovaginal hematoma, resulting from a significant bleed, can cause patients to be hemodynamically unstable and go into hemorrhagic shock. After placing these patients on prophylactic, broad-spectrum antibiotics, some hematomas can be treated conservatively (if they are small and not expanding); others will have to be treated more aggressively. For large and rapidly expanding hematomas, consideration can be given to incision and drainage. However, this may result in more bleeding from an injured vessel because the "tamponade" created by the large and tense hematoma, has now been "lifted." On the other hand, once the hematoma has been opened and the clots removed, a bleeding vessel can be potentially identified and ligated. If bleeding is seen, and the vessel cannot be identified, then the patient may require emergent hysterectomy or embolization.

If the above techniques fail to control the bleeding, then a hysterectomy is indicated. Hysterectomy for intractable PPH occurs in 0.5 to 0.8 per 1000 deliveries.[5,51] Today, this should be considered the option of last resort in the management of PPH secondary to uterine causes.[13] Although a total abdominal hysterectomy can be considered, a supracervical or subtotal hysterectomy is often preferred because it is quicker, simpler, safer, and associated with less blood loss than a total hysterectomy.[13,52] Bleeding after hysterectomy will likely require the use of interventional therapy.[53]

Interventional Treatment of Postpartum Hemorrhage

Since Brown et al[54] reported the use of embolization as a treatment option for patients with postpartum hemorrhage in 1979, there have been several reports confirming that this procedure can be an effective way to address the bleeding seen in these patients. Given the anecdotal and literature-based experience that exists surrounding the use of embolization in this setting, it is certainly fair to say that embolization has a role in treating patients with PPH. The questions that come up revolve around the most appropriate timing and indications for the use of embolization in this patient population and with the safety of transferring a patient from labor and delivery to an interventional radiology suite.[11] Although some believe that embolization should only be applied in the care of patients failing both medical and surgical management, others believe that obstetrician-gynecologists should turn to embolization once patients fail medical or conservative management.[54] This can be done in lieu of surgery or before surgery is performed.[55] Still others believe that catheter-based therapy has a role in offering prophylaxis to patients at high risk for postpartum hemorrhage, which can enable the rapid performance of an embolization procedure if needed.

Technically, an angiogram and embolization performed in a patient with postpartum hemorrhage is not significantly different from pelvic embolization procedures performed for other indications. Unilateral femoral access is typically achieved and the internal iliac arteries and subsequently the uterine arteries are selectively catheterized. With the performance of a diagnostic angiogram, it is possible to identify extravasation, pseudoaneurysm formation, or other findings compatible with traumatic injury to the uterine vasculature. Embolization of both uterine arteries is then performed, most commonly with Gelfoam (Pfizer, Inc., New York, NY), until stasis of flow in the target artery is achieved.

The use of coils or polyvinyl (PVA) particles as the embolic agent for this procedure has been reported. Microcoils can be used when there is visible, active bleeding.[56] The use of PVA particles has been associated with uterine necrosis after embolization.[57] Selective internal iliac angiography and nonselective abdominal aortography are both recommended at some point during these procedures because it is possible that the source of bleeding can be from a vessel other than the uterine artery, including the vaginal, ovarian, and/or inferior epigastric arteries.[53,58–60] Once both uterine arteries are embolized, the catheter and sheath are removed and the patient is followed to determine their response to the procedure.

Several articles have been published supporting the use of embolization in this setting. Ojala et al[61] found that emergent embolization successfully addressed postpartum bleeding in 75% of patients. In addition, it addressed bleeding in all patients who had persistent bleeding after hysterectomy. In this study, complications associated with emergency embolization included thrombosis of the popliteal artery, vaginal necrosis, and paresthesia of the right leg. Pelage et al reviewed their experience with embolization performed for both primary (n = 27) and secondary (n = 14) PPH.[62,63] Bleeding in the secondary PPH group was caused by retained portions of placenta, endometritis, and genital tract tears. Only two patients in the group with primary PPH ultimately required a hysterectomy; no patients with secondary PPH required a hysterectomy after embolization. No complications associated with embolization were reported in either group. Cheng et al[64] reported their success with this technique, but also mentioned that repeat embolization was of value in one patient with retained fragments of placenta after delivery.

Several other studies have reported on the success of emergent embolization to treat PPH due to uterine atony, abnormal placentation, and genital tract injuries.[65–68] Ornan et al[69] reported perforation of an internal iliac artery during the embolization procedure, resulting in a retroperitoneal hematoma. They also reported transient buttock numbness in two of their patients. In no patients were the side effects severe enough to seek further medical attention. Boulleret et al[70] reported complications after embolization including a false aneurysm at the femoral puncture site (treated by ultrasound-guided compression), two cases of lower extremity paraesthesia, one femoral vein deep vein thrombosis (DVT), and nonsignificant puncture site hematomas. Uterine necrosis has also been reported with embolization performed in this setting.[57]

Because patients in this situation are obviously in their childbearing years, one question that arises frequently is whether embolization can preserve a patient's future fertility. Although there is no definite answer to this question, it is known that most patients have resumed normal menstruation and that successful, uneventful pregnancies have occurred.[54,55,61–63,71,72] Importantly, Ornan et al[69] stated that all patients wishing to get pregnant after embolization were able to do so. In all of the reported pregnancies after embolization for PPH, Gelfoam was the embolic agent used; hence, Gelfoam is considered the preferred agent to use for embolization in this clinical setting.

Interventional radiology may be used prophylactically in patients at risk for postpartum hemorrhage (particularly in patients with abnormal placentation). To maximize the degree of preparedness to perform an embolization procedure if needed, place angiographic catheters in the abdominal aorta or internal iliac arteries, or balloon catheters in the internal iliac arteries (**Fig. 8.4**). This way the arterial system has been accessed and catheters are virtually ready so that with only a slight amount of additional catheter manipulation under fluoroscopic guidance, an embolization procedure can be performed emergently. The use of both standard occlusion balloons and angioplasty balloons has been described. If balloons are in place, then they can be inflated after delivery to limit blood flow to the uterus, which can potentially reduce the incidence of significant bleeding.

Several studies have supported the use of prophylactic arterial catheterization in patients felt to be at high risk for postpartum hemorrhage. Alvarez et al compared two small groups of patients who underwent embolization due to PPH.[73] One group (n = 4) underwent emergent embolization after PPH was recognized and the other group (n = 5) had catheters placed in the internal iliac arteries prior to elective cesarean section followed by embolization as needed. Three of the patients in the second group ultimately required embolization. When the groups were compared, the group undergoing emergent embolization all had a coagulopathy at the time of embolization, had a greater degree of blood loss, and had an increased rate of postpartum complications. Alvarez et al and others have concluded that in patients felt to be at risk for PPH, prophylactic catheter placement is a safe and effective way to reduce blood loss, transfusion requirements, and maternal morbidity.[61,67,74–76]

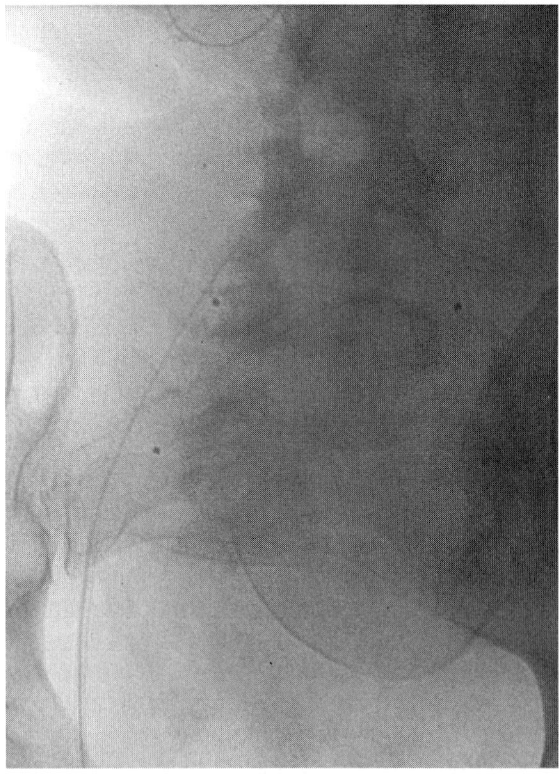

Fig. 8.4 Angiographic balloon catheters in place within the internal iliac arteries prior to cesarean delivery of a pregnancy felt to be at high risk for postpartum hemorrhage.

These studies support the idea that prophylactic placement of internal iliac artery catheters can assist with rapid performance of an embolization to address bleeding on its own or can provide the time needed to safely perform a cesarean hysterectomy in these patients. However, sporadic reports have questioned the value of the placement of such balloons in decreasing the intraoperative blood loss.[77] In a large series of patients (n = 28), Bodner et al[78] found no differences in intraoperative blood loss, transfusion and fluid replacement requirements, operating room time, or postoperative recovery time when prophylactic catheter placement is performed in this patient population.

Clearly, there is disparity in published results when it comes to the value of placing catheters prophylactically in the internal iliac arteries prior to a high-risk delivery. In part, this disparity can be explained by the following: (1) unforeseen movement of the catheter during the delivery, (2) use of the wrong size balloon catheter, and (3) a failure to account for significant collateral circulation. Significant collateral vessels are present during a normal pregnancy, but the vasculature becomes even more hypertrophied when there is an abnormal invasion of the trophoblast into the myometrium. Shih et al[79] has attempted to account for this by placing balloon catheters in the common iliac arteries as opposed to the internal iliac arteries, and then proceeding to a cesarean hysterectomy, but this can place the lower extremities at risk for ischemia.

■ Cervical Ectopic Pregnancies

Cervical ectopic pregnancy is a very rare form of ectopic pregnancy with an incidence that has been reported anywhere from 1 to 1000 to 1 to 95,000.[80,81] This occurs when the pregnancy implants into the cervical mucosa, below the level of the internal os. The etiology of cervical ectopic pregnancy remains unknown. One theory attributes this to damage to the cervix and endometrium during operative uterine procedures.[82] Risk factors include previous surgical termination of pregnancy, Asherman syndrome, and assisted reproductive techniques including intrauterine and intrafallopian tube embryo transfers.[82–85]

This extremely rare event can be disastrous due to the excessive bleeding that occurs prior or during evacuation of the abnormal pregnancy. In light of this risk of bleeding, and in light of the fact that cervical pregnancies are being diagnosed at an early gestational age with ultrasound and MRI (**Fig. 8.5**), therapies that are more conservative have been used in these patients. Conservative therapy has been successful at avoiding hysterectomy in 95.6% of patients.[86]

The hallmark of conservative management of cervical ectopic pregnancies is the administration of systemic or intraamniotic methotrexate, especially in a clinically stable patient in her first trimester.[86,87] This was first described in 1983.[88] Methotrexate is a folic acid antagonist

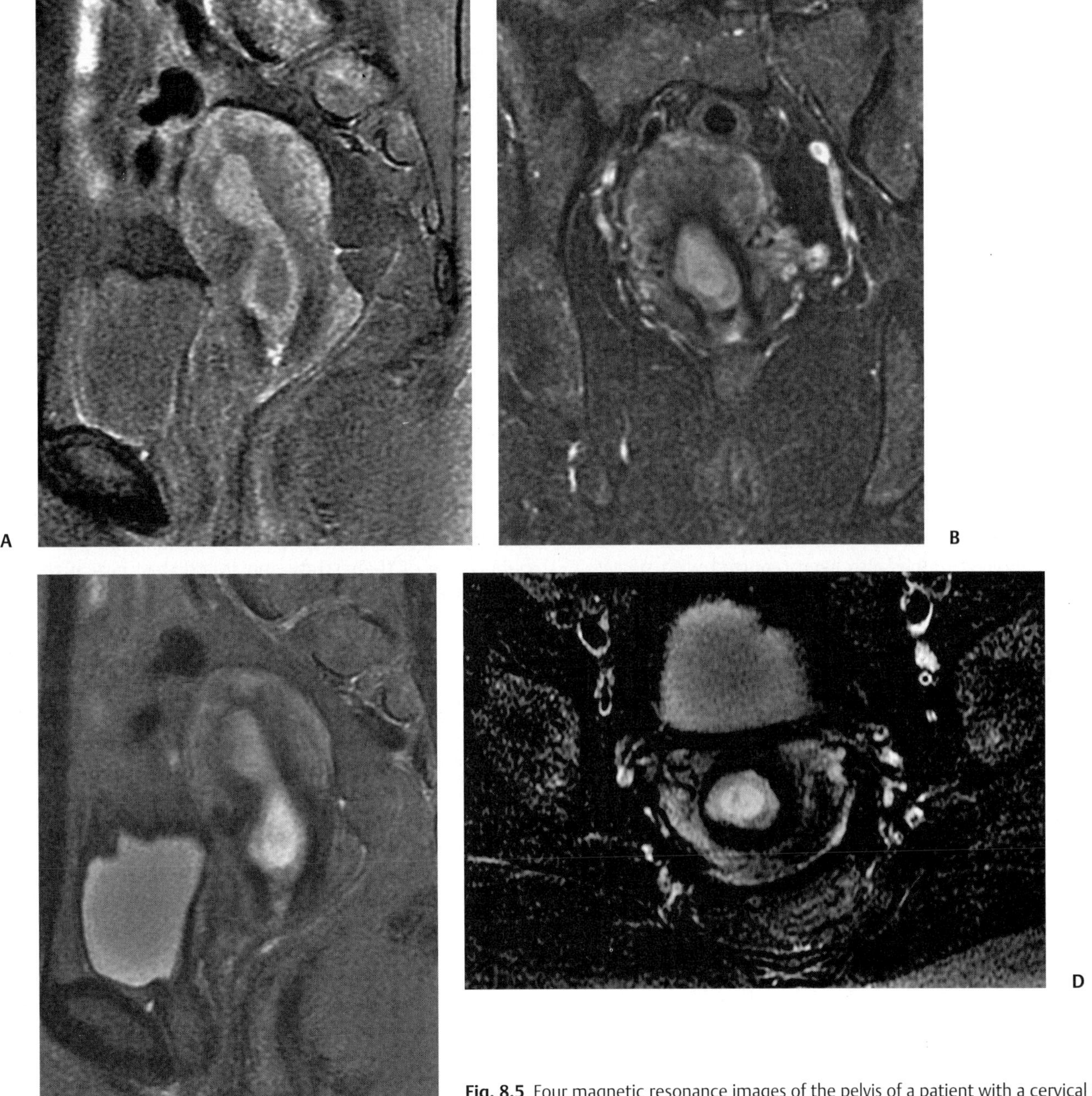

Fig. 8.5 Four magnetic resonance images of the pelvis of a patient with a cervical ectopic pregnancy.

that is highly toxic to rapidly dividing tissue.[89] The contraindications to methotrexate therapy are listed in **Table 8.4**. An intraamniotic injection of methotrexate is felt to be more effective than systemic administration in stopping cardiac activity within the embryo and decreasing the risk for treatment failure.[90–93] The success rate of methotrexate therapy has been reported at 55 to 83%.[86,92,94] Failure of methotrexate therapy is more likely to occur when there is fetal cardiac activity, when the serum human chorionic gonadotropin (HCG) level is >10,000 IU/L, when the gestational age is older than 9 weeks, and when the crown-rump length is longer than 10 mm.[86,92]

Despite the success of methotrexate therapy, 21% of women will need an additional procedure to control bleeding.[85,90] Uterine artery embolization (UAE) is one of those procedures that has been used with success in combination with methotrexate therapy. Its use in practice is either as a planned adjunct to methotrexate therapy[95] or as an unplanned addition when there is significant bleeding after medical therapy. Kung et al[96] reported that the need for (or another procedure such as simple curettage, dilation and curettage, or cervical blocking) in conjunction with methotrexate was significantly higher when there is fetal cardiac activity. Mesogitis et al described the use of cervical evacuation curettage after methotrexate due to the inability to predict the occurrence of massive bleeding and need to eradicate the aberrant trophoblastic tissue.[90,96] Several others have reported on the success of embolization after failed methotrexate therapy (continued bleeding).[97–99] The use of embolization has also been reported with success before the administration of methotrexate.[100]

UAE has also been used as a stand-alone treatment for cervical ectopic pregnancies, most commonly in patients presenting with significant bleeding. Trambert et al[101] reported the success of embolization to address both emergent and nonemergent bleeding associated with cervical ectopic pregnancies. In this series, β-HCG levels persisted in three of the nonemergent cases. All three patients had additional episodes of bleeding, two of which were treated with methotrexate and the third was treated with repeat embolization. Normal menses returned in the seven patients available for follow-up and there were two subsequent pregnancies. This prompted the recommendation that embolization should be used in all patients with cervical ectopic pregnancies presenting with bleeding.

Takano et al[102] presented a cervical ectopic pregnancy case treated by UAE without methotrexate. Following embolization, the β-HCG levels decreased and the cervical mass disappeared within 31 days. Several others have also reported the successful use of embolization without methotrexate or surgery.[103,104] In these cases and in cases when embolization was used after methotrexate or before surgery, normal menstruation is generally the rule and successful pregnancies have been reported.[90,97,101] However, a case of premature amenorrhea has been reported in association with this procedure.[105]

It should always be kept in mind that there is a risk of rebleeding when UAE is used to treat a cervical ectopic pregnancy.[106] This is due to the fact that once the uterine arteries have been embolized, collateral vessels to the cervix are established which can potentially perfuse the gestation. This at the very least makes it possible for rebleeding to occur, which is why some have advocated that surgical removal of the aberrant pregnancy should be performed after embolization to decrease or prevent hemorrhage and to prevent the need for a hysterectomy.[107,108] Ushakov et al[109] reviewed the published cases prior to publication of their study and found that 71% of the 41 published cases that had surgical treatment without selective embolization resulted in massive hemorrhage, with several patients requiring either hysterectomy or internal iliac or uterine artery ligation. When surgery is planned, it has been suggested that it be performed within 24 hours of embolization to control heavy bleeding and avoid recurrent bleeding associated with a cervical ectopic pregnancy, especially when future fertility is desired.[106] Even in these cases, rebleeding can occur because the gestational tissue may implant deeply in the cervix, which makes it difficult to be removed completely by curettage.[106] Should this occur, a repeat embolization can be considered.

Table 8.4 Contraindications to Methotrexate Therapy for Cervical Ectopic Pregnancy

Intrauterine pregnancy
Evidence of immunodeficiency
Moderate to severe anemia, leucopenia, or thrombocytopenia
Active pulmonary disease
Active peptic ulcer disease
Clinically significant hepatic or renal dysfunction
Breast feeding
Known sensitivity to methotrexate

Source: From the Practice Committee for the American Society for Reproductive Medicine. Medical treatment of ectopic pregnancy. Fertil Steril 2006; 86(Suppl 4): S96–S102.

■ Uterine Arteriovenous Malformations

Uterine arteriovenous malformations (AVM) are very rare events. Since Dubreuil reported the first case in 1926, there have been ~100 cases reported in the literature.[110] Histologically, uterine AVMs consist of arteries and veins without intervening capillaries.[111] In a manner similar to vascular malformations in other parts of the body, uterine

AVMs can be classified as high-flow or low-flow malformations. Low-flow uterine AVMs are probably due to subinvolution of a placenta after pregnancy.[112] They can also be classified as congenital or acquired, with acquired lesions being more common. Congenital lesions are typically due to abnormal angiogenesis, with anomalous differentiation or developmental arrest in the primitive capillary plexus.[113] They are often high-flow AVMs and tend to extend beyond the uterus into the pelvis.[114] Acquired lesions can be attributed to instrumentation (cesarean section, dilatation and curettage, other uterine surgery) or to conditions such as infection, retained products of conception, fibroids, endometriosis, diethylstilbestrol exposure, gestational trophoblastic disease, choriocarcinoma, and other gynecologic malignancies.[113,115] Gestational trophoblastic disease may be the most common cause of an acquired AVM.[116] Acquired AVMs of the uterus are typically single, large connections between the artery and vein; congenital AVMs consist of multiple small vascular connections that may invade surrounding structures.[117]

Most uterine AVMs are found in women between 20 to 40 years of age. Hormonal changes, such as those seen with pregnancy and menstruation, may play a role in the pathogenesis of an AVM and may also trigger the associated bleeding.[118] Clinically, these patients may present acutely with abnormal, possibly very heavy bleeding, which may require a transfusion in one-third of cases. This can present as a postpartum hemorrhage as well. Uterine AVMs have also been associated with recurrent pregnancy loss.[119] Unless the diagnosis of an AVM is suspected, the diagnosis is often missed. As a result, these patients are either instrumented or taken to the operating room for more invasive diagnostic testing such as a dilation and curettage or an operative hysteroscopy. This may be catastrophic because patients may bleed excessively, resulting in hypotension and anemia.[120]

If the diagnosis of an AVM is suspected then all efforts should be made to obtain noninvasive imaging such as Doppler ultrasound or MRI with contrast. Color Doppler images reveal hypoechoic areas in the myometrium that exhibit vascular flow.[121] Other findings include low pulsatility and irregular spectral broadening of the waveform, low-resistance index measurements, and mixing of arterial and venous waveforms.[113,122] On MRI, one can see a focal mass, disruption of the junctional zone, multiple serpiginous flow-related signal voids within the lesion, and prominent parametrial vessels.[113,115,121] MRI and CT can both be helpful in determining if there is suspected involvement of the bladder and rectum.[113]

Once the diagnosis is confirmed, hysterectomy can be considered for definitive treatment. Surgical removal of the AVM can also be performed, and has been reported as a surgical option with uterine preservation.[113] However, selective UAE is a procedure that can effectively address the arterial inflow and nidus of an arterial malformation potentially providing definitive therapy. This was first reported by Forssman et al in 1982.[123] Since that time, it has been used successfully in emergent and less-urgent circumstances and is now often the first option to consider when treating a patient with a symptomatic AVM who wishes to preserve her future fertility options.

In published reports, 96% of patients who underwent UAE had significant improvement in terms of symptom control.[112,114,116,122,124,125] Different embolic agents have been used with success including PVA particles, tris-acryl gelatin microspheres, microcoils, Gelfoam, and glue (*N*-butyl cyanoacrylate). Based on the experience of Ghai et al, the use of glue is preferable whenever a catheter position can be achieved that allows for safe deposition into the nidus and feeding vessels of the AVM.[114] One always has to remember when treating AVMs that recurrence may occur due to recruitment of new vasculature.[115] Care must always be taken to try and identify feeding vessels other than the uterine arteries to be certain that the malformation is addressed in its entirety. Although often effective, there have been reports of symptom recurrence in patients treated with embolization for a uterine AVM.[126,127]

Pregnancies have been reported after particulate or liquid UAE performed for an AVM in multiple studies.[119,128–130] Normal vaginal deliveries have taken place after embolization procedures for AVMs, which provides confidence in making this recommendation to patients.[112] Potential complications related to pregnancy after embolization of an AVM include postpartum hemorrhage secondary to uterine atony, intrauterine growth retardation, malpresentation, and uterine rupture.[112]

■ Gynecologic Malignancies

Most, if not all gynecological malignancies are usually managed surgically. At times, however, medical comorbidities may make a patient a poor surgical candidate. Additionally, there can be advanced disease that may also make a patient a poor candidate for surgery. In these cases, conservative management may be used. Vaginal packing, radiation, or chemotherapy can all be used as temporizing measures for these patients. However, the bleeding associated with these tumors may necessitate other treatment given the acute compromise that can result in the patient's clinical condition.

In these cases, embolization procedures can and should be considered as a procedure that can safely and effectively address the bleeding associated with these advanced gynecologic malignancies.[131] Embolization of the uterine arteries and of the internal iliac arteries has been reported in this setting. Several studies are now available describing the success seen after embolization is performed to treat the bleeding associated with cervical cancer,[132–136] endometrial cancer,[134,136] choriocarcinoma,[134] gestational trophoblastic disease,[135,137,138] and vulvovaginal metastatic disease.[134–136] During these cases, Gelfoam, coils, and PVA particles have all been used as the embolic agent.[132,136,139,140] Most embolization cases performed for this indication are associated with a postembolization syndrome consisting of nausea, vomiting, and fever due to tissue necrosis.[141]

■ Conclusions

Uterine artery embolization has been a valuable addition to the treatment options available to patients with a wide variety of obstetric and gynecologic indications. The ability to treat patients with this minimally invasive procedure has enabled many women who at one time required hysterectomy to be treated with a uterine sparing option. With improvements in technique and in the catheters and embolic agents being used for these procedures, it is not difficult to imagine the indications for this procedure increasing in the future.

References

1. Ronsmans C, Graham WJ; Lancet Maternal Survival Series Steering Group. Maternal mortality: who, when, where, and why. Lancet 2006;368:1189–1200
2. McCormick ML, Sanghvi HC, Kinzie B, McIntosh N. Preventing postpartum hemorrhage in low-resource settings. Int J Gynaecol Obstet 2002;77:267–275
3. El-Refaey H, Rodeck C. Post-partum hemorrhage: definitions, medical and surgical management. A time for change. Br Med Bull 2003; 67:205–217
4. World Health Organization. Maternal Mortality A Global Factbook. Geneva: WHO; 1991: 3–16
5. Glaze S, Ekwalanga P, Roberts G, et al. Peripartum hysterectomy 1999–2006. Obstet Gynecol 2008;111:732–738
6. Singla AK, Lapinski RH, Berkowitz RL, Saphier CJ. Are women who are Jehovah's Witnesses at risk of maternal death? Am J Obstet Gynecol 2001;185:893–895
7. World Health Organization (WHO). The Prevention and Management of Postpartum Haemorrhage. Report of a Technical Working Group. World Health Organization/Maternal and Child Health 90.7. Geneva: WHO; 1990
8. American College of Obstetricians and Gynecologists. ACOG Practice Bulletin: Clinical Management Guidelines for Obstetrician-Gynecologists. Postpartum Hemorrhage. Obstet Gynecol 2006;108:1039–1047
9. Combs CA, Murphy EL, Laros RK Jr. Factors associated with postpartum hemorrhage with vaginal birth. Obstet Gynecol 1991;77:69–76
10. Clark SL, Yeh SY, Phelan JP, Bruce S, Paul RH. Emergency hysterectomy for obstetric hemorrhage. Obstet Gynecol 1984;64:376–380
11. Sundaram R, Brown AG, Koteeswaran SK, Urquhart G. Anaesthetic implications of uterine artery embolisation in management of massive obstetric hemorrhage. Anaesthesia 2006;61:248–252
12. Combs CA, Murphy EL, Laros RK. Factors associated with postpartum haemorrhage with vaginal birth. Obstet Gynecol 1991;77:69–76
13. Tamizian O, Arulkumaran S. The surgical management of postpartum haemorrhage. Curr Opin Obstet Gynecol 2001;13:127–131
14. Mousa HA, Walkinshaw S. Major postpartum haemorrhage. Curr Opin Obstet Gynecol 2001;13:595–603
15. Stanco LM, Schrimmer DB, Paul RH, Mishell DR Jr. Emergency peripartum hysterectomy and associated risk factors. Am J Obstet Gynecol 1993;168:879–883
16. Bakshi S, Meyer BA. Indications for and outcomes of emergency peripartum hysterectomy: a five-year review. J Reprod Med 2000;45:733–737
17. Clark SL, Koonings PP, Phelan JP. Placenta previa/accrete and prior cesarean section. Obstet Gynecol 1985;66:89–92
18. Baudo F, Caimi TM, Mostarda G, De Cataldo F, Morra E. Critical bleeding in pregnancy: a novel therapeutic approach to bleeding. Minerva Anestesiol 2006;72:389–393
19. James AH. Von Willebrand disease. Obstet Gynecol Surv 2006;61:136–145
20. Chong YS, Su LL, Arulkumaran S. Current strategies for the prevention of postpartum haemorrhage in the third stage of labour. Curr Opin Obstet Gynecol 2004;16:143–150
21. Anderson JM, Etches D. Prevention and management of postpartum hemorrhage. Am Fam Physician 2007;75:875–882
22. Jackson KW Jr, Allbert JR, Schemmer GK, Elliot M, Humphrey A, Taylor J. A randomized controlled trial comparing oxytocin administration before and after placental delivery in the prevention of postpartum hemorrhage. Am J Obstet Gynecol 2001;185:873–877
23. Lalonde A, Daviss BA, Acosta A, Herschderfer K. Postpartum hemorrhage today ICM/FIGO initiative 2004–2006. Int J Gynaecol Obstet 2006;94:243–253
24. Ceriani Cernadas JM, Carroli G, Pellegrini L, et al. The effect of timing of cord clamping on neonatal venous hematocrit values and clinical outcome at term: a randomized, controlled trial. Pediatrics 2006;117: e779–e786
25. Nordstrom L, Fogelstam K, Fridman G, Larsson A, Rydhstroem H. Routine oxytocin in the third stage of labour: a placebo controlled randomized trial. Br J Obstet Gynaecol 1997;104:781–786
26. Prendiville WJ, Harding JE, Elbourne DR, Stirrat GM. The Bristol third stage trial: active vs physiological management of the third stage of labour. BMJ 1988;297:1295–1300
27. Rogers J, Wood J, McCandlish R, et al. Active vs expectant management of the third stage of labour: the Hinchingbrooke randomised controlled trial. Lancet 1998;351:693–699
28. Prendiville WJ, Elbourne D, McDonald S. Active versus expectant management in the third stage of labour. Cochrane Database Syst Rev 2000;3:CD000007
29. Daro AF, Gollin HA, Lavieri V. Management of postpartum hemorrhage by prolonged administration of oxytocics. Am J Obstet Gynecol 1952;64:1163–1164
30. Chua S, Chew SL, Yeoh CL, et al. A randomized controlled study of prostaglandin 15-methyl F2 alpha compared with syntometrine for prophylactic use in the third stage of labour. Aust N Z J Obstet Gynaecol 1995;35:413–416
31. Gulmezoglu AM. Prostaglandins for prevention of postpartum haemorrhage. Cochrane Database Syst Rev 2000; (2):CD000494
32. Goldberg AB, Greenberg MB, Darney PD. Misoprostol and pregnancy. N Engl J Med 2001;344:38–47
33. Bamigboye AA, Merrell DA, Hofmeyr GJ, Mitchell R. Randomized comparison of rectal misoprostol with syntometrine for management of third stage of labor. Acta Obstet Gynecol Scand 1998;77:178–181
34. El Refaey H, Nooh R, O'Brien P, et al. The misoprostol third stage of labour study: a randomised controlled comparison between orally administered misoprostol and standard management. BJOG 2000;107:1104–1110
35. Surbek DV, Fehr PM, Hosli I, Holzgreve W. Oral misoprostol for third stage of labor: a randomized placebo-controlled trial. Obstet Gynecol 1999;94:255–258
36. Villar J, Gulmezoglu AM, Hofmeyr GJ, Forna F. Systematic review of randomized controlled trials of misoprostol to prevent postpartum hemorrhage. Obstet Gynecol 2002;100:1301–1312
37. Chong YS, Chua S, Arulkumaran S. Severe hyperthermia following oral misoprostol in the immediate postpartum period. Obstet Gynecol 1997;90:703–704

38. Bouwmeester FW, Jonkhoff AR, Verheijen RH, van Geijn HP. Successful treatment of life-threatening postpartum hemorrhage with recombinant activated factor VII. Obstet Gynecol 2003;101:1174–1177
39. Boehlen F, Morales MA, Fontaana P, Ricou B, Irion O, de Moerloose P. Prolonged treatment of massive postpartum haemorrhage with recombinant factor VIIa: case report and review of the literature. BJOG 2004;111:284–287
40. O'Connell KA, Wood JJ, Wise RP, Lozier JN, Braun MM. Thromboembolic adverse events after use of recombinant human coagulation factor VIIa. JAMA 2006;295:293–298
41. Franchini M, Franchi M, Bergamini V, Salvagno GL, Montagnana M, Lippi G. A critical review on the use of recombinant factor VIIa in life-threatening obstetric postpartum hemorrhage. Semin Thromb Hemost 2008;34:104–112
42. Maier RC. Control of postpartum hemorrhage with uterine packing. Am J Obstet Gynecol 1993;169:317–321
43. Johanson R, Kumar M, Obhrai M, Young P. Management of massive postpartum haemorrhage: use of a hydrostatic balloon catheter to avoid laparotomy. BJOG 2001;108:420–422
44. Bakri YN, Amri A, Abdul Jabbar F. Tamponade-balloon for obstetrical bleeding. Int J Gynaecol Obstet 2001;74:139–142
45. Moriarty KT, Premila S, Bulmer PJ. Use of FloSeal haemostatic gel in massive obstetric hemorrhage: a case report. BJOG 2008;115:793–795
46. O'Leary JA. Uterine artery ligation in the control of postcesarean hemorrhage. J Reprod Med 1995;40:189–193
47. O'Leary JL, O'Leary JA. Uterine artery ligation for control of postcesarean section hemorrhage. Obstet Gynecol 1974;43:849–853
48. Nizard J, Barrinque L, Frydman R, et al. Fertility and pregnancy outcomes following hypogastric artery ligation for severe post-partum haemorrhage. Hum Reprod 2003;18:844–848
49. Lynch BC, Coker A, Laval AH, et al. The B-lynch surgical technique for control of massive postpartum haemorrhage: an alternative to hysterectomy? Five cases reported. Br J Obstet Gynaecol 1997;104:372–376
50. Cho JH, Jun HS, Lee CN. Hemostatic suturing technique for uterine bleeding during cesarean delivery. Obstet Gynecol 2000;96:129–131
51. Bai SW, Lee HJ, Cho JS, Park JW, Kin SK, Park KH. Peripartum hysterectomy and associated factors. J Reprod Med 2003;48:148–152
52. Chanrachakul B, Chaturachinda K, Phuapradit W, Roungsipragarn R. Cesarean and postpartum hysterectomy. Int J Gynaecol Obstet 1996; 54:109–113
53. Naydich M, Friedman A, Aaron G, Silberzweig J. Arterial embolization of vaginal arterial branches for severe postpartum hemorrhage despite hysterectomy. J Vasc Interv Radiol 2007;18:1047–1050
54. Brown BJ, Heaston DK, Poulson AM, Gabert HA, Mineau DE, Miller EJ. Uncontrolled postpartum bleeding: a new approach to hemostasis through angiographic arterial embolization. Obstet Gynecol 1979;54: 361–365
55. Hansch E, Chitkara U, McAlpine J, El-Sayed Y, Dake MD, Razavi MK. Pelvic arterial embolization for control of obstetric hemorrhage: a five-year experience. Am J Obstet Gynecol 1999;180(6 Pt 1):1454–1460
56. Chung JW, Jeong HJ, Joh JH, Park JS, Jun JK, Kim SH. Percutaneous transcatheter angiographic embolization in the management of obstetric hemorrhage. J Reprod Med 2003;48:268–276
57. Hong TM, Tseng HS, Lee RC, Wang JH, Chang CY. Uterine artery embolization: an effective treatment for intractable obstetric hemorrhage. Clin Radiol 2004;59:96–101
58. Cottier JP, Fignon A, Tranquart F, Herbreteau D. Uterine necrosis after arterial embolization for postpartum hemorrhage. Obstet Gynecol 2002;100(5 Pt 2):1074–1077
59. Ko SF, Lin H, Ng SH, Lee TY, Wan YL. Postpartum hemorrhage with concurrent massive inferior epigastric artery bleeding after cesarean delivery. Am J Obstet Gynecol 2002;187:243–244
60. Rathod KR, Deshmukh HL, Asrani A, Salvi VS, Prabhu S. Successful embolization of an ovarian artery pseudoaneurysm complicating obstetric hysterectomy. Cardiovasc Intervent Radiol 2005;28:113–116
61. Ojala K, Perala J, Kariniemi J, Ranta P, Raudaskoski T, Tekay A. Arterial embolization and prophylactic catheterization for the treatment for severe obstetric hemorrhage. Acta Obstet Gynecol Scand 2005;84:1075–1080
62. Palacios Jaraquemada JM. Life-threatening primary postpartum hemorrhage: treatment with emergency selective arterial embolization. Radiology 1999;210:876–878
63. Pelage JP, Soyer P, Repiquet D, et al. Secondary postpartum hemorrhage: treatment with selective arterial embolization. Radiology 1999;212:385–389
64. Cheng YY, Hwang JI, Hung SW, et al. Angiographic embolization for emergent and prophylactic management of obstetric hemorrhage: a four-year experience. J Chin Med Assoc 2003;66:727–734
65. Alanis M, Hurst BS, Marshburn PB, Matthews ML. Conservative management of placenta increta with selective arterial embolization preserves future fertility and results in a favorable outcome in subsequent pregnancies. Fertil Steril 2006;86(5):1514
66. Soncini E, Pelicelli A, Larini P, Marcato C, Monaco D, Grignaffini A. Uterine artery embolization in the treatment and prevention of postpartum hemorrhage. Int J Gynaecol Obstet 2007;96:181–185
67. Vegas G, Illescas T, Munoz M, Perez-Pinar A. Selective pelvic arterial embolization in the management of obstetric hemorrhage. Eur J Obstet Gynecol Reprod Biol 2006;127:68–72
68. Yamashita Y, Takahashi M, Ito M, Okamura H. Transcatheter arterial embolization in the management of postpartum hemorrhage due to genital tract injury. Obstet Gynecol 1991;77:160–163
69. Ornan D, White R, Pollak J, Tal M. Pelvic embolization for intractable postpartum hemorrhage: long-term follow-up and implications for fertility. Obstet Gynecol 2003;102(5 Pt 1):904–910
70. Boulleret C, Chahid T, Gallot D, et al. Hypogastric arterial selective and superselective embolization for severe postpartum hemorrhage: a retrospective review of 36 cases. Cardiovasc Intervent Radiol 2004;27:344–348
71. Descargues G, Mauger Tinlot F, Douvrin F, Clavier E, Lemoine JP, Marpeau L. Menses, fertility and pregnancy after arterial embolization for the control of postpartum haemorrhage. Hum Reprod 2004;19:339–343
72. Wang H, Garmel S. Successful term pregnancy after bilateral uterine artery embolization for postpartum hemorrhage. Obstet Gynecol 2003;102:603–604
73. Alvarez M, Lockwood CJ, Ghidini A, Dottino P, Mitty HA, Berkowitz RL. Prophylactic and emergent arterial catheterization for selective embolization in obstetric hemorrhage. Am J Perinatol 1992;9:441–444
74. Kidney DD, Nguyen AM, Ahdoot D, Bickmore D, Deutsch LS, Majors C. Prophylactic perioperative hypogastric artery balloon occlusion in abnormal placentation. AJR Am J Roentgenol 2001;176:1521–1524
75. Dubois J, Garel L, Grignon A, Lemay M, Leduc L. Placenta percreta: balloon occlusion and embolization of the internal iliac arteries to reduce intraoperative blood losses. Am J Obstet Gynecol 1997;176:723–726
76. Mitty HA, Sterling KM, Alvarez M, Gendler R. Obstetric hemorrhage: prophylactic and emergency arterial catheterization and embolotherapy. Radiology 1993;188:183–187
77. Butt K, Gagnon A, Delisle MF. Failure of methotrexate and internal iliac balloon catheterization to manage placenta percreta. Obstet Gynecol 2002;99:981–982
78. Bodner LJ, Nosher JL, Gribbin C, Siegel RL, Beale S, Scorza W. Balloon-assisted occlusion of the internal iliac arteries in patients with placenta accreta/percreta. Cardiovasc Intervent Radiol 2006;29:354–361
79. Shih JC, Liu KL, Shyu MK. Temporary balloon occlusion of the common iliac artery: new approach to bleeding control during cesarean hysterectomy for placenta percreta. Am J Obstet Gynecol 2005;193:1756–1758
80. Celik C, Bala A, Acar A, Gezgine K, Akyurek C. Methotrexate for cervical pregnancy. A case report. J Reprod Med 2003;48:130–132
81. Yankowitz J, Leake J, Huggins G, Gazaway P, Gates E. Cervical ectopic pregnancy. Review of the literature and report of a case treated by single-dose methotrexate therapy. Obstet Gynecol Surv 1990;45:405–414

82. Studdiford WE. Cervical pregnancy: a partial review of the literature and a report of two probable cases. Am J Obstet Gynecol 1945;49:169–185
83. Dicker D, Feldberg D, Samuel N, Goldman JA. Etiology of cervical pregnancy. Association with abortion, pelvic pathology, IUDs, and Asherman's syndrome. J Reprod Med 1985;30:25–27
84. Qasim SM, Bohrer MK, Kemmann E. Recurrent cervical pregnancy after assisted reproduction by intra-fallopian transfer. Obstet Gynecol 1996;87:831–832
85. Shinagawa S, Nagayama M. Cervical pregnancy as a possible sequela of induced abortion. Report of 19 cases. Am J Obstet Gynecol 1969;105:282–284
86. Kirk E, Condous G, Haider Z, Syed A, Ojha K, Bourne T. The conservative management of cervical ectopic pregnancies. Ultrasound Obstet Gynecol 2006;27:430–437
87. Benson CB, Doubilet PM. Strategies for conservative treatment of cervical ectopic pregnancy. Ultrasound Obstet Gynecol 1996;8:371–372
88. Farabow WS, Fulton JW, Fletcher V, Velat CA, White JT. Cervical pregnancy treated with methotrexate. N C Med J 1983;44:91–93
89. The Practice Committee for the American Society for Reproductive Medicine. Medical treatment of ectopic pregnancy. Fertil Steril 2006;86:S96–S102
90. Mesogitis S, Pilalis A, Daskalakis G, Papantoniou N, Antsaklis A. Management of early viable cervical pregnancy. BJOG 2005;112:409–411
91. Kung FT, Chang S, Tsai YC, Hwang FR, Hsu TY, Soong YK. Subsequent reduction and obstetric outcome after methotrexate treatment of cervical pregnancy: a review of original literature and international collaborate follow-up. Hum Reprod 1997;12:591–595
92. Hung TH, Shau WY, Hseih TT, Hsu JJ, Soong YK, Jeng CJ. Prognostic factors for an unsatisfactory primary methotrexate treatment of cervical pregnancy: a quantitative review. Hum Reprod 1998;13:2636–2642
93. Mitra AG, Harris-Owens M. Conservative medical management of advanced cervical ectopic pregnancies. Obstet Gynecol Surv 2000;55:385–389
94. Kim TJ, Seong SJ, Lee KJ, et al. Clinical outcomes of patients treated for cervical pregnancy with or without methotrexate. J Korean Med Sci 2004;19:848–852
95. Yitzhak M, Orvieto R, Nitke S, Neuman-Levin M, Ben-Rafael Z, Schoenfeld A. Cervical pregnancy – a conservative stepwise approach. Hum Reprod 1999;14:847–849
96. Kung FT, Chang SY. Efficacy of methotrexate treatment in viable and nonviable cervical pregnancies. Am J Obstet Gynecol 1999;181:1438–1444
97. Sherer DM, Lysikiewicz A, Abulafia O. Viable cervical pregnancy managed with systemic methotrexate, uterine artery embolization, and local tamponade with inflated Foley catheter balloon. Am J Perinatol 2003;20:263–267
98. Gun M, Mavrogiorgis M. Cervical ectopic pregnancy: a case report and literature review. Ultrasound Obstet Gynecol 2002;19:297–301
99. Cosin JA, Bean M, Grow D, Wiczyk H. The use of methotrexate and arterial embolization to avoid surgery in a case of cervical pregnancy. Fertil Steril 1997;67:1169–1171
100. Frates MC, Benson CB, Doubilet PM, et al. Cervical ectopic pregnancy: results of conservative treatment. Radiology 1994;191:773–775
101. Trambert JJ, Einstein MH, Banks E, Frost A, Goldberg GL. Uterine artery embolization in the management of vaginal bleeding from cervical pregnancy: a case series. J Reprod Med 2005;50:844–850
102. Takano M, Hasegawa Y, Matsuda H, Kikuchi Y. Successful management of cervical pregnancy by selective uterine artery embolization: a case report. J Reprod Med 2004;49:986–988
103. Lambert P, Marpeau L, Jannet D, et al. Cervical pregnancy: conservative treatment with primary embolization of the uterine arteries. A case report. Review of the literature. J Gynecol Obstet Biol Reprod (Paris) 1995;24:43–47
104. Saliken JC, Normore WJ, Pattinson HA, Wood S. Embolization of the uterine arteries before termination of a 15-week cervical pregnancy. Can Assoc Radiol J 1994;45:399–401
105. Has R, Balci NC, Ibrahimglu L, Rozanes I, Topuz S. Uterine artery embolization in a 10-week cervical pregnancy with coexisting fibroids. Int J Gynaecol Obstet 2001;72:253–258
106. Xu B, Wang YZ, Zhang YH, Wang S, Yang L, Dai SZ. Angiographic uterine artery embolization followed by immediate curettage: an efficient treatment for controlling heavy bleeding and avoiding recurrent bleeding in cervical pregnancy. J Obstet Gynaecol Res 2007;33:190–194
107. Yao M, Tulandi T. Surgical and medical management of tubal and non-tubal ectopic pregnancies. Curr Opin Obstet Gynecol 1998;10:371–374
108. Nakao Y, Yokoyama M, Iwasaka T. Uterine artery embolization followed by dilatation and curettage for cervical pregnancy. Obstet Gynecol 2008;111(2 Pt 2):505–507
109. Ushakov FB, Elchalal U, Aceman PJ, Schenker JG. Cervical pregnancy: Past and future. Obstet Gynecol Surv 1997;52:45–59
110. Dubreuil GLE. Anevrysme cirsoide de l'uterus. Ann Anat Pathol (Paris) 1926;3:697–718
111. Fleming H, Ostor AG, Pickel H, Fortune DW. Arteriovenous malformations of the uterus. Obstet Gynecol 1989;73:209–214
112. Maleux G, Timmerman D, Heye S, Wilms G. Acquired uterine vascular malformations: radiological and clinical outcome after transcatheter embolotherapy. Eur Radiol 2006;16:299–306
113. Grivell RM, Reid KM, Mellor A. Uterine arteriovenous malformations: a review of the current literature. Obstet Gynecol Surv 2005;60:761–767
114. Ghai S, Rajan DK, Asch MR, Muradali D, Simons ME, TerBrugge KG. Efficacy of embolization in traumatic uterine vascular malformations. J Vasc Interv Radiol 2003;14:1401–1408
115. Rangarajan RD, Moloney JC, Anderson HJ, et al. Diagnosis and nonsurgical management of uterine arteriovenous malformation. Cardiovasc Intervent Radiol 2007;30(6):1267–1270
116. Lim AK, Agarwal R, Seckl MJ, et al. Embolization of bleeding residual uterine vascular malformations in patients with treated gestational trophoblastic tumors. Radiology 2002;222:640–644
117. Aziz N, Lenzi TA, Jeffrey RB, et al. Postpartum uterine arteriovenous fistula. Obstet Gynecol 2004;103:1076–1078
118. Hoffman MK, Meilstrup JW, Shackelford DP, et al. Arteriovenous malformations of the uterus: an uncommon cause of vaginal bleeding. Obstet Gynecol Surv 1997;52:736–740
119. Gopal M, Goldberg J, Klein TA, Fossum GT. Embolization of a uterine arteriovenous malformation followed by a twin pregnancy. Obstet Gynecol 2003;102:696–698
120. Manolitsas T, Hurley V, Gilford E. Uterine arteriovenous malformation – a rare cause of uterine hemorrhage. Aust N Z J Obstet Gynaecol 1994;34:197–199
121. Torres WE, Sones PJ Jr, Thames FM. Ultrasound appearance of a pelvic arteriovenous malformation. J Clin Ultrasound 1979;7:383–385
122. Clarke MJ, Mitchell PJ. Uterine arteriovenous malformation: a rare cause of uterine bleeding. Diagnosis and treatment. Australas Radiol 2003;47:302–305
123. Forssman L, Lundberg J, Schersten T. Conservative treatment of uterine arteriovenous fistula. Acta Obstet Gynecol Scand 1982;61:85–87
124. Vogelzang RL, Nemcek AA, Skrtic Z, Gorell J, Lurain JR. Uterine arteriovenous malformations: primary treatment with therapeutic embolization. J Vasc Interv Radiol 1991;2:517–521
125. Wilms GE, Favril A, Baert AL, Poppe W, Van Assche F. Transcatheter embolization of an uterine arteriovenous malformation. Cardiovasc Intervent Radiol 1986;9:61–64
126. Takeuchi K, Yamada T, Iwasa M, Maruo T. Successful medical treatment with danazol after failed embolization of uterine arteriovenous malformation. Obstet Gynecol 2003;102:843–844
127. Bagga R, Verma P, Aggarwal N, Suri V, Bapuraj JR, Kalra N. Failed angiographic embolization in uterine arteriovenous malformation: a case report and review of the literature. Medscape J Med 2008;10:12
128. Delotte J, Chevallier P, Benoit B, Castillon JM, Bongain A. Pregnancy after embolization therapy for uterine arteriovenous malformation. Fertil Steril 2006;85:228

129. McCormick CC, Kim HS. Successful pregnancy with a full-term vaginal delivery one year after *N*-butyl cyanoacrylate embolization of a uterine arteriovenous malformation. Cardiovasc Intervent Radiol 2006;29:699–701
130. Armagada JO, Karankgaokar V, Wood A, et al. Successful pregnancy following two uterine artery embolization procedures for arteriovenous malformation. J Obstet Gynaecol 2004;24:86–87
131. Vedantham S, Goodwin SC, McLucas B, Mohr G. Uterine artery embolization: an underused method of controlling pelvic hemorrhage. Am J Obstet Gynecol 1997;176:938–948
132. Hayashi M, Murakami A, Iwasaki N, Yaoi Y. Effectiveness of arterial embolization procedure in uterine cancer patients. J Med 1999;30:225–234
133. Yalvac S, Kayikcioglu F, Boran N, et al. Embolization of the uterine artery in terminal stage cervical cancers. Cancer Invest 2002;20:754–758
134. Wilms G, Peene P, Baert AL. Transcatheter embolization in the management of gynaecological bleeding. J Belge Radiol 1990;73:21–25
135. Dehaeck CM. Transcatheter embolization of pelvic vessels to stop intractable hemorrhage. Gynecol Oncol 1986;24:9–16
136. Mihmanli I, Cantasdemir M, Kantarci F, Hallit Yilmaz M, Numan F, Mihmanli V. Percutaneous embolization in the management of intractable vaginal bleeding. Arch Gynecol Obstet 2001;264:211–214
137. Tse KY, Chan KK, Tam KF, Ngan HY. 20 year experience of managing profuse bleeding in gestational trophoblastic disease. J Reprod Med 2007;52:397–401
138. Moodley M, Moodley J. Transcatheter angiographic embolization for the control of massive pelvic hemorrhage due to gestational trophoblastic disease: a case series and review of the literature. Int J Gynecol Cancer 2003;13:94–97
139. Miller FJ, Mortel R, Mann WJ, Jahshan AF. Selective arterial embolization for control of hemorrhage in pelvic malignancy: femoral and brachial catheter approaches. AJR Am J Roentgenol 1976;126:1028–1032
140. Suvorova IV, Tarazov PG, Zharinov GM, Naklasova NI. Arterial embolization in chronic hemorrhage from uterine neoplasms. Vopr Onkol 1996;42:59–62
141. Pisco JM, Martins JM, Correia MG. Internal iliac artery embolization to control hemorrhage from pelvic neoplasms. Radiology 1989;172:337–339

9 Clinical Perspective: Uterine Fibroid Embolization (Gynecology)

Jay Goldberg

Until the late 1990s, the primary reason for obstetrician/gynecologists (Ob/Gyns) to involve interventional radiologists (IRs) in the care of their patients was focused in primarily two Ob/Gyn treatment areas: (1) the drainage of pelvic/abdominal fluid collections, and (2) embolization for acute pelvic hemorrhage. The 1995 publication in *Lancet* authored by Jacque Ravina, M.D., a French gynecologist and colleagues, which presented uterine artery embolization (UAE) as an effective primary fibroid therapy, completely and permanently revolutionized the interventional radiologist's involvement in women's health, as well as their relationship with the Ob/Gyn.[1]

■ Embolization for Indications Other Than Uterine Fibroids

Embolization aimed at stopping bleeding in the acute setting may be a uterine sparing and a potentially life-saving treatment option for both gynecologic and obstetric patients. For gynecologic patients, the most common scenario would be having declining hemoglobin levels in the first 24 hours postoperatively. A specific example might be a woman with delayed arterial bleeding at the cervical stump following hysterectomy. Selective arterial embolization may be preferable to surgical reexploration to both identify the origin of and treat the bleeding. This approach may be especially desirable in the patient with complicated medical conditions, extensive adhesive disease or with bleeding that might be difficult to control surgically, such as in the Space of Retzius following a Burch procedure for urinary incontinence. Postcesarean delivery patients may similarly benefit from selective embolization in the same clinical situation of declining hemoglobin levels thought to be due to arterial bleeding soon following delivery.

The more common scenario when embolization might be considered in obstetrics is the patient with an immediate postpartum uterine hemorrhage following vaginal delivery. This is usually caused by uterine atony that has been nonresponsive to the usual interventions of uterine massage, uterotonic medications (pitocin, carboprost tromethamine, misoprostol, and/or methylergonovine), and possibly uterine curettage. Rather than directly proceeding to laparotomy for the specific purpose of obtaining surgical access for uterine artery ligation, uterine compression suturing (B-Lynch), hypogastric artery ligation (rarely performed and not currently a recommended intervention), or hysterectomy, the obstetrician may attempt uterine packing followed by UAE. The uterus is tightly packed with gauze, placed transcervically until it hopefully leads to compression that is sufficient to stop or significantly decrease bleeding. A decision must then be made to just observe the patient or to proceed with UAE, during which time blood products might be given, depending upon the hemodynamic stability, estimated blood loss, and starting hematocrit. The goal of embolization of both uterine arteries for such patients would be to decrease overall uterine perfusion and arterial pressure by blocking its major blood supply, hopefully leading to decreased uterine bleeding. Collateral blood supply to the uterus almost always supplies perfusion sufficient to prevent uterine necrosis.

In theory, embolization of the uterine arteries in the postpartum patient bleeding from a nonresponsive uterine atony sounds like a better option than laparotomy and vessel ligation or hysterectomy. However, there are several factors that may limit its clinical effectiveness and practicality. Most obstetrical areas do not have the fluoroscopy equipment necessary for embolization, requiring an often hemodynamically unstable patient to be transferred to another area of the hospital. If the patient becomes more unstable during transport or in the radiology suite, a potential disaster could occur. Additionally, with most births occurring after usual work hours or on weekends, an IR may not be readily available, delaying the embolization. Also, in cases of postpartum uterine atony not responding to embolization attempt, surgical intervention has been further delayed with additional blood loss, putting the woman at greater risk for disseminated intravascular coagulopathy (DIC), hemorrhagic shock, and death.

Patients that are hemodynamically unstable are usually best served by being quickly taken to the operating room. However, not all patients are candidates for this type of intervention. Most IRs prefer the patient to have an international normalized ratio (INR) <2, often requiring time to sufficiently replace blood products. Even in postpartum patients with bleeding successfully abated following bilateral uterine artery embolization, there may be significant morbidity, including the risk of complete uterine necrosis. The majority of patients stable enough for the time required to transfer them to the radiology suite and for the embolization procedure would probably have been sufficiently treated with uterine packing and blood transfusion alone. Obviously, it would be impossible to have the power sufficient for a randomized trial assessing the added benefit of UAE added to uterine packing in severe postpartum uterine atony.

One final consideration for the Ob/Gyn is that a patient who requires an exploratory laparotomy to correct a surgical complication will be much more likely to file a lawsuit than one whose condition was effectively treated by minimally invasive transcutaneous or transvaginal techniques performed by an IR. This is another reason why embolization in this setting has become an increasingly accepted option for treatment.

■ Uterine Fibroid Embolization

Uterine fibroids are the most common tumors of the female reproductive tract, occurring in 20 to 70% of women between the ages 30 to 50 years. Black women are most frequently affected, whereas white women, Asians, and Scandinavians have lower incidences. Tumor size varies widely and many women have multiple fibroids. Patients may be asymptomatic with diagnosis on palpation of a firm, enlarged uterus on routine examination or on an incidental finding at imaging. Others may present symptoms such as menorrhagia, intermenstrual bleeding, pelvic pain/pressure, dyspareunia, urinary frequency, abdominal distension, infertility, and pregnancy complications. Given the nature and severity of these symptoms, fibroids can have a significant impact on quality of life.[2]

Most symptomatic women eventually seek medical treatment. There are many fibroid treatments available, their selection based on many factors, including bulk symptoms, bleeding symptoms, and desire for future fertility/uterine preservation (**Fig. 9.1**). Medications used to treat fibroids include analgesics, usually nonsteroidal antiinflammatory drugs (NSAIDs), and combination estrogen/progestin oral contraceptives (OCPs). Gonadotropin-releasing hormone agonists (e.g., leuprolide) can temporarily reduce fibroid volume by up to 40% while also decreasing vaginal bleeding.[3] However, their significant side-effect profile (e.g., vasomotor instability, mood swings, bone loss) and the fibroids' quick return to baseline upon discontinuation of therapy primarily restrict use to temporary tumor reduction prior to surgery.

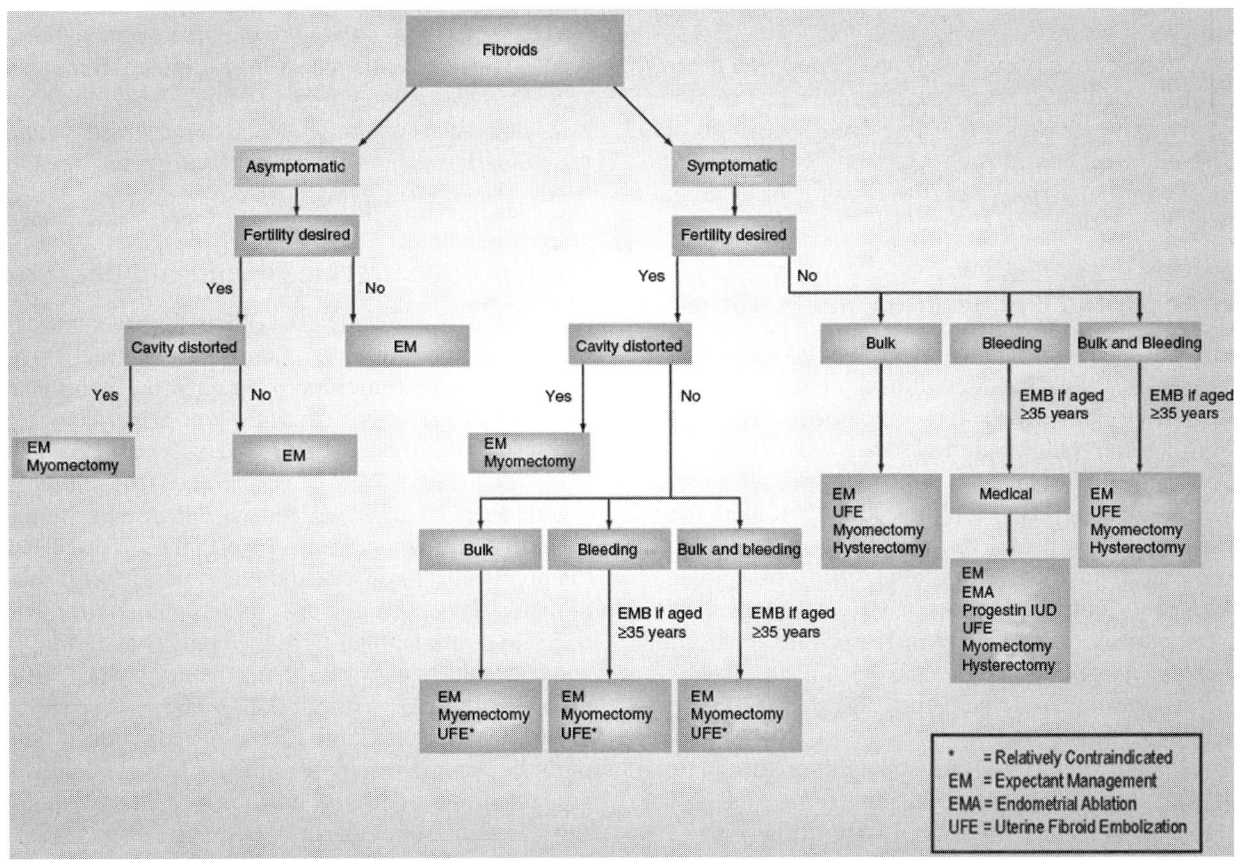

Fig. 9.1 Algorithm for the treatment of uterine fibroids. (Image courtesy of Jefferson Fibroid Center, www.jeffersonhospital.org/fibroid)

Women with symptomatic uterine fibroids refractory to medical management have traditionally undergone surgical resection via hysterectomy or myomectomy. In the United States ~250,000 women undergo hysterectomy annually for symptomatic fibroids, with ~35,000 undergoing myomectomy. While preserving the uterus, many women undergoing myomectomy may require additional procedures due to persistent symptoms or the growth of new fibroids. The desire for uterine/fertility preservation and avoidance of surgery has increased the demand for alternative treatments. Uterine fibroid embolization has emerged over the last decade as an increasingly popular and effective nonsurgical option. In its first decade of usage, UFE has treated ~150,000 women with symptomatic fibroids worldwide. It is estimated that ~40,000 additional women will undergo treatment in 2009 (25,000 in the United States and 25,000 elsewhere) (Personal communication, Jim Kelly, BioSphere Medical, Inc., Rockland, MA).

As reviewed in Chapter 5, UFE has shown to be a safe and effective treatment for symptomatic uterine fibroids[4–6] with improvement in more recent studies noted on a long-term basis.[7–9] Additional data on the long-term safety and efficacy of UFE will continue to be published from the UAE Fibroid Registry for Outcomes Data project. The project is a longitudinal study developed by the Society of Interventional Radiology that follows UFE procedures performed at 72 centers with enrollments of more than 3,000 patients. This is the largest prospective fibroid study ever done. Unfortunately, there are no similar studies in the Ob/Gyn literature of myomectomy or hysterectomy for comparison.

Uterine Fibroid Embolization and Fertility

Whether or not UFE should be performed in women desiring future fertility has been a much debated question between both Ob/Gyns, IRs, and within the IR community itself. Our series, published in *Obstetrics & Gynecology* in 2002, was the first to calculate risks associated with pregnancies following UFE. Its most clinically important finding was an increased rate of preterm delivery compared with the general population.[10] In a follow-up study comparing pregnancy outcomes following UFE and laparoscopic myomectomy, we also found an increased rate of preterm delivery following UFE, whereas the rate following laparoscopic myomectomy was no higher than that seen in the general population.[11]

More recent studies have also reported increased rates of preterm delivery following UFE, but they have not demonstrated an increase in premature, preterm delivery (<32 weeks). Most pregnancies in these studies did well overall. Importantly, however, there are no studies available with power sufficient to reliably calculate pregnancy rates following UFE. In addition, the limited number of these pregnancies following UFE has not allowed performance of a subanalysis to determine which fibroid characteristics are most important in evaluating whether UFE is a good option for certain fertility desiring patients. The American College of Obstetricians and Gynecologists (ACOG), though presenting a much more positive attitude toward UFE in Committee Opinion #293 (February 2004), regards it as relatively contraindicated for women desiring future fertility for the above reasons.[12]

Still, UFE procedures are being performed in patients desiring future fertility. Studies of women undergoing in vitro fertilization (IVF) have shown that fibroids that distort the endometrial cavity decrease pregnancy rates. A meta-analysis by Donnez and Jadoul of six studies demonstrated that women with submucosal and intramural fibroids distorting the uterine cavity undergoing IVF had lower pregnancy rates compared with women with fibroids not distorting the cavity and women without fibroids.[13] Myomectomy in this setting has been helpful because it reconstructs normal uterine anatomy. UFE, on the other hand, merely decreases fibroid volume. Therefore, in a woman with multiple fibroids distorting her cavity, UFE may make the fibroids smaller, but it is likely that they will still distort her cavity. This, in theory, will potentially lead to subfertility with lower pregnancy and higher miscarriage rates in women desiring future fertility following UFE. Thus, for women desiring future fertility, although it may be reasonable to offer UFE to those with a nondistorted uterine cavity, those with distorted cavities should be advised to undergo myomectomy.

Preoperative Uterine Fibroid Embolization

Ravina et al[1] had initially used UFE as a preoperative treatment prior to myomectomy in massively enlarged uteri (>20 weeks size) in attempt to decrease the risk for hemorrhage. UFE performed several weeks prior to myomectomy can accomplish this goal by reducing fibroid volume and vascularity (**Fig. 9.2**). Ravina and colleagues noted that several women cancelled their scheduled surgery after receiving satisfactory symptom relief in the interval between the premyomectomy UFE and the day of surgery. This led to their study of UFE as a primary fibroid therapy.[1]

Ob/Gyns are familiar with the benefits of preoperative gonadotropin-releasing hormone therapy agonist (GnRHa) therapy to decrease surgical risk during myomectomy or hysterectomy for large fibroid uteri. Although temporarily decreasing uterine volume up to 40%, GnRHa therapy requires 3 months for maximum benefit, is expensive, and has significant and unpleasant side effects from the induced menopausal state.

Premyomectomy UFE is currently an underutilized surgical adjuvant that can decrease the risk for the mas-

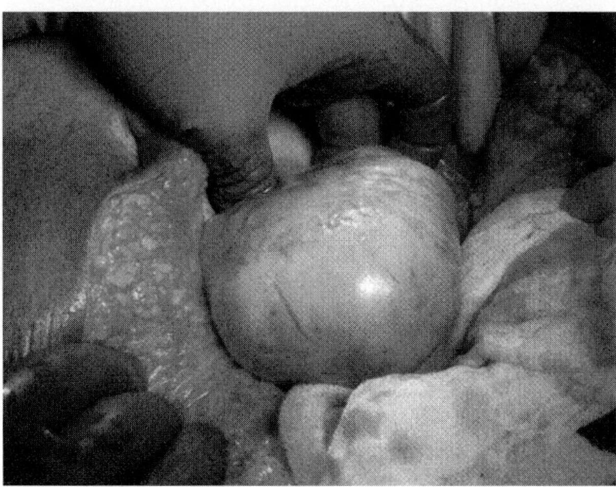
A

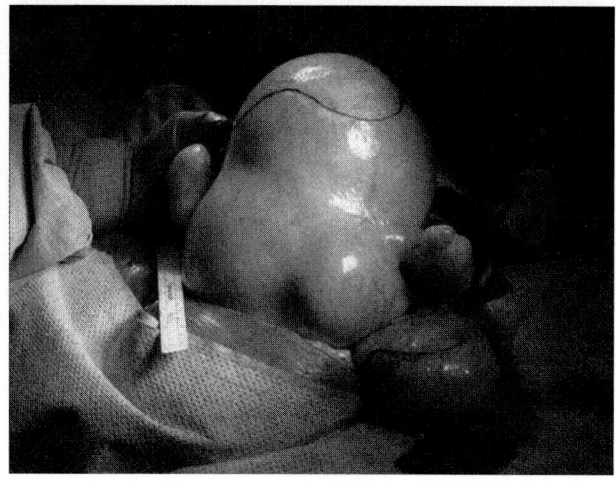
B

Fig. 9.2 Appearance of an embolized fibroid at myomectomy. (Image courtesy of Jefferson Fibroid Center, www.jeffersonhospital.org/fibroid)

sively enlarged fibroid uterus. These benefits, especially the decreased risk of intraoperative hemorrhage, may also outweigh potential risks in women desiring future fertility. The optimal interval for performing myomectomy following adjuvant UFE remains to be established. Compared with GnRHa therapy, the interval until surgery is much shorter and the systemic side effects are avoided. Premyomectomy UFE does confer substantial additional cost (e.g., a 48% increase from $5,676 for a myomectomy alone to $8,383 in Philadelphia, PA). However, these expenses must be weighed against the potential savings via complication reduction in this high-risk subgroup of patients with massively enlarged uteri.[14]

■ Economic Issues

There is at present a financial "turf war" between gynecologists and interventional radiologists regarding the treatment of fibroids. With 250,000 women undergoing hysterectomy yearly, primarily for uterine fibroids, in addition to the large number undergoing myomectomy, the relative number of UFE procedures has remained relatively low, with only 5 to 8% recent yearly growth. It had been implied that gynecologists, often acting as "gatekeepers," were not referring or even discussing the option of UFE with appropriate patients due to financial self-interest.[15] Although this negative insinuation may unfortunately be true for a few gynecologists, there are certainly other factors contributing to gynecologists previously not discussing UFE with patients being offered myomectomies or hysterectomies for fibroids. Many Ob/Gyns, as well as primary care providers (PCPs), were previously unfamiliar with the procedure. They may have had misconceptions regarding its risks and who are potential candidates or awaited long-term outcome data.[16] Additionally, the gynecology community was initially put off by many IRs not properly taking responsibility for early UFE complications and their cavalier approach to recommending UFE to patients desiring future fertility.

In response to the gatekeeper issue, UFE became a procedure that is heavily marketed by IRs directly to the public through the Internet and print media, as an increasingly popular, safe, nonsurgical alternative to myomectomy and hysterectomy. Most women undergoing UFE are self-referrals to IRs or are referred by their gynecologist or PCP only after specifically inquiring about the procedure. Especially given the recent long-term outcome data, a proper informed consent for patients being offered myomectomy or hysterectomy should also include the option of UFE unless otherwise contraindicated.[17,18] Over the past 2 to 3 years, it has been my experience that UFE is becoming more accepted and increasingly offered to patients by gynecologists as a mainstream treatment option for appropriate candidates.

■ Conclusions

The role of the interventional radiologist in women's health has recently expanded from primarily draining pelvic/abdominal fluid collections and embolizing acute obstetrical and gynecologic hemorrhage to providing a primary treatment for symptomatic uterine fibroids. As an increasingly utilized alternative to hysterectomy and myomectomy, UFE is a safe and effective option for improving bleeding and bulk symptoms in most patients with symptomatic uterine fibroids (**Table 9.1**). In addition to uterine preservation, UFE offers the benefits of avoidance of a surgery, shorter hospitalization, decreased morbidity, quicker return to work, and potential financial savings for the health care system. Not all fibroids are best treated with UFE.

Table 9.1 Major Advantages and Disadvantages of Uterine Fibroid Treatments

Treatment	Advantages	Disadvantages
Hysterectomy	Definitive therapy End of menses	4 to 6 Week recovery Loss of fertility Higher complication rate
Myomectomy	Future fertility Uterine preservation	4 to 6 Week recovery Higher complication rate
Uterine fibroid embolization	7- to 10-day recovery Lower complication rate Uterine preservation	Increases future pregnancy risks Higher treatment failure rate

Myomectomy may be a better option in the woman desiring future fertility, especially if fibroid-related distortion of the uterine cavity is present. As both patients and Ob/Gyns become more familiar with the benefits and accepting of UFE, its utilization will continue to increase.

Acknowledgment

Dr. Goldberg is a consultant for BioSphere Medical (Rockland, MA) and Repros Therapeutics (The Woodlands, TX).

For additional embolization and fibroid educational information and images, please visit the Web site of the Jefferson Fibroid Center, www.jeffersonhospital.org/fibroid

References

1. Ravina JH, Herbreteau D, Ciraru-Vigneron N, et al. Arterial embolization to treat uterine myomata. Lancet 1995;346(3976):671–672
2. Goldberg J. Uterine artery embolization for symptomatic leiomyomata. Female Patient 2006;31:45–50
3. Friedman AJ, Hoffman DI, Comite F, Browneller RW, Miller JD. Treatment of leiomyomata uteri with leuprolide acetate depot: a double-blind, placebo-controlled, multicenter study. The Leuprolide Study Group. Obstet Gynecol 1991;77(1):720–725
4. Spies JB, Ascher SA, Roth AR, Kim J, Levy EB, Gomez-Jorge J. Uterine artery embolization for leiomyomata. Obstet Gynecol 2001;98(1):29–34
5. Pron G, Bennett J, Common A, Wall J, Asch M, Sniderman K. The Ontario Uterine Fibroid Embolization Trial. Part 2. Uterine fibroid reduction and symptom relief after uterine artery embolization for fibroids. Fertil Steril 2003;79(1):120–127
6. Spies JB, Cooper JM, Worthington-Kirsch R, Lipman JC, Mills BB, Benenati JF. Outcome of uterine embolization and hysterectomy for leiomyomas: results of a multicenter study. Am J Obstet Gynecol 2004;191(1):22–31
7. Spies JB, Bruno J, Czeyda-Pommersheim F, Magee ST, Ascher SA, Jha RC. Long-term outcome of uterine artery embolization of leiomyomata. Obstet Gynecol 2005;106:933–939
8. Walker WJ, Barton-Smith P. Long-term follow up of uterine artery embolisation – an effective alternative in the treatment of fibroids. BJOG 2006;113:464–468
9. Katsumori T, Kasahara T, Akazawa K. Long-term outcomes of uterine artery embolization using gelatin sponge particles alone for symptomatic fibroids. AJR Am J Roentgenol 2006;186:848–854
10. Goldberg J, Pereira L, Berghella V. Pregnancy after uterine artery embolization. Obstet Gynecol 2002;100(5 Pt 1):869–872
11. Goldberg J, Pereira L, Diamond J, et al. Pregnancy outcomes following treatment for fibroids: uterine artery embolization versus laparoscopic myomectomy. Am J Obstet Gynecol 2004;191(1):18–21
12. Committee on Gynecologic Practice, American College of Obstetricians and Gynecologists. ACOG Committee Opinion. Uterine artery embolization. Obstet Gynecol 2004;103(2):403–404
13. Donnez J, Jadoul P. What are the implications of myomas on fertility? A need for debate? Hum Reprod 2002;17:1424–1430
14. Goldberg J, Cothran S, Bonn J. Pre-myomectomy uterine fibroid embolization for a massively enlarged fibroid uterus. Female Patient 2006;31:1–3
15. Hysterectomy alternative goes unmentioned to many women. Wall Street Journal. August 24, 2004:1
16. Goldberg J, Pereira L, Mude-Nochumson H. Uterine artery embolization for symptomatic fibroids. OBG Management 2003; 4:69–79
17. Goldberg J. Uterine fibroid embolization: a hidden alternative? Obstet Gynecol Surv 2005;60:209–210
18. Goldberg J, Ness A, Fossum G. Does uterine fibroid embolization need to be offered as a treatment alternative? Pros and cons. Contemp Ob Gyn 2005;6:78–84

10 Clinical Perspective: Uterine Fibroid Embolization (Interventional Radiology)

James Spies

Given the frequency that uterine fibroid embolization (UFE) is being performed in today's interventional practice, it is hard to believe that just 10 years ago the first experience in the United States was reported by Goodwin at the 1997 Society of Cardiovascular and Interventional Radiology (now the Society of Interventional Radiology [SIR]) Annual Meeting in Washington, DC.[1] Although the procedure had been published in the English literature in 1995 by Ravina et al,[2] it was Goodwin's report that triggered the media's and scientific community's interest that led to UFE's rapid adoption into practice in the United States.

A decade is a very brief time for a new therapy to become so firmly established in the care of patients with a given clinical condition. With this in mind, it is remarkable that UFE has progressed so far in its assessment. We have a very detailed understanding of this therapy and are now exploring its last frontiers, which include long-term outcome, comparative outcomes, and reproductive impact of the procedure.

Lessons from the Development of Uterine Fibroid Embolization

It is worth a few moments to discuss the development of UFE because it is a somewhat atypical procedure in comparison to what has been developed by interventional radiologists (IRs) over the past 40 years. For most IR procedures there are typically a few initial reports in small groups of patients and usually one or two larger follow-on case series. Perhaps there will be one study of outcomes of up to 12 to 24 months or a case series on complications. The procedure is accepted into practice and investigations into various aspects of the treatment are then few and far between. In contrast, the story for UFE has been much different. There are dozens of case series reporting on UFE; with at least 10 larger than 100 patients. There is a registry that enrolled 3000 patients,[3] there have been four randomized studies published,[4–7] and now outcomes at 5 years have been reported for three series.[8–10]

There are several reasons for this remarkable research productivity related to UFE. The first is that reimbursement for the procedure was available from its introduction. Most new therapies require several years of poorly reimbursed or nonreimbursed experience before insurers are willing to accept the treatment. However, the availability of a nonspecific, noncentral nervous system embolization current procedural terminology (CPT) code of 37204 for the billing of the procedure allowed investigators to rapidly recruit patients to their studies. Unknowingly, insurers funded the research that allowed the procedure to be validated. It is extraordinarily fortunate that this was the case, as this procedure was directed at patients typically treated only by gynecologists who would be unlikely to support reimbursement for this procedure early on.

The insurers who recognized this procedure as a new therapy for fibroids often developed policies refusing coverage based on assessment by the gynecology members of their medical advisory committees. There were some insurers who took a progressive view of this procedure and allowed it to be reimbursed for patients on research protocols. I am referring to the leadership of Arnold Cohen, M.D. of Aetna (Aetna, Inc., Hartford, CT), a gynecologist in charge of the company's national policy in this area. He recognized the potential of UFE as an alternative to hysterectomy for the treatment of fibroids and encouraged its evaluation. There is no doubt that insurance coverage for UFE was a key factor in the success of early treatment studies.

A second reason for this procedure's rapid acceptance is that this treatment only required minimal additional training for interventionalists to perform the procedure successfully. A similar method had been in use for the management of postpartum hemorrhage for at least 15 years. In addition, interventionalists were already well versed in subselective catheterization techniques, and the use of microcatheters and particulate embolic agents. The very high technical success rates and low rates of procedural complications were likely due to the skill set broadly available in the community. This is not to say that there was not a need for new knowledge and skills to care optimally for patients undergoing this procedure; I will discuss the unmet needs in this regard in a later section. However, the average interventionalist could easily succeed in this therapy and this fact stimulated its acceptance.

A third factor in UFE's success is that the procedure did not require the development of any new devices. All the tools were on the shelf in most interventional suites. Although there certainly has been innovation in the materials and catheters available for this technique (several embolics had been developed specifically for the procedure), there were excellent outcomes from the materials that had been in historic use within IR. The sudden growth in sales of these products has stimulated interest among investors and start-up companies to join the market in this procedure. Biosphere Medical (Rockland, MA), Biocompatibles (Farnham, UK), and other corporations were formed, in large part, based on a mission of developing and marketing new products for UFE. The contributions of the companies in this field should not be underestimated.

In particular, Biosphere Medical and Boston Scientific (Natick, MA) have been instrumental in the development of new products. They have also been the primary supporters of educating the physicians interested in performing the procedure, informing gynecologists and patients about the benefits of UFE, and perhaps most importantly, supporting the research that has helped validate the treatment. The comparative studies supported by these two companies were among the first to place the outcomes of UFE in the context of surgical alternatives. They also provided the lion's share of the funding for the FIBROID Registry, a collaborative effort between the SIR Foundation, industry supporters, the Food and Drug Administration (FDA), and the Agency for Health Research and Quality (AHRQ).[11] The collaboration between these parties represents an unusual effort to better understand a new intervention as it diffuses into practice. It is rare that such an effort is made for new therapies and it has played a substantial role in the broad acceptance of the treatment by regulators and insurers both.

A fourth factor in the rapid acceptance of UFE is the Internet. UFE is one of the first therapies to be developed in the Internet Age. Just as it was becoming common for an individual to access the Internet for health care information, this new therapy was featured on a dozen different sites for review; in some cases, the Web sites were advertising the procedure.[12] Detractors might say the Internet allowed patients to be convinced to accept an unproven treatment but this ignores the obvious: gynecologists were not likely to consider referring patients for uterine embolization in the early years, even when the patients were part of a research protocol. If it had been left to gynecologists to approve each patient's decision to undergo UFE, the procedure would never have developed. Patients wanted more choice in the approach to their fibroid therapy. In truth, there seems to have been a developing demand among patients for years prior to UFE for an alternative to hysterectomy for fibroids. The appearance of an appealing procedure such as UFE fulfilled that unmet need. If it had not been UFE, it would have been another minimally invasive approach.

This enthusiasm among patients promoted their participation in research studies. This along with the fact that fibroids are ubiquitous, made the rapid accrual of study participants for investigators much easier than it might have been. The fact that this procedure was performed on a population of patients with benign conditions and were otherwise healthy provided for the perfect circumstances to assess outcomes. There were a few comorbidities to complicate the assessment of symptoms and quality of life afterward yet these patients were in the prime of their adult lives, which allowed patients to assess their own status.

UFE also benefited from an organized approach to the research agenda. In 1999, a research consensus panel of the Cardiovascular and Interventional Radiology Foundation (CIRREF, now the SIR Foundation) met in conjunction with the RAND Corporation (Santa Monica, CA) and identified a research agenda for the procedure.[13] The recommendations included a randomized controlled trial comparing UFE to surgery, a large broad-based registry to determine outcome in general practice, a cost-effectiveness study, and the development of a fibroid-specific symptom and quality of life questionnaire. Each of these projects has since been achieved.

In the case of the Registry, the study was organized and coordinated by the SIR Foundation; the UFS-QOL, the fibroid-specific symptom and quality of life questionnaire, was funded by the SIR Foundation.[14] In addition, SIR created a task force on UFE to coordinate educational activities for its members, patient information via brochures and the Internet, outreach to the gynecology community and to insurers regarding reimbursement. The SIR's efforts were undertaken to ensure that this procedure was promoted in a scientifically sound manner.

There is another factor that drove the scientific agenda that is implicit in some of the discussion above. We had developed a therapy for fibroids – a condition that had exclusively been the purview of a different specialty – gynecology. This may have initially appeared to be an impediment to our progress in gaining the acceptance of our therapy, but in the long run it was of benefit to us and to our patients. It was in this challenged environment that we needed to produce evidence. In many of our interventional therapies, we offered procedures for which there were no alternatives or for which therapies provided by other specialties had already failed. For UFE, we were offering an alternative to the standard, well-accepted treatment. If we were to gain any measure of acceptance we needed to provide evidence that would be beyond argument. We needed rigorous research methods and clear data in support of our positions. And we, as a group of researchers, have risen to the challenge. There have been dozens of case series reporting outcomes, comparative studies, including randomized studies. There are very detailed studies of adverse events, technical aspects of the treatment, and quality of life improvements after UFE. Although we certainly might have achieved some of these research milestones without another specialty to convince, the level of research has been higher as a result of this challenge.

■ The Next Steps for Uterine Fibroid Embolization

Therefore, through a fortuitous convergence of circumstances, UFE has developed based on sound clinical data. This procedure is effective and safe for the majority of women treated and will be lasting for most. This community of researchers and clinicians has achieved a great deal and, to many, the procedure is firmly established and has proven effectiveness. The question then arises as to whether there are any remaining questions that need study. In other words, have all our questions been answered and if not, which questions are the next to be answered?

From my perspective, no procedure is ever completely proven, understood or above further study. This is clearly true of embolization. The most pressing questions surround the potential impacts, both good or bad, to future fertility and childbearing. Is this procedure safe for women who would like to become pregnant? Will it improve or harm their fertility? What about fertile women who would like to have additional children? Is a myomectomy better for improving fertility than embolization? If it is, on average, is this always the case? How will the procedure affect women who have already had a myomectomy? Is it safe in infertile women?

Separate from fertility, does UFE have a systematic negative effect on ovarian functions in women? If there is an effect, does it occur at all reproductive ages or only in later reproductive life? What about the durability of embolization? Although we have several long-term studies, which patients are most likely to have fibroids that recur? Can this be predicted with sufficient accuracy to provide useful criteria for triaging patients? What about new approaches to fibroid therapy, such as magnetic resonance-guided focused ultrasound (MRgFUS) and some of the other therapies discussed in this section of the text? Are these and other developing therapies complementary or competitive to UFE and what role will they play in the care of these patients?

It is clear to see that our exploration of UFE and more broadly, exploration of our role in fibroid therapy has not yet been completed. In 2005, the SIR Foundation, recognizing the research needs that were still unmet, set an agenda for research in UFE.[15] Although we have come a long way, we have not yet reached the end of the journey on UFE. The years of investigation that lay ahead may be the most exciting yet.

References

1. Goodwin SC, Vedantham S, McLucas B, Forno A, Perrella R. Preliminary experience with uterine artery embolization for uterine fibroids. J Vasc Interv Radiol 1997;8:517–526
2. Ravina JH, Herbreteau D, Ciraru-Vigneron N, et al. Arterial embolisation to treat uterine myomata. Lancet 1995;346:671–672
3. Worthington-Kirsch R, Spies J, Myers E, et al. The Fibroid Registry for Outcomes Data (FIBROID) for Uterine Artery Embolization: Short term outcomes. Obstet Gynecol 2005;106:52–59
4. Edwards RD, Moss JG, Lumsden MA, et al. Uterine-artery embolization versus surgery for symptomatic uterine fibroids. N Engl J Med 2007;356(4):360–370
5. Hehenkamp WJ, Volkers NA, Donderwinkel PF, et al. Uterine artery embolization versus hysterectomy in the treatment of symptomatic uterine fibroids (EMMY trial): peri- and postprocedural results from a randomized controlled trial. Am J Obstet Gynecol 2005;193(5):1618–1629
6. Mara M, Fucikova Z, Maskova J, Kuzel D, Haakova L. Uterine fibroid embolization versus myomectomy in women wishing to preserve fertility: preliminary results of a randomized controlled trial. Eur J Obstet Gynecol Reprod Biol 2006;126(2):226–233
7. Pinto I, Chimeno P, Romo A, et al. Uterine fibroids: uterine artery embolization versus abdominal hysterectomy for treatment – a prospective randomized, and controlled clinical trial. Radiology 2003;226:425–431
8. Katsumori T, Kasahara T, Akazawa K. Long-term outcomes of uterine artery embolization using gelatin sponge particles alone for symptomatic fibroids. AJR Am J Roentgenol 2006;186:848–853
9. Spies JB, Bruno J, Czeyda-Pommersheim F, Magee S, Ascher S, Jha R. Long-term outcome of uterine artery embolization of leiomyomas. Obstet Gynecol 2005;106:933–939
10. Walker WJ, Barton-Smith P. Long-term follow up of uterine artery embolization – an effective alternative in the treatment of fibroids. BJOG 2006;113(4):464–468
11. Myers ER, Goodwin S, Landow W, et al. Prospective data collection of a new procedure by a specialty society: The FIBROID Registry. Obstet Gynecol 2005;106:44–51
12. Goldberg J, Pereira L, Mude-Nochumson H. Uterine artery embolization for symptomatic fibroids: pros and cons. OBG Management 23;15:69–79
13. Broder MS, Landow W, Goodwin S, Brook R, Sherbourne C, Harris K. An agenda for research into uterine artery embolization: results of an expert panel conference. J Vasc Interv Radiol 2000;11(4):509–515
14. Spies JB, Coyne K, Guaou Guaou N, Boyle D, Skyrnarz-Murphy K, Gonzalves S. The UFS-QOL, a new disease-specific symptom and health-related quality of life questionnaire for leiomyomata. Obstet Gynecol 2002;99:290–300
15. Spies JB, Cornell C, Worthington-Kirsch R, Lipman JC, Benenati JF. Long-term outcome from uterine fibroid embolization with tris-acryl gelatin microspheres: results of a multicenter study. J Vasc Interv Radiol 2007;18(2):203–207

III Fallopian Tube Interventions

11 Clinical Review: Infertility

Stephen Cohen

Preservation of the species is the most basic instinct of every animal species. The ability to have offspring is desired by most of the population. Unfortunately, many couples are unable to conceive. Infertility has been defined as the inability to become pregnant after a year of attempting conception.[1] It is estimated that 10 to 15% of reproductive age couples in the United States are infertile.[2] The incidence of infertility rises significantly as a woman ages, rising to 35% when she is 40 years old. Her eggs become more resistant to fertilization and the incidence of chromosome anomalies increases, raising the likelihood of early pregnancy loss.

The treatment of infertility is relatively unique in medicine because the practitioner is treating two patients together. During the last two decades, significant progress has been made in the prevention, diagnosis, and treatment of infertility. The American Society of Reproductive Medicine has been conducting a campaign to inform patients of preventable causes of infertility and describes ways to lower that risk. Research has provided evidence-based data that has better defined the clinical tests and treatments most likely to help infertile couples. Certain tests that were performed in the past have been abandoned, while new tests have been discovered. There have also been significant improvements in diagnostic imaging, which have allowed practitioners to better diagnose and understand the clinical condition of the patient.

Improvements in technology, pharmaceuticals, and imaging have revolutionized infertility treatments. New advances in surgical instrumentation allow the surgeon to use less invasive techniques and obtain better results. Medical therapy has improved our ability to treat ovulatory dysfunction and endometriosis. Advanced ultrasound imaging, in particular, has improved success rates with in vitro fertilization and intrauterine inseminations.

Traditionally, the infertility workup consists of a comprehensive multiple system evaluation of the many complex processes of reproduction that must be performed precisely so that conception will occur. Areas of study include semen viability, cervical mucus, the endometrial cavity, the uterus, the fallopian tubes, the ovaries, and the peritoneal cavity. A basic infertility workup usually takes 2 to 3 months. Often more than one problem is discovered.

■ Ovarian Factors

The most common cause of female infertility is problems with ovulation. Ovulatory dysfunction is found in ~15 to 20% of all infertile couples and accounts for up to 40% of infertility in women.[3] Ovulatory dysfunction can be classified as anovulation (absent ovulation) or oligoovulation (infrequent ovulation defined as less than 8 periods/year or cycles that are longer than 35 days), which can cause either gross or subtle menstrual disturbances.[4] There are many causes for ovulatory dysfunction including elevated androgens, polycystic ovary syndrome, thyroid disease, elevated prolactin, low body fat (due to eating disorders, extreme weight loss, extreme exercise, etc.), obesity, Cushing syndrome, and chronic medical problems. Polycystic ovary syndrome is one of the most common endocrine disorders in women of reproductive age and the most frequent cause of oligoovulation or anovulation.[5] Ovulation induction with clomiphene citrate or gonadotropins can be effective for these patients.[5]

A standard infertility laboratory evaluation will be diagnostic in most of these conditions. This includes obtaining progesterone, urinary luteinizing hormone (LH), thyroid-stimulating hormone (TSH), prolactin, and follicle-stimulating hormone (FSH) levels.[4] Basal body temperature charting is a simple way to document ovulation; a rise in temperature is generally noted 2 days after a surge in LH occurs.[6] Women older than 35 years of age may benefit from testing FSH levels on day 3 of the menstrual cycle to assess ovarian reserve.[7] Stimulation and suppression tests can be added when clinically appropriate. If a specific condition is discovered, directed treatment, such as administration of exogenous hormones, will often be successful at restoring ovulation. Similarly, evaluation of a patient with ovulatory dysfunction may lead a practitioner to recommend oocyte donation.[4]

In patients who are anovulatory without a medical problem that can be specifically addressed, ovulation induction is the recommended treatment. This can be achieved by administration of exogenous gonadotropins or by augmenting endogenous FSH with clomiphene citrate.[8] This drug blocks the negative estrogen feedback on the hypothalamus. Clomiphene is given once a day for

5 days shortly after a period to stimulate ovulation. The cycle can be monitored with ultrasound to evaluate the effects of the dose chosen. The information that ultrasound provides helps to fine-tune the timing and dose of clomiphene prescribed. The follicle size seen with this drug is usually slightly larger (22 to 24 mm) than those seen with spontaneous ovulation (20 mm). Clomiphene often produces two dominant follicles and so the twinning rate is increased in these patients (~25%). Adding the drug human chorionic gonadotropin (HCG) to create a timed ovulation is particularly useful in patients who need intrauterine inseminations. When unmonitored clomiphene cycles fail to produce a pregnancy, more aggressive intervention can improve the pregnancy rate. Ultrasound is the critical part of this more aggressive approach. The leading ovarian follicle is followed with ultrasound beginning approximately 2 days prior to the expected ovulation, usually day 12. When the follicle reaches a size of 18 to 20 mm, an injection of HCG, which acts like LH, is given. Ovulation will occur 36 to 44 hours later. Eighty percent of appropriately selected patients will ovulate with this treatment.[6] Aromatase-inhibitors, such as letrozole, may have the potential to replace clomiphene as an ovulation-inducing drug.[8]

Certain ovarian cysts decrease the fertility of women. Although any cyst may create infertility, an endometrioma is most likely to cause this problem. Disruption of ovarian function and ovum pickup are created by an endometrioma. In addition, severe pelvic adhesions involving the ovary, fallopian tube, and cul-de-sac are often associated with this type of cyst. The diagnosis of an endometrioma is confirmed via laparoscopy, but the condition is often first suggested by the pelvic ultrasound or magnetic resonance imaging (MRI) (**Fig. 11.1**). Not only is the ovarian cyst revealed, but these imaging modalities can usually demonstrate the unique characteristics of an endometrioma. Treatment of the benign ovarian cyst, regardless of the etiology, is surgical excision and in these cases, a cystectomy or oophorectomy will need to be performed. Depending on the pathology and condition of the patient, this surgery is either performed via operative laparoscopy or laparotomy.

■ Tubal Factors

Fallopian tube disease can account for up to 25 to 35% of all infertility cases.[9] The fallopian tube is an extremely complex organ that performs a vast array of physiologic processes, including ovum pickup, ovum transport, sperm transport, environmental support for the early embryo, and deposition of the embryo into the uterus. Even subtle changes of the fallopian tubal mucosa, such as those seen with ciliary immotility, can disrupt these complex processes. Any bacterial infection that can ascend into the fallopian tube might create structural damage which can inhibit the function of this fragile organ. The entire mucosal surface can be damaged by these infections. The most common infection creating tubal damage is *Chlamydia*, although many other bacteria can also damage the tube. The two areas of the tube that are most susceptible to an ascending infection are the intramural tube and the fimbrial portion. In the most severe situation, the infection creates a complete obstruction of the tube. An obstructed fallopian tube can therefore be due to an infection, can occur due to intraabdominal or pelvic surgery, or can be attributed to

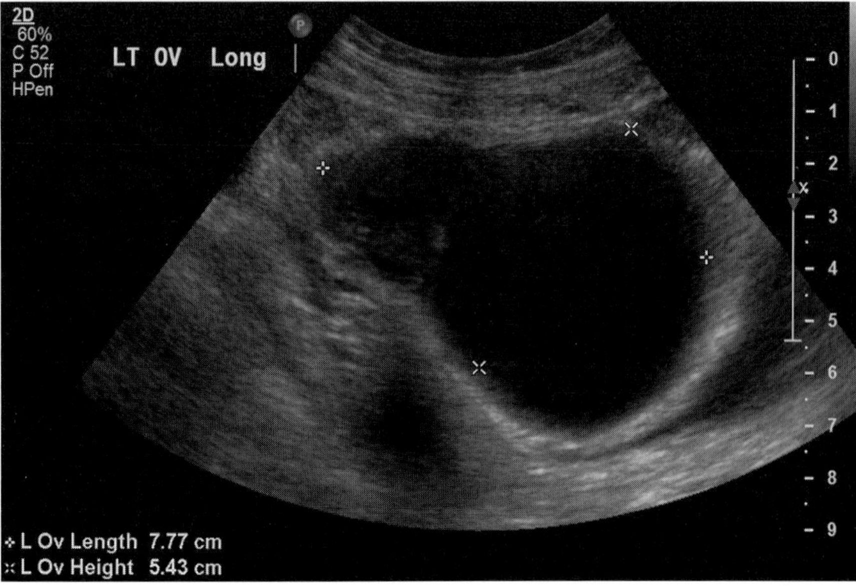

Fig. 11.1 Longitudinal ultrasound image of the left ovary in a 37-year-old patient with infertility. This image reveals a largely anechoic cyst within the left ovary that contains multiple internal echoes. On laparoscopy, this was found to represent an endometrioma.

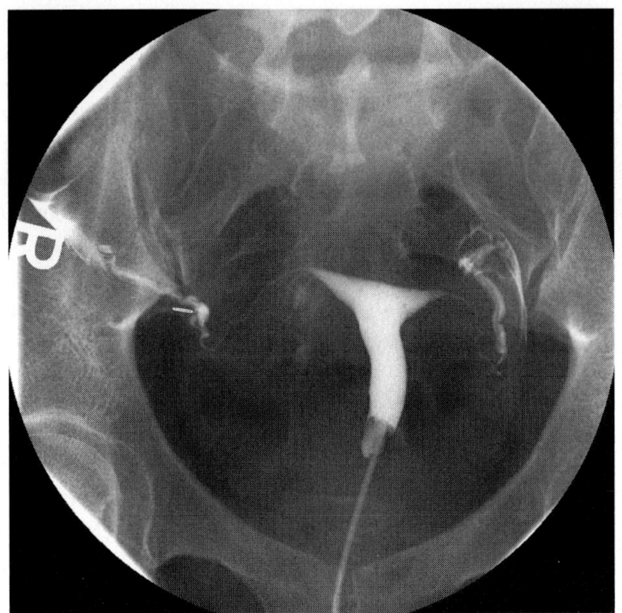

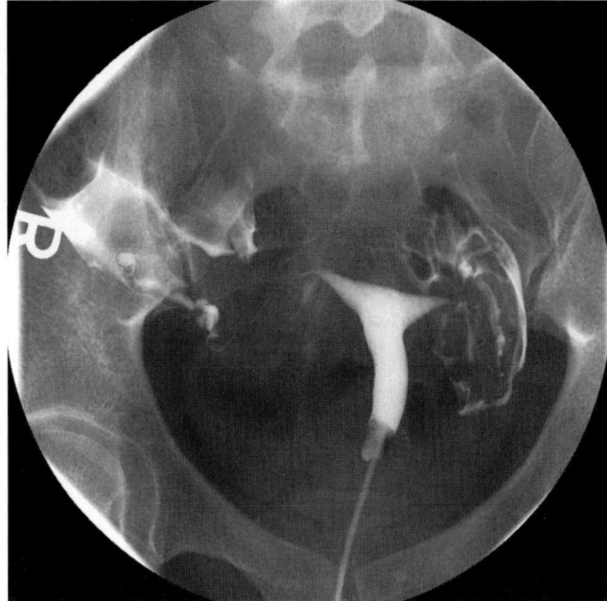

Fig. 11.2 (A) Early and **(B)** late view from a hysterosalpingogram in a 29-year-old patient with infertility. These images reveal a normal endometrial cavity and bilateral fallopian tube patency.

salpingitis isthmica nodosa or peritubal adhesions.[9] Many patients with fallopian tube disease will require either tubal reconstructive surgery or in vitro fertilization.[10]

The diagnosis of tubal damage or obstruction in an infertile woman is made initially by the hysterosalpingogram. During this procedure, water soluble contrast is administered into the endometrial cavity via a catheter or cannula. As the contrast is slowly infused, fluoroscopic monitoring enables the practitioner to demonstrate whether the fallopian tubes are patent by directly visualizing them and by demonstrating free spill of contrast into the peritoneal cavity (**Fig. 11.2**). During the initial slow filling of the tube, mucosal folds should be demonstrated. Alterations or absence of these folds implies prior tubal infection. If contrast enters the fallopian tube but free spill into the peritoneal cavity cannot be demonstrated, then distal tubal disease can be diagnosed. A large collection of contrast at the distal end of the tube, occurring with a gentle infusion, is indicative of a hydrosalpinx, which is important to diagnose in an infertile patient. Recent studies have demonstrated that a hydrosalpinx decreases the pregnancy rate in women undergoing in vitro fertilization cycles. It is now recommended that a tube containing a hydrosalpinx be excised via laparoscopy prior to attempting in vitro fertilization. The practitioner performing the hysterosalpingogram must gently infuse the contrast into the uterus. Excessive pressure or volume can create an iatrogenic-produced hydrosalpinx. The distal fallopian tube may also be damaged by infections occurring from inflammation or perforation of a nearby organ, such as the appendix or colon. In these situations, the tube itself is usually not damaged, but surrounded by extensive adhesions limiting ovum pickup.

Bilateral proximal tubal obstruction may be demonstrated on hysterosalpingogram during the infertility workup (**Fig. 11.3**). Although this finding may be accurate, one must consider that tubal spasm has caused a false-positive result. Visualization of only one patent fallopian tube on a hysterosalpingogram may possibly be because the contrast followed the path of least resistance through

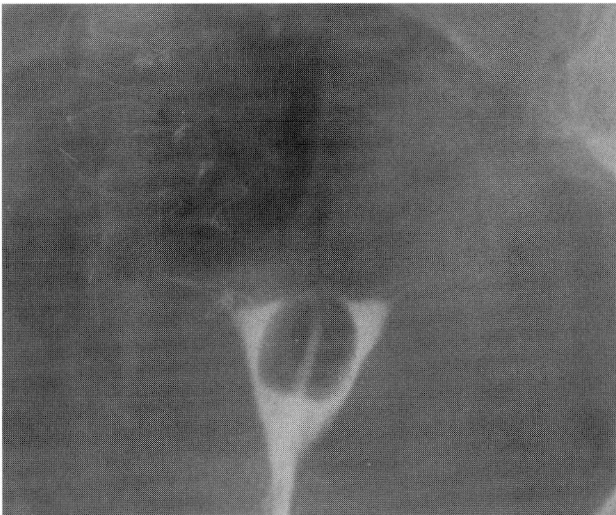

Fig. 11.3 Single anteroposterior (AP) view from a hysterosalpingogram in a 30-year-old patient with infertility. This image reveals bilateral proximal fallopian tube occlusion.

the fallopian tube that first demonstrated patency. Some studies have demonstrated an increased fecundity rate in patients who have undergone a hysterosalpingogram using oil-based contrast medium. The reason that this might be true is not known, but correction of structural abnormalities or changes in the immune response have been postulated as possibilities. If oil-based contrast is to be used, one should first demonstrate patency of the tubes with water-soluble contrast. Oil-based contrast has been shown to create granulation formation in the tube, and so it is important to demonstrate distal patency allowing egress of the contrast from the tube. In addition, oil-based contrast should be infused slowly under fluoroscopic control, so that intravascular infusions do not occur. Fatal outcomes during infusion of oil-based contrast were reported prior to the use of fluoroscopic monitoring. Women with proximal tubal obstruction may be treated with catheterization of the tubal ostia performed under fluoroscopic or hysteroscopic guidance. The technique of proximal fallopian tube recanalization using fluoroscopic guidance is addressed with more detail later in this section of the text.

■ Uterine Factors

Uterine abnormalities are commonly diagnosed in infertile women. These abnormalities, which include congenital uterine deformities, leiomyomata, endometrial polyps, and intrauterine adhesions (Asherman syndrome) impact fertility when they interfere with normal implantation and placentation.[11]

Congenital uterine abnormalities can range from subtle (arcuate or septate) deformities of the endometrial cavity to complex (bicornuate or didelphys) deformities of the entire uterus. Arcuate and septate uteri are contained within a single uterine cavity, whereas bicornuate and didelphys uteri have abnormalities of the walls with partial or complete duplication of the uterus. Each of these conditions can be associated with infertility, spontaneous abortion, and most frequently with premature labor and second-trimester deliveries. A septate uterus is the most common congenital abnormality of the uterus and also has the poorest reproductive outcome. It develops when the septum between the fused mullerian ducts fails to get resorbed early in fetal development. This disorder is associated with a fetal survival rate of 6 to 28% and a spontaneous abortion rate of >60%.[11] Imaging modalities such as hysterosalpingography, ultrasound, and MRI have all been shown to effectively diagnose each of these congenital abnormalities of the uterus (**Fig. 11.4**). Laparoscopy and/or hysteroscopy can be performed as well if there is doubt about the diagnosis based on the above imaging studies. Surgical correction of these arcuate and septate deformities can be performed via hysteroscopy. In patients who have had prior pregnancy losses, significantly improved delivery results will occur after the metroplasty is performed.[12–14] The repair of a bicornuate uterus usually requires a laparotomy, although laparoscopic repairs have been reported in the literature. Uterine didelphys rarely causes recurrent pregnancy loss, and thus surgery is not indicated in these patients.

Intrauterine adhesions (Asherman syndrome) usually occur following dilation and curettage (D&C) associated with a recent pregnancy, but can also occur in the presence of an estrogen-deficient state or after any endometrial injury (such as cesarean section, myomectomy, or endometrial tuberculosis).[11] Adhesions range from irrelevant to severe with severe adhesions associated with amenorrhea and infertility. Ultrasound, saline-infused ultrasound, hysterosalpingogram, and hysteroscopy are used to diagnose and classify the severity of these adhesions. Hysteroscopic lysis of these adhesions can be performed to relieve the menstrual abnormalities and improve fertility in these patients.[15,16]

Fibroids and polyps are often discovered during the workup of an infertility patient. Although many women with these problems will conceive without removal, others will need surgical removal to improve their likelihood of conception. Submucosal fibroids are more likely to create infertility than intramural or subserosal fibroids. The diagnosis of fibroids and polyps can be made with a hysterosalpingogram, ultrasound, or MRI (**Fig. 11.5** and **Fig. 11.6**); MRI is more accurate than ultrasound in the preoperative assessment of submucosal fibroids prior to hysteroscopic resection. Operative hysteroscopy is the surgical technique of choice for excising submucosal fibroids and polyps with the goal of preserving fertility, with uterine artery embolization having possible utility in patients not felt to be candidates for hysteroscopic resection. This is discussed in more detail earlier in this text. Hysteroscopic polypectomy does appear to improve pregnancy rates in patients with endometrial polyps and infertility.[17]

Endometrial factors can also impact fertility. Histological changes of the endometrium occur throughout the menstrual cycle in preparation for the arrival of the embryo. During the early phase of the cycle (proliferative phase) the vascularity and thickness of the endometrium increases. During the second half of the cycle (secretory phase), the endometrium shrinks, compacts, and becomes more glandular. This change is very important for normal implantation and embryo support. During the luteal phase, the endometrium demonstrates specific daily changes that can be recognized under the microscope. The endometrium that is "out of phase" may reject the early embryo and create infertility. This so-called luteal phase defect can be diagnosed by a timed office endometrial biopsy obtained a few days prior to menses. Adding supplemental progesterone during this phase of the cycle may correct this condition.

The endometrial biopsy may also show evidence of infection (chronic endometritis), which can be treated with antibiotics. The thickness of the endometrium is useful to monitor by ultrasound during cycles in which drugs have been used to stimulate ovulation. Commonly, the endometrium is noted to be thinner than in a spontaneous cycle. Progesterone support should be considered in these patients.

■ Cervical Factors

The cervix is critical to the fertilization process as it provides the mucus that stores and transmits the sperm to the upper genital tract. Normal cervical mucus, which is a

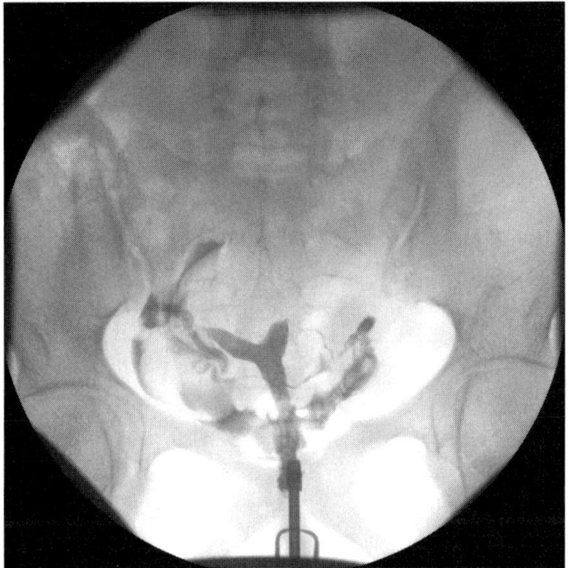

A

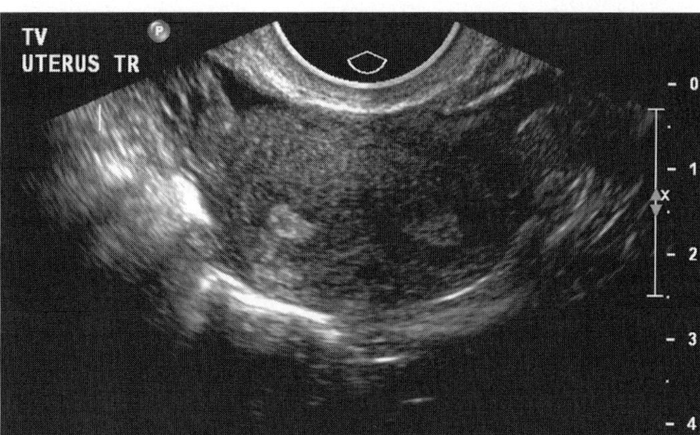

B

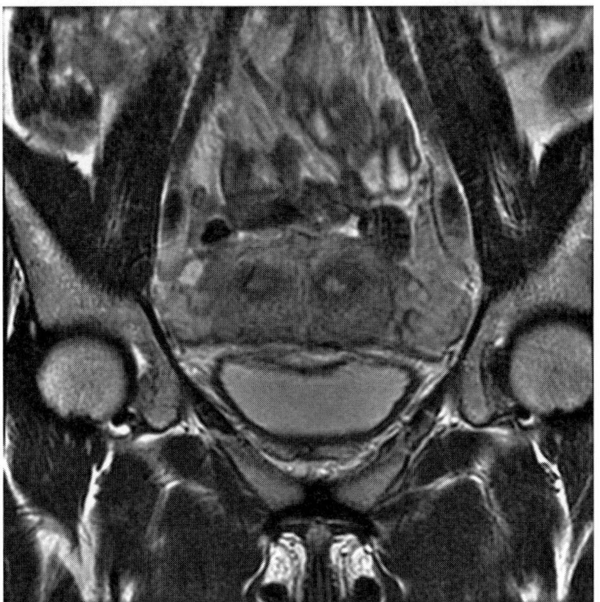

C

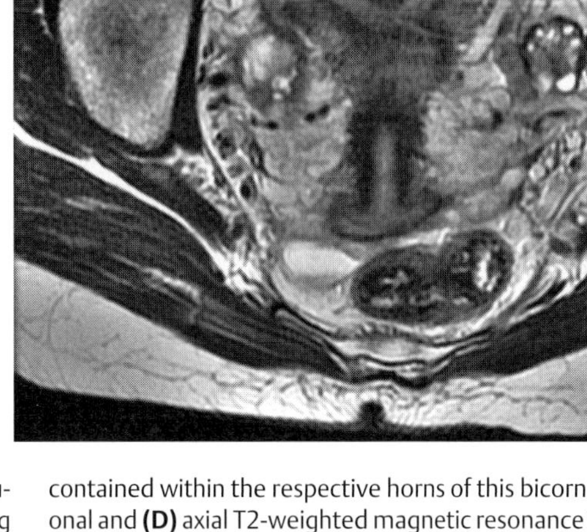

D

Fig. 11.4 Multiple images demonstrating the appearance of a bicornuate uterus. **(A)** Single image from a hysterosalpingogram demonstrating a single cervix and two distinct uterine horns. Bilateral fallopian tube patency is also seen on this image. **(B)** Single transverse image from a pelvic ultrasound demonstrating two distinct echogenic endometrial cavities contained within the respective horns of this bicornuate uterus. **(C)** Coronal and **(D)** axial T2-weighted magnetic resonance images of the uterus demonstrating the two horns of this bicornuate uterus, each containing a distinct endometrial cavity.

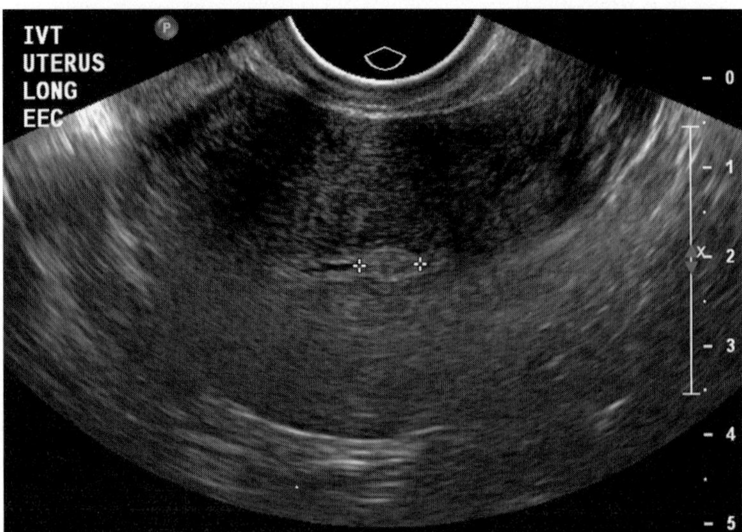

Fig. 11.5 Single transvaginal ultrasound image of the uterus demonstrating a small echogenic polyp within the endometrial cavity.

hydrogel consisting of water, proteins, and electrolytes, is produced in response to the secretion of estrogen immediately before ovulation. This mucus can facilitate fertilization by keeping normal sperm active for 48 hours or longer after intercourse, creating a much wider window for fertilization to occur. Motile sperm have been recorded in the cervical mucus for 5 days following ejaculation. After ovulation, mucus production by the cervical epithelium is inhibited by progesterone.

Abnormalities of cervical mucus production or sperm/mucus interaction prevent this process from occurring and are considered to be a significant problem in 10% of infertility cases.[4] All forms of vaginitis and cervicitis, can lead to a change in the pH of the cervical mucus, which might retard or prevent sperm transport.[18] Infection or sperm antibodies in the mucus may immobilize sperm, also hindering the fertilization process. Prior surgical procedures performed on the cervix, such as cone biopsy, loop electrical excision procedure (LEEP), laser or cryocautery of the cervix, often damage the cervix and reduce cervical mucus production.

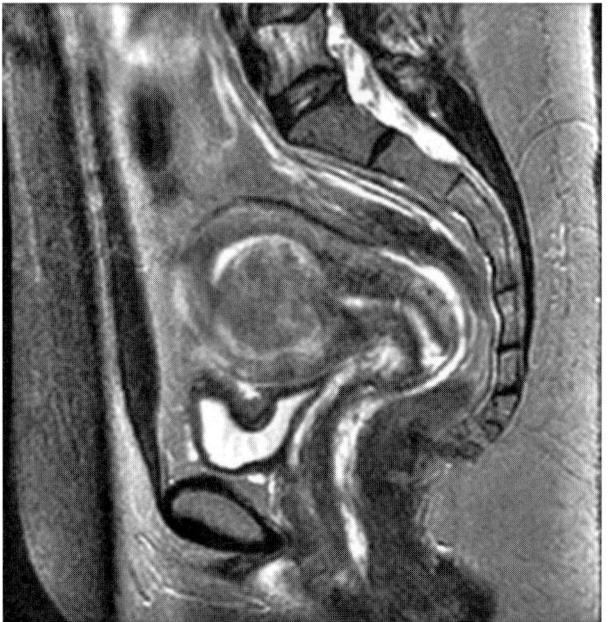

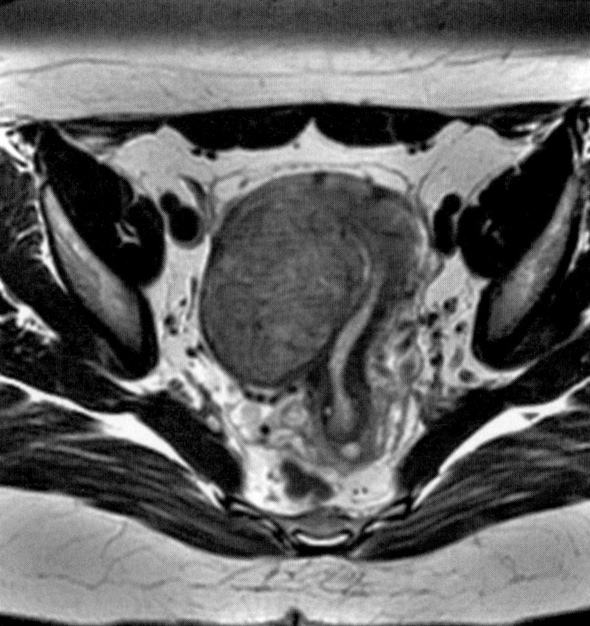

Fig. 11.6 **(A)** Sagittal and **(B)** axial T2-weighted magnetic resonance images of the uterus demonstrating a right-sided submucosal fibroid that is deviating the endometrial cavity to the left side of the uterus.

The postcoital test (PCT), an examination of the cervical mucus under the microscope after intercourse for surviving sperm, can be performed to diagnose cervical function.[19] This test is performed in close proximity to ovulation and can detect motile sperm within the mucus and assess the quality of the mucus. If a problem with cervical mucus is discovered, intrauterine inseminations can be performed to bypass the cervix and place the prepared sperm directly into the endometrial cavity. The PCT, which has been performed for over 100 years, is considered controversial as the results have not been shown to correlate well with pregnancy rates.[20]

■ Peritoneal Factors

Infertile women are often discovered to have intraabdominal pathology that can potentially explain their infertility. Endometriosis and pelvic adhesions are often found during the diagnostic workup of infertile patients. Both of these conditions can more typically cause chronic pelvic pain, but many patients diagnosed with these conditions do not have any symptoms, even when these processes are considered severe. Studies have suggested that 25 to 50% of infertile women have endometriosis and that 30 to 50% of women with endometriosis are infertile.[21] Although considered controversial, several mechanisms have been proposed to explain the association between endometriosis and infertility, including distorted pelvic anatomy, altered peritoneal function, altered endocrine function, and impaired implantation.[22–24] The diagnosis of both these conditions is made by laparoscopy. Prior to laparoscopy, one may get a sense of adhesive disease during a transvaginal ultrasound examination, if decreased mobility of the pelvic structures is demonstrated. Endometriosis and adhesions can be excised during laparoscopy. Endometriosis can be treated medically using gonadotropin agonists to lower the estrogen level. In addition, infertility related to endometriosis can potentially be addressed with clomiphene or gonadotropins with intrauterine insemination, or in vitro fertilization.[22]

■ Male Factors

Thirty to forty percent of couples are infertile because of a male factor and in 20% of cases, male and female factors can coexist.[25] These problems include hormonal abnormalities, chromosomal abnormalities (such as Y-chromosome microdeletions and cystic fibrosis), cryptorchidism, testicular cancer, abnormal spermatogenesis due to environmental exposures (such as industrial solvents, radiation, heavy metals, tobacco, etc.) or medications (e.g., cimetidine, ketoconazole), varicoceles, erectile dysfunction, premature ejaculation, neurologic disease (e.g., multiple sclerosis, diabetes mellitus), and genital tract obstruction (due to pediatric hernia repair, sexually transmitted diseases, etc.).[25–29] Certainly, the approval of new medical treatments for erectile dysfunction has made a significant impact in overcoming this problem. In patients who do not respond or are unable to use these drugs, the practitioner can perform vaginal inseminations or intrauterine inseminations with ejaculated and prepared sperm. Patients with spinal cord lesions and neurologic disease can be made to ejaculate with electroejaculation techniques (**Table 11.1**).

A semen analysis is typically used to determine the male contribution to infertility to assess sperm concentration, motility, and morphology. Low sperm counts, decreased sperm motility, and abnormal sperm form or morphology are the most common laboratory findings in these patients. A varicocele can explain many of these findings and is a common finding among males with an abnormal semen

Table 11.1 Causes of Male Infertility

Causes
Primary hypogonadism
Androgen insensitivity
Congenital or developmental testicular disorders
Cryptorchidism
Medications (including cimetidine, ketoconazole, spironolactone)
Orchitis
Radiation
Systemic disorders
Testicular trauma
Varicocele
Y Chromosome defects/microdeletions
Altered sperm transport
Absent vas deferens or obstruction
Epididymal absence or obstruction
Erectile dysfunction
Retrograde ejaculation
Secondary hypogonadism
Androgen excess state (such as exogenous administration)
Congenital idiopathic hypogonadotropic hypogonadism
Estrogen excess state
Infiltrative disorder (including sarcoidosis, tuberculosis)
Medication effect
Multiorgan genetic disorder
Pituitary adenoma
Trauma
Unknown (40–50%)

Source: From Jose-Miller AB, Boyden JW, Frey KA. Infertility. Am Fam Physician 2007;75:849–858. Reprinted by permission.

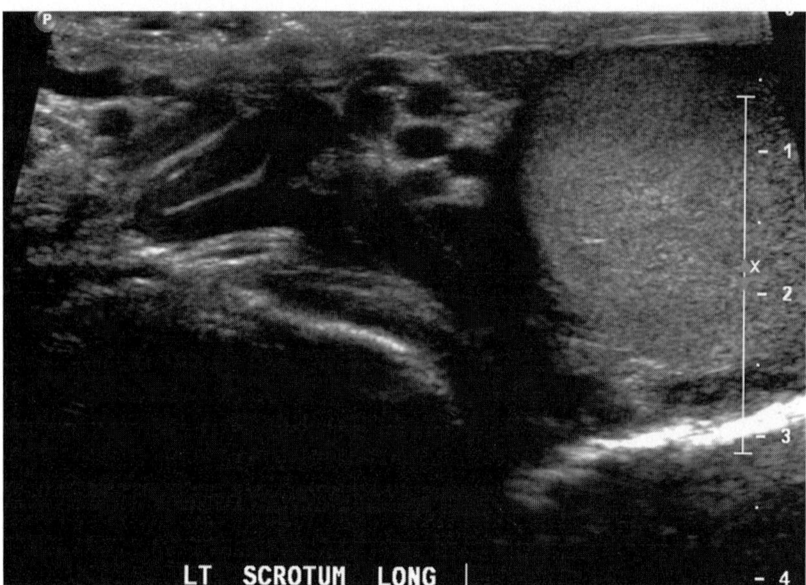

Fig. 11.7 Gray-scale image from a scrotal ultrasound demonstrating multiple vessels adjacent to the left testicle, which is consistent with a varicocele.

analysis. Therefore, all of these men should have a physical examination with special emphasis on testicular and scrotal anatomy and endocrine abnormalities. An ultrasound examination is recommended if a varicocele is suspected based on physical examination (**Fig. 11.7**). However, it is not recommended routinely because varicoceles that cannot be detected clinically are unlikely to be a cause of male infertility. If a varicocele is found, both surgical ligation and embolization of the gonadal vein are recognized treatment options in an effort to improve sperm motility. In males with azoospermia, endocrine assays and a testicular biopsy should be performed to determine if sperm production is absent or arrested. In those men with no identifiable or correctable cause of male subfertility, intracytoplasmic sperm injection offers one treatment option.[25]

■ Other Causes of Infertility

There are other causes of infertility and recurrent pregnancy loss including coagulation and clotting disorders, connective tissue abnormalities, sperm antibodies, and chromosome abnormalities and infections. Importantly, an age-related decline in female fertility has been demonstrated and is playing an increasing role in the evaluation and management of infertility as more women delay having children. This decline in fertility begins for women in their late twenties or early thirties and becomes more pronounced after the age of 35.[9,30] This is most likely attributable to abnormalities in the oocyte that appear to be more common in older women, including an abnormal meiotic spindle, an increased rate of single chromatid abnormalities, and increased mitochondrial DNA deletions.[9]

■ Conclusions

The diagnosis and treatment of the infertile couple is a complex process, requiring patience on behalf of the patients and physician. Often, many specialists become involved in the treatment, including gynecologists, urologists, endocrinologists, internists, and radiologists. Recent discoveries and advancements in pharmacology, embryology, and technology have significantly improved the likelihood that the infertile couple will be able to have a family. The interventional radiologist has become a vital member of the medical team working to improve results for the infertile couple.

References

1. The Practice Committee of the American Society for Reproductive Medicine. Definition of "infertility". Fertil Steril 2006;86(Suppl 4):S228
2. Mosher WD, Bachrach CA. Understanding U.S. fertility: continuity and change in the National Survey of Family Growth 1988–1995. Fam Plann Perspect 1996;28:4–12
3. Mosher WD, Pratt WF. Fecundicity and infertility in the United States: incidence and trends. Fertil Steril 1991;56:192–193
4. The Practice Committee of the American Society for Reproductive Medicine. Optimal evaluation of the infertile patient. Fertil Steril 2006;86(suppl 4):S264–S267
5. Norman RJ, Dewaillyu D, Legro RS, Hickey TE. Polycystic ovary syndrome. Lancet 2007;370:685–697
6. Jose-Miller AB, Boyden JW, Frey KA. Infertility. Am Fam Physician 2007;75:849–858
7. The Practice Committee of the American Society for Reproductive Medicine. Aging and infertility in women. Fertil Steril 2004;82(Suppl 1):S123–S130
8. Kafy S, Tulandi T. New advances in ovulation induction. Curr Opin Obstet Gynecol 2007;19:248–252
9. Adamson GD, Baker VL. Subfertility: causes, treatment, and outcome. Best Pract Res Clin Obstet Gynaecol 2003;17:169–185

10. The Practice Committee of the American Society for Reproductive Medicine. The role of tubal reconstructive surgery in the era of assisted reproductive technologies. Fertil Steril 2006;86(Suppl 4):S31–S34
11. Sanders B. Uterine factors and infertility. J Reprod Med 2006;51:169–176
12. Daly DC, Walters CA, Soto-Abors CE, et al. Hysteroscopic metroplasty: six years' experience. Obstet Gynecol 1989;73:201–205
13. Pabuccu R, Atay V, Urman B, et al. Hysterscopic treatment of septate uterus. Gynaecol Endosc 1995;4:213–215
14. Venturoli S, Colombo FM, Vianello F, et al. A study of hysteroscopic metroplasty in 141 women with a septate uterus. Arch Gynecol Obstet 2002;266:157–159
15. Capella-Allouc S, Morsad F, Rongieres-Bertrand C, et al. Hysteroscopic treatment of severe Asherman's syndrome and subsequent fertility. Hum Reprod 1999;14:1230–1233
16. Valle RF, Sciarra JJ. Intrauterine adhesions: hysteroscopic diagnosis, classification, treatment, and reproductive outcome. Am J Obstet Gynecol 1988;158:1459–1470
17. Varasteh NN, Neuwirth RS, Levin B, et al. Pregnancy rates after hysteroscopic polypectomy and myomectomy in infertile women. Obstet Gynecol 1999;94:168–171
18. Forti G, Krausz C. Clinical review 100: evaluation and treatment of the infertile couple. J Clin Endocrinol Metab 1998;83:4177–4188
19. Glatstein IZ, Harlow BL, Hornstein MD. Practice patterns among reproductive endocrinologists: further aspects of the infertility evaluation. Fertil Steril 1998;70:263–269
20. Oei SG, Helmerhorst FM, Bloemenkamp KW, et al. Effectiveness of the postcoital test: randomized controlled trial. BMJ 1998;317:502–505
21. Verkauf BS. The incidence, symptoms, and signs of endometriosis in fertile and infertile women. J Fla Med Assoc 1987;74:671–675
22. The Practice Committee of the American Society for Reproductive Medicine. Endometriosis and infertility. Fertil Steril 2006;86(Suppl 4):S156
23. Schenken RS, Asch RH, Williams RF, Hodgen GD. Etiology of infertility in monkeys with endometriosis: luteinized unruptured follicles, luteal phase defects, pelvic adhesions, and spontaneous abortions. Fertil Steril 1984;41:122–130
24. Lebovic DI, Mueller MD, Taylor RN. Immunobiology of endometriosis. Fertil Steril 2001;75:1–10
25. Chow V, Cheung AP. Male infertility. J Reprod Med 2006;51:149–156
26. Sigman M, Jarow JP. Endocrine evaluation of infertile men. Urology 1997;50:659–664
27. Pryor JL, Kent-First M, Muallem A, et al. Microdeletions in Y chromosome of infertile men. N Engl J Med 1997;336:534–539
28. Burrows PJ, Schrepferman G, Lipshultz LI. Comprehensive office evaluation in the new millennium. Urol Clin North Am 2002;29:873–894
29. Gorelick JI, Goldstein M. Loss of fertility in men with varicocele. Fertil Steril 1993;519:613–636
30. Dunson DB, Colombo B, Baird D. Changes with age in the level and duration of fertility in the menstrual cycle. Hum Reprod 2002;17:1399–1403

12 Fallopian Tube Recanalization

David M. Hovsepian and Gary P. Siskin

For nearly two decades, scientific studies have clearly demonstrated the role of selective salpingography and fallopian tube recanalization (FTR) in the evaluation and management of infertile patients.[1–23] The American Society for Reproductive Medicine (ASRM) recommends that selective salpingography should be the next step when a diagnostic hysterosalpingogram (HSG) reveals blockage of one or both fallopian tubes.[24] However, these techniques remain vastly underutilized for a variety of reasons. The number of FTRs performed annually in the United States represents only a small fraction of the 300,000 or so women who have blockage of their fallopian tubes that should be amenable to catheter-based intervention.[25,26]

The reasons for this are multiple. Foremost is a lack of familiarity with the ASRM guidelines by referring physicians and radiologists alike. There are also several practical issues related to circumstances and physician preferences. For instance, gynecologists who see infertile patients often perform diagnostic sonography or sonohysterography in their offices and perhaps proceed to in vitro techniques directly, avoiding radiologic tests altogether. Others may recommend laparoscopy from the start, with the goal of investigating any and all possible causes of infertility, buoyed by a handful of articles from a confusing literature. Patients usually have little choice in the matter. Additionally, on the radiology side, FTR may not be available or appropriate in some outpatient settings. Enthusiastic radiologists may find themselves frustrated, even when offering "one-stop shopping," by insurance, referral patterns, or other issues.

In university teaching hospitals, physical and logistical constraints often impede the ability to provide a comprehensive service. A division between diagnostic and interventional services frequently necessitates that FTRs be performed at a separate time and place by radiologists who routinely perform catheter-based procedures. Most interventional radiologists are at least familiar with the techniques involved and many have amassed considerable experience. All should be fundamentally aware, however, of the fertility benefits and low risk of complications.

In this chapter, fallopian tube recanalization will be reviewed, from patient selection to techniques, results and outcomes, and potential complications. Our intention is that most readers will readily come to appreciate that the techniques involved are straightforward and can easily be incorporated into practice. The results for this otherwise healthy and well-motivated group of patients can be quite gratifying.

■ Background Information

Fallopian tube recanalization is not a new or experimental technique. Radiologically speaking, it is prehistoric. In 1849, a London surgeon named W. Tyler Smith was among the first to describe the use of a whalebone bougie to reopen women's fallopian tubes using only tactile feedback to guide the procedure.[27] Over a century would pass before nonsurgical methods to reopen fallopian tubes that had become occluded would again be presented.

In 1977, a French radiologist, Dr. J-P Rouanet, published a case report describing the use of standard angiographic equipment to catheterize blocked fallopian tubes.[14] This was followed in 1985 by Platia and Krudy, who used a 3F catheter to clear proximally occluded fallopian tubes to treat infertile women.[28] A short time later, Dr. Amy Thurmond and her colleagues at the University of Oregon published a series of articles that established the methods and scientific validity of the procedure we know today as fallopian tube recanalization.[19,20,29–32] In the years that followed, the list of published series grew and FTR passed beyond the experimental stage into maturity, although many insurance companies still fail to reimburse treatments for infertility, FTR included, based on the perception that tubal occlusion is not truly a disease.

Much of the success of FTR rests on the fact that a proximal tubal occlusion is commonly caused by the accumulation of mucus and/or inflammatory debris, although the reason that mucus "plugs" develop remains a source of speculation.[33,34] Retrograde menstrual flow can occur[35] (which has also been suggested to be a cause of endometriosis, *Chlamydia* infection,[36] and impaired ciliary function[37,38] have all been implicated. More recently, work has focused on the influence of hormonally regulated mechanisms that control muscular contractions at the uterotubal junction and ciliary activity. Estrogen and progesterone affect direction and flow of tubal secretions, which may accumulate, inspissate, and eventually calcify.[33,34,39] Early intervention may restore a normal luminal interior, whereas chronic blockage can lead to irreversible damage.

Once the blockage is cleared, many fallopian tubes appear entirely normal and will resume function and allow conception.[40] However, endometriosis, prior surgery and severe pelvic infection can all produce transmural fibrosis and alter normal biological function (fallopian tubes are not just plumbing), so that even after successful recanalization, fertility is still impaired.

■ Patient Selection

Primary infertility is defined as the inability to conceive after 12 months of unprotected intercourse. Secondary infertility is the inability to conceive after previously being able to do so, and referred for FTR fall equally into both categories. Patients with secondary infertility often have had prior surgery or instrumentation and generally present more of a technical challenge to recanalization, but by no means should be excluded on this basis.

Most women referred for FTR have had a prior HSG documenting occlusion of one or both tubes. Sometimes laparoscopy with chromopertubation (dye injection into the uterus) has demonstrated the blockage. In a study sponsored by the World Health Organization that compared methods for evaluating tubal patency, the findings at laparoscopy and HSG were frequently discordant.[41] Nine percent of bilateral occlusions at laparoscopy were found to be patent at HSG, whereas 18% of unilaterally blocked tubes were found to actually be patent. However, false-negatives occurred as well; that is, tubes not visualized at HSG demonstrated spillage of dye at laparoscopy. Overall, the conclusions were that weight of the evidence supported dye injection during laparoscopy as the gold standard to document not only tubal patency, but also for uncovering other significant disease.[41] However, HSG remains a useful, low-cost screening tool.

Another study, published in 2006, found that the cumulative pregnancy rate did not change whether HSG was performed prior to laparoscopy and intervention, or if patients skipped the HSG and underwent the latter directly.[42] Unfortunately, the ASRM guidelines were not followed and no patient underwent selective catheterization after discovery of tubal blockage at the HSG. Therefore, the benefit of transcatheter therapy versus laparoscopic intervention remains an open question. In approximately one-quarter of the patients in that study, endometriosis was found and treated, which is a high proportion relative to the general infertile population, and FTR might be expected to have had less overall success in this group. Over 40% of patients in both arms of the study also underwent adjunctive fertility treatment (intrauterine insemination [IUI) or in vitro fertilization [IVF]), making it difficult to ascertain which aspects of treatment were responsible for the success.

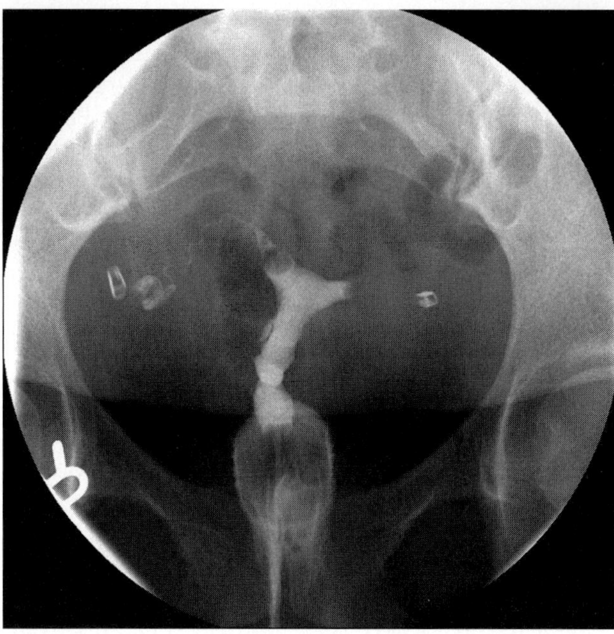

Fig. 12.1 This is a single image from a hysterosalpingogram demonstrating a patent right fallopian tube and a proximally occluded left fallopian tube.

Although one patent tube alone should be sufficient for conception, the side of ovulation varies month-to-month and the open tube will not regularly correspond to the side bearing the ovum. There are no consistent recommendations regarding what to do when an HSG shows that one tube is patent and the other is not (**Fig. 12.1**). However, unilateral spill on an HSG can be the result of asymmetric resistance to flow and be an artifact rather than represent an actual obstruction, so one should be careful not to jump to conclusions. Hayashi et al[5] evaluated the strategy of proceeding with FTR in 11 patients who had persistent occlusion of only one tube on two successive HSGs. They found that recanalization of the one blocked tube still added benefit, resulting in six pregnancies (55%) on the treated side, confirmed by preovulatory ultrasound examinations identifying a dominant follicle. Hovsepian et al[6] also found that having two patent tubes appeared to double the rate of conception, although their study was not sufficiently powered to observe statistical significance nor was the side of conception noted.

■ Technique

The patient is placed in the lithotomy position and the pelvis is elevated with a foam cushion or similar padding to allow room to maneuver the speculum (because most fluoroscopy tables cannot accommodate stirrups). The cervix is often located up along the anterior wall of the vagina, not straight ahead, with a posterior orientation that requires the speculum to be angled upward. Elevating the pelvis allows the handle of the speculum to clear the table. The perineum is cleaned with Betadine (Purdue Pharma, Stamford, CT), the patient is draped, and the speculum is inserted. Before cannulation, the cervix is also cleaned with Betadine. The procedure is usually done under sterile technique, with varying adherence to strict guidelines depending on the institution.

There are three principal styles of cervical catheterization that employ different equipment, two of which place an acorn-tip catheter on the exterior cervix. One, the Thurmond-Rösch Hysterocath (Cook, Inc., Bloomington, IN), uses a vacuum cup to maintain traction on the cervix, and the other, the Tenacath (Cook, Inc.), secures the cervix with a tenaculum. The third alternative, and there are a variety of products, is a form of balloon-tipped catheter that is advanced across the cervix into the endocervical canal or lower uterine segment.

All three styles have their advantages and disadvantages. The vacuum cup is often a challenge to advance through the speculum without contacting the vaginal walls (which can be very uncomfortable) and it is impossible to visualize the cervix as you are advancing it. The axis of the cervix can also deform the cup and interfere with the ability to maintain an adequate vacuum, whether using the manufacturer's pump or even wall suction. The Tenacath and balloon-tipped catheters have a lower profile and are easier than the vacuum cup to advance through a speculum.

Insertion of any of these devices can be greatly facilitated by advancing them coaxially over a catheter and guide wire. The catheter and wire together will help support passage of a balloon-tipped catheter through the cervix or help center an acorn-tipped catheter on the external os. A floppy guide wire, such as a 0.035" Bentson (Cook, Inc.) and an angled 5F catheter, such as a Kumpe or MPA (Cook, Inc.) make a good combination that will pass through any of the above devices. The same combination can also be used for fallopian tube catheterization once inside the uterine cavity.

The equipment is preloaded inside the outer cannula before insertion into the cervix. The external os is first engaged with the 5F catheter, then the guide wire is passed up, and the 5F catheter is advanced over the guide wire into the uterine cavity. The catheter and wire serve as the guide for the larger outer cannula. Insertion of a balloon-tipped catheter can be difficult into a nulliparous cervix, and the result can be to push the cervix away and potentially lose access. Often one is only able to position it just inside the endocervical canal. If the balloon is successfully advanced up to the lower uterine segment, gentle traction can be applied that can help to straighten out severe angles. Air is used to inflate the balloon, because saline or contrast will exert greater pressure on the tissues, which can be uncomfortable for hours afterward. Inflation of the balloon is also desirable for sealing the uterine cavity to allow continued visualization during catheterization of the tubal ostia.

Occasionally, the angles created by anteversion, retroversion, or flexion will preclude easy cannulation of the tubal ostia. Procedure time may become inadvisably long, translating to increased x-ray dose, so if traction with a balloon-tipped catheter is not an option, the use of a tenaculum is advisable. Using a tenaculum can cause more discomfort for the operator than it does for the patient, especially when anesthetic spray has been applied liberally to the cervix beforehand. Traction on the tenaculum not only gives better visualization of the uterine cavity, it usually makes selective catheterization of the fallopian tubes far easier. The natural shape of the 5F catheter engages the fallopian tube ostia easily and with less discomfort because the uterine fundus is not being stretched by a catheter pressing on it as it loops around.

Another advantage of the Hysterocath and Tenacath is the ability to perform a "push–pull" maneuver. By pushing forward and pulling back on the cervix, contrast that has emerged from the tubes into the peritoneal cavity can move to cover the outer surface of the uterus. This is extremely helpful for trying to differentiate a bicornuate from a septate uterus, by demonstrating contrast flowing over a rounded fundal surface or into a cleft between the uterine horns.

Once the cervix and endometrial cavity have been accessed, a hysterosalpingogram is performed to delineate the anatomy and identify the cornual regions of the uterus (**Fig. 12.2**). Not uncommon, proximal fallopian tube occlusion at a prior HSG is no longer evident. This is probably due, in part, to sedatives and narcotics, but can also be attributed to tubal spasm at the time of the initial HSG, which is a well-recognized phenomenon that can account for tubal patency when the examination is repeated at another time. Al-Jaroudi et al[1] demonstrated that 27% of patients will have tubal patency when a repeat hysterosalpingogram is performed immediately before a planned recanalization procedure. Conversely, a hysterosalpingogram immediately after recanalization can demonstrate pseudoobstruction due to spasm, and is a practice to avoid.

To catheterize the fallopian tubes, there are a variety of techniques and equipment available. It is important to remember that the uterus is a muscle that responds to stretching by contracting, producing interstitial occlusion and contractions that are similar to intense menstrual cramps by the patient. Pushing against the fundus of the

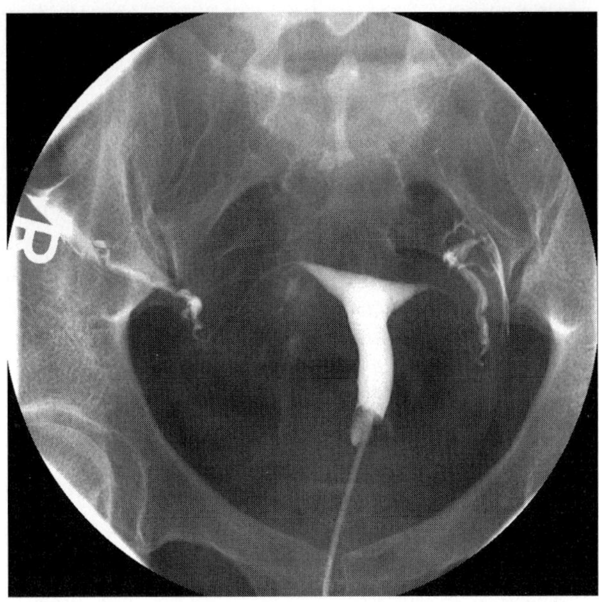

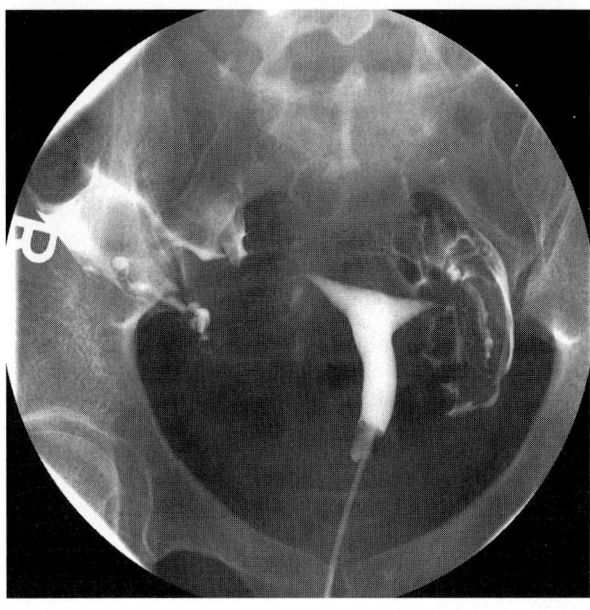

Fig. 12.2 This is an **(A)** early and **(B)** late image from a hysterosalpingogram performed in a patient presenting with infertility believed to be secondary to a proximal tubal occlusion observed on a previous hysterosalpingogram. This study demonstrated bilateral fallopian tube patency as evidenced by free spill of contrast into the peritoneal cavity on the late image.

uterus with any effort can cause unsedated patients to remember that aspect of the procedure to the exclusion of positive outcome.

The 5F catheter is advanced over a guide wire until it is pointing to the cornu. Often, the guide wire will then "funnel" into the tube and effectively recanalize it. Sometimes, the plug of debris requires a stiffer guide wire to dislodge it. An angled glide wire (Terumo Medical Corp., Somerset, NJ) is ideal for this purpose and Thurmond[30] showed no harmful effect of the hydrophilic coating on spermatic function.

The guide wire should not be advanced much beyond the interstitial portion of the fallopian tube because subintimal passage becomes more likely as one proceeds toward the fimbriated end. Only the interstitial segment is contained strictly within the myometrium. Beyond that point (1 to 1½ cm), the tube is much more delicate. If occlusion is encountered past the interstitial segment, use of a coaxial 3F microcatheter is recommended. Unfortunately, at this point, the cause of obstruction is more often fibrosis and recanalization is less likely to be successful and normal ciliary function is probably already compromised. Recanalization after tubal ligation reversal is similarly affected, but successful pregnancies have been reported, so it is still worth a try.[31,43]

Once the guide wire has traversed the obstruction and contrast injection shows patency has been restored, there is no advantage to trying to expand the tubal lumen ("Dottering" it) by advancing the catheter over the guide wire. Despite early reports describing successful balloon tuboplasty,[44] no definite advantage has been demonstrated. The process which causes tubal occlusion is not at all similar to atherosclerosis, so not only is that type of intervention unwarranted, it could also be potentially harmful.

Manometry of the tube has been suggested to correlate with conception rates,[45–47] but the technical factors involved in obtaining an accurate reading are significant, and the catheter itself is likely to take up much if not all of the submillimeter lumen. Tubal pressures in the range of 300 to 500 mm Hg have been considered indicative of an increased likelihood of tubal impairment,[48] but it is difficult to understand how such elevation above the normal systolic blood pressure can be achieved by the thin layer of smooth muscle cells surrounding the fallopian tubes.

■ Results, Outcomes, and Complications

When evaluating outcomes after selective salpingography and fallopian tube recanalization, it is important to consider procedural and clinical outcomes as separate measures. Technical success is often described in terms of the ability to restore patency to a fallopian tube that was found to be occluded by HSG or chromopertubation (**Fig. 12.3**). Once patency has been reestablished, the outcomes that are of interest are the rates of conception, intrauterine pregnancy, ectopic pregnancy, and live birth. These values can vary significantly depending on whether the denominator of the equation represents only the technical successes or an intent-to-treat cohort.

In 1987, Thurmond et al[19] were the first to publish their experience with FTR in seven infertile patients. In 1990, they summarized their experience with 100 consecutive patients, reporting a high technical success rate (95%) and a rate of conception of 26%.[20] In a well-defined subset in that series that included 20 patients who had nothing in their history to indicate the possibility of tubal disease, the conception rate climbed to 47% and there were no ectopic pregnancies. This result again attests to the fact noted by Dr. Smith and his contemporaries almost 160 years ago that, once cleared of debris, many tubes are essentially normal.

This was the case, too, for Lang and Dunaway in 1996, whose series of 400 patients included 213 whose obstruction on a prior HSG resolved with only prostaglandin antagonist and nonselective uterine injection or by selective salpingography.[43] (The authors did not record the pregnancy outcomes in this group, unfortunately.). The outcomes of the 145 who underwent guide wire recana-

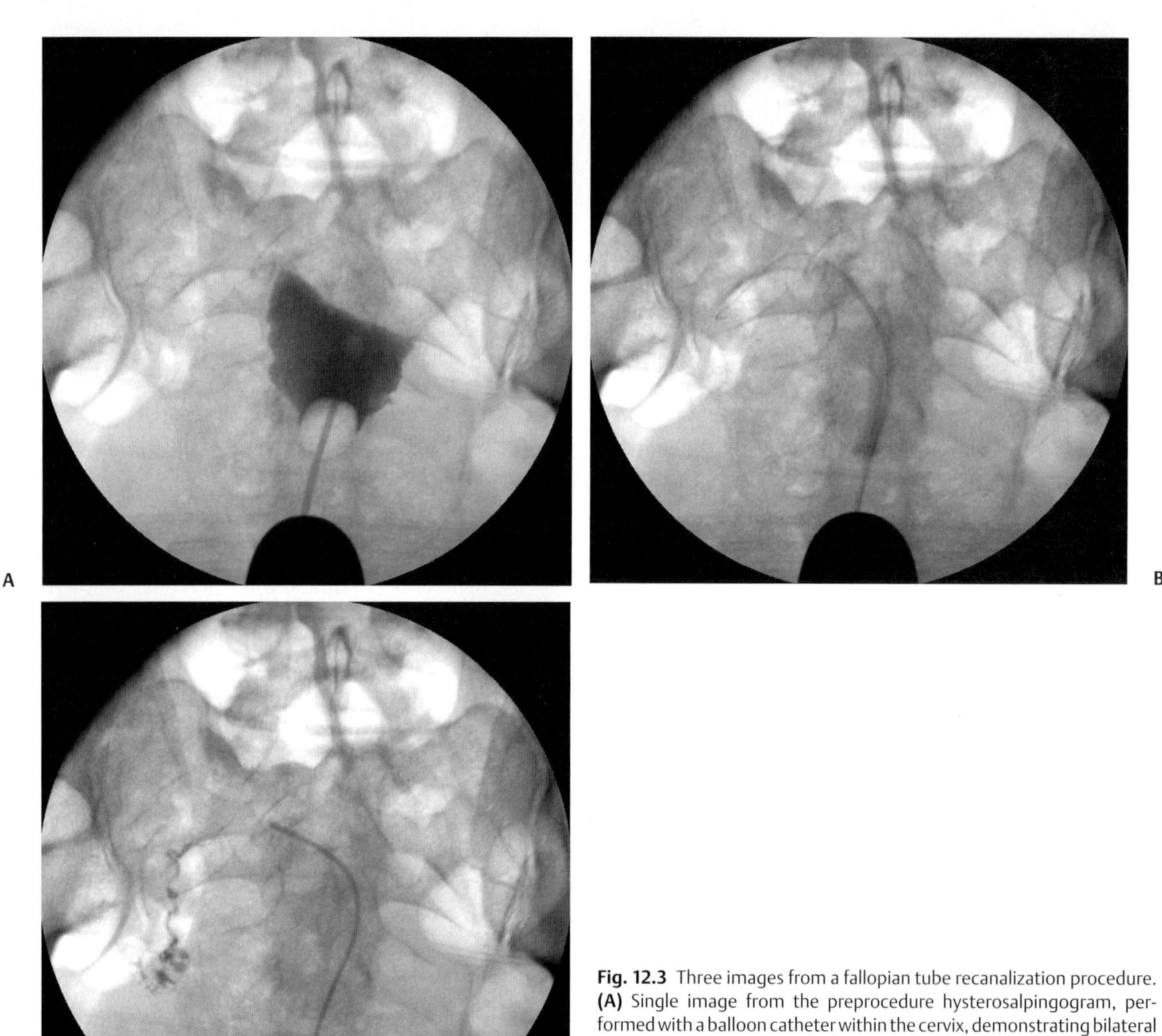

Fig. 12.3 Three images from a fallopian tube recanalization procedure. **(A)** Single image from the preprocedure hysterosalpingogram, performed with a balloon catheter within the cervix, demonstrating bilateral proximal fallopian tube occlusion. **(B)** Image demonstrating passage of a coaxial catheter and 0.018" guidewire into the proximal portion of the occluded right fallopian tube. **(C)** Single image from a contrast injection via the microcatheter within the right fallopian tube, demonstrating patency of the mid- and distal portions of this tube.

lization included 24 who became pregnant, 19 of whom had significant tubal disease, which is a below-average conception rate, perhaps reflecting more severe disease.

The reports by other investigators that followed the pioneering work by Thurmond et al confirmed the safety and effectiveness of this procedure, but some studies excluded patients for whom a positive outcome was thought to be unlikely. In 1994, Hovsepian et al[6] performed FTR in an unselected patient population. Forty-two procedures were performed in 37 patients, more than half of whom were found to have significant tubal disease. They were technically successful in reopening 71% of the occluded fallopian tubes, resulting in 14 conceptions (33%). There were 11 intrauterine pregnancies – five spontaneous first trimester abortions, five fullterm deliveries, and one ongoing pregnancy). There were three ectopic pregnancies, which occurred in three women who were noted to have had ectopic pregnancies before their procedure.

In the same year as Thurmond and Rösch published their landmark article, Kumpe et al reported their results for FTR in 22 infertile patients. With a technical success rate of 98%, five of their patients successfully conceived (23%). There were three intrauterine and two ectopic pregnancies. In 2004, Schmitz-Rode et al[49] reviewed their experience in 42 patients. Their technical success rate was 88% and the resulting fertility rate was 30%. In contrast to the experience of Kumpe et al,[8] but similar to Thurmond and Rösch, no ectopic pregnancies were reported.

In 2005, Al-Jaroudi et al[1] reviewed their experience in 98 patients referred for tubal obstruction by HSG. Of the 72 women with occlusion of both tubes at the start of the FTR procedure, they were able to open at least one tube in 25 patients (35%) and both in 44 (61%). The cumulative probability of conception was 28%, 59%, and 73% at 12, 18, and 24 months of follow-up. The median interval between the procedure and conception was 16.2 months. In contrast, much shorter times-to-conception were noted by Thurmond and Rösch[20] (4 months) and Pinto et al[50] (4.4 months).

In the largest series to date, Li et al retrospectively reviewed their experience in 1,006 patients.[11] The technical success rate was 88% among those patients with complete tubal occlusion. Approximately one-third of tubes were opened with selective salpingography, whereas two-thirds required passage of a guide wire to restore patency. The pregnancy rate was 40%, with an ectopic pregnancy rate of 3%. In the first year after the procedure, there was a 2% rate of reocclusion. This stands in contrast to Thurmond and Rösch, who found that four of eight patients studied between 2 and 10 months after FTR were found to have reocclusion of both tubes and two had reocclusion of one of two tubes recanalized earlier. In a later review, Dr. Thurmond quoted an average reocclusion rate of 30%.[51]

Although the indication for FTR is often primary infertility, many patients will present with secondary infertility due to a variety of causes. One interesting subset of these is women who have had tubal ligation reversal surgery. In 1994, Lang and Dunaway[52] described their early results with FTR in 19 such patients. The procedure succeeded most commonly when strictures developed focally at the site of reanastomosis. Three patients became pregnant after recanalization, but reocclusion occurred in 2 of 10 women who were reexamined between 6 and 36 months after the procedure.

In 1999, Thurmond et al[31] reported their results for 24 women in this same subgroup of FTR patients. Patency was reestablished in 68% of tubes. In the 13 patients who could only have conceived via a recanalized tube, the pregnancy rate was 46%. Of the six women who conceived, there were two intrauterine pregnancies (IUP), two early spontaneous abortions, and two tubal pregnancies. The mean time from procedure to conception was 2 months. In 2000, Houston et al[53] reported their experience in eight patients. They were able to recanalize at least one tube in five of eight patients (57%), which resulted in one IUP. Therefore, whereas FTR is technically feasible, the results reflect a much more abnormal substrate than that of the general population.

The complications associated with fallopian tube recanalization are rare and are often of minor clinical significance when they occur.[54] Tubal perforation is perhaps the most common and has been reported to occur on average in 2% of procedures.[54] Through-and-through perforation is rare. More commonly, what is perceived as perforation is actually submucosal passage of a hydrophilic guide wire that has encountered an obstruction beyond the interstitial portion of the tube. The event is usually imperceptible to the patient and rarely leads to more serious sequelae.

Complications such as bleeding or infection are extremely rare.[7,49] Peritonitis can occur, although at a frequency well below 1%,[55] particularly if prophylactic antibiotics are used, which is the current recommendation. Inoculation of the peritoneal cavity happens in much the same fashion that a diagnostic HSG transits perineal or vaginal flora via a patent fallopian tube into the peritoneal cavity. Pyosalpinx can result if a hydrosalpinx becomes contaminated during injection. Endometritis is also a rare possibility, although pinkish vaginal discharge is common for a day or two afterward, which is simply due to chemical irritation of the uterine lining.

Intravasation of contrast can occur if the catheter is not well seated in the tubal ostium or excessive force is used; although sometimes abnormalities of the uterus or tube at the point of obstruction may predispose to intravasation with only minimal effort. When opacification of any pelvic veins is appreciated, further injection should be discontinued, just as when early filling of a hydrosalpinx is suspected. Adverse outcomes are unlikely, but there is always the possibility of a contrast reaction, and if using an oil-based agent, lipid pneumonia can ensue, so proper informed consent is essential.

Ectopic pregnancy has been referred to previously, but deserves mention here as well. Although it may be considered a complication of FTR, occurring on average in 3% of cases,[54,55] the likelihood of ectopic pregnancy in tubes that appear normal after FTR should not be any higher than for the general population.[55] Kumpe et al[8] reported two ectopic pregnancies in 17 patients (12%), which is much higher than expected and probably signifies more severely diseased tubes. In our own experience, women who have had an ectopic pregnancy after FTR frequently have had another ectopic pregnancy prior to their FTR that did not always result in salpingectomy.

In general, FTR does not reopen tubes that are predisposed to ectopic pregnancy, especially when they appear normal, but after FTR many tube show evidence of lasting damage.[10,15,17] In fact, Sowa et al[17] felt that only 23% of fallopian tubes were truly normal after recanalization. The most common discovery in this unusually diseased population was peritubal adhesions, but other abnormalities included hydrosalpinx, salpingitis isthmica nodosa, and intratubal adhesions were noted.

Since the early days of FTR, many authors have added a total of ~3000 cases to the worldwide experience with FTR. Issues such as the use of oil-based versus water-soluble contrast, the need for bilateral recanalization, and reocclusion rates after FTR are important, and the following section examines these.

■ Discussion

Although FTR enjoys a high rate of technical success, the factors that impede successful outcome(s) are not always easy to understand. Clearly, there are anatomic as well as technical constraints. For instance, although the interstitial segment of the tube is generally straight or gently curved, coursing a centimeter or two before transitioning to the isthmic portion, that is not always the case. In a landmark article published in 1962, Sweeney examined 50 hysterectomy specimens and found that the intramural portion varied in length up to 3.5 cm and was often quite tortuous.[56] This report unfortunately deterred a generation from exploring catheter-based therapies, branding them as either misguided or experimental.

The pathological processes leading to occlusion of the fallopian tubes will also influence technical success. It has been well demonstrated that the further away from the interstitial segment that an occlusion is encountered, the less favorable the outcome because the blockage is more likely to be due to scarring and not a mucus plug. Hayashi et al[54] also reported an increase in the incidence of perforation or subintimal injury in patients with more distal disease and, as mentioned earlier, ectopic pregnancy may be more likely as well.

The large series by Li et al[11] attributed many technical failures to scarring and fibrosis in the distal tubes, which in general is commonly the result of pelvic inflammatory disease, although their series included cases of tuberculosis. They also reported technical failures with salpingitis isthmica nodosum (SIN). In contrast, other investigators have had some measure of success with FTR in these patients. For instance, Houston and Machan[58] reported their results in 1998 with 22 patients with SIN, which represented 6% of their overall population (349 patients). They achieved technical success in 69% of tubes, with encouraging results. Their rates of conception (23%), IUP (18%), and ectopic pregnancy (4.5%) were not significantly different from the average results with FTR in general.

Thurmond et al[58] reported similarly high technical success in patients with SIN (72%). Among the 19 women who were able to conceive only via a recanalized tube, there were six live births (32%) and two tubal pregnancies (10%). Based on these results, it would seem warranted to attempt FTR before embarking on microsurgery or in vitro techniques in patients known to have SIN by HSG or when SIN is discovered after proximal recanalization.

The most important outcome measure is successful pregnancy, and some diagnostic HSG series have suggested an improvement in pregnancy rates by the use of oil-based contrast agents,[21] but does this translate to improved results for FTR? Pinto et al[50] reviewed pregnancy outcomes after using a water-soluble agent followed by ETHIODOL (ethiodized oil; an oil-based, iodinated contrast) in 43 patients and water-soluble contrast alone in 50 patients. They found a weak trend toward a higher pregnancy rate in the oil-based contrast group, but this was not statistically significant. The mean time to pregnancy of 4.4 months was shorter for the oil-based agent, compared with the 7.7 months for water-soluble contrast.

■ Conclusions

FTR is a straightforward adjunct to diagnostic hysterosalpingography that most medical practices should be able to incorporate. Providing this service hinges mainly on whether conscious sedation is available for those patients who need it, not specialized skills or equipment. Technical success is gratifyingly routine, with almost no risk of significant complication. Most patients are otherwise healthy and infertile couples are understandably daunted by the expense and logistics accompanying the assortment of assisted reproductive technologies to choose from. FTR, a simple outpatient procedure, has the capacity to change lives.

References

1. Al-Jaroudi D, Herba MJ, Tulandi T. Reproductive performance after selective tubal catheterization. J Minim Invasive Gynecol 2005;12(2):150–152
2. Capitanio GL, Ferraiolo A, Croce S, Gazzo R, Anserini P, de Cecco L. Transcervical selective salpingography: a diagnostic and therapeutic approach to cases of proximal tubal injection failure. Fertil Steril 1991;55(6):1045–1050
3. Deaton JL, Gibson M, Riddick DH, Brumsted JR. Diagnosis and treatment of cornual obstruction using a flexible tip guidewire. Fertil Steril 1990;53(2):232–236
4. Ferraiolo A, Ferraro F, Remorgida V, Gorlero F, Capitanio GL, de Cecco L. Unexpected pregnancies after tubal recanalization failure with selective catheterization. Fertil Steril 1995;63(2):299–302
5. Hayashi M, Hoshimoto K, Ohkura T. Successful conception following fallopian tube recanalization in infertile patients with a unilateral proximally occluded tube and a contralateral patent tube. Hum Reprod 2003;18(1):96–99
6. Hovsepian DM, Bonn J, Eschelman DJ, Shapiro MJ, Sullivan KL, Gardiner GA Jr. Fallopian tube recanalization in an unrestricted patient population. Radiology 1994;190(1):137–140
7. Isaacson KB, Amendola M, Banner M, Glassner M, Sondheimer SJ. Transcervical fallopian tube recanalization: a safe and effective therapy for patients with proximal tubal obstruction. Int J Fertil 1992;37(2):106–110
8. Kumpe DA, Zwerdlinger SC, Rothbarth LJ, Durham JD, Albrecht BH. Proximal fallopian tube occlusion: diagnosis and treatment with transcervical fallopian tube catheterization. Radiology 1990;177(1):183–187
9. LaBerge JM, Ponec DJ, Gordon RL. Fallopian tube catheterization: modified fluoroscopic technique. Radiology 1990;176(1):283–284
10. Lang EK, Dunaway HE Jr. Efficacy of salpingography and transcervical recanalization in diagnosis, categorization, and treatment of fallopian tube obstruction. Cardiovasc Intervent Radiol 2000;23(6):417–422
11. Li QY, Zhou XL, Qin HP, Liu R. Analysis of 1006 cases with selective salpingography and fallopian tube recanalization. Zhonghua Fu Chan Ke Za Zhi 2004;39(2):80–82
12. Martensson O, Nilsson B, Ekelund L, Johansson J, Wickman G. Selective salpingography and fluoroscopic transcervical salpingoplasty for diagnosis and treatment of proximal fallopian tube occlusions. Acta Obstet Gynecol Scand 1993;72(6):458–464
13. Maubon A, Rouanet JP, Cover S, Courtieu C, Mares P. Fallopian tube recanalization by selective salpingography: an alternative to more invasive techniques? Hum Reprod 1992;7(10):1425–1428
14. Rouanet JP, Chalut J. An application of selective catheterization: salpingography: preliminary note. Nouv Presse Med 1977;6(31):2785
15. Sato M, Yamada R, Kimura M, et al. Transvaginal fallopian tube catheterization–diagnostic and therapeutic usefulness. Radiat Med 1993; 11(2):49–52
16. Segars JH, Herbert CM III, Moore DE, Hill GA, Wentz AC, Winfield AC. Selective fallopian tube cannulation: initial experience in an infertile population. Fertil Steril 1990;53(2):357–359
17. Sowa M, Shimamoto T, Nakano R, Sato M, Yamada R. Diagnosis and treatment of proximal tubal obstruction by fluoroscopic transcervical fallopian tube catheterization. Hum Reprod 1993;8(10):1711–1714
18. Thompson KA, Kiltz RJ, Koci T, Cabus ET, Kletzky OA. Transcervical fallopian tube catheterization and recanalization for proximal tubal obstruction. Fertil Steril 1994;61(2):243–247
19. Thurmond AS, Novy M, Uchida BT, Rosch J. Fallopian tube obstruction: selective salpingography and recanalization. Work in progress. Radiology 1987;163(2):511–514
20. Thurmond AS, Rosch J. Nonsurgical fallopian tube recanalization for treatment of infertility. Radiology 1990;174(2):371–374
21. Watson A, Vandekerckhove P, Lilford R, Vail A, Brosens I, Hughes E. A meta-analysis of the therapeutic role of oil soluble contrast media at hysterosalpingography: a surprising result? Fertil Steril 1994;61(3):470–477
22. Woolcott R, Petchpud A, O'Donnell P, Stanger J. Differential impact on pregnancy rate of selective salpingography, tubal catheterization and wire-guide recanalization in the treatment of proximal fallopian tube obstruction. Hum Reprod 1995;10(6):1423–1426
23. Zagoria RJ, Regan SW, Dyer RB. Nonsurgical fallopian tube recanalization for treatment of infertility. N C Med J 1991;52(10):491–493
24. The Practice Committee of the American Society for Reproductive Medicine. The role of tubal reconstructive surgery in the era of assisted reproductive technologies. Fertil Steril 2006;86:531–534
25. Serafini P, Batzofin J. Diagnosis of female infertility. A comprehensive approach. J Reprod Med 1989;34(1):29–40
26. Wadin K, Lonnemark M, Rasmussen C, Magnusson A. Frequency of proximal tubal obstruction in patients undergoing infertility evaluation. Acta Radiol 1994;35(4):357–360
27. Smith W. New method of treating sterility by removal of obstructions of the fallopian tubes. Lancet 1849;20(1):529–530
28. Platia MP, Krudy AG. Transvaginal fluoroscopic recanalization of a proximally occluded oviduct. Fertil Steril 1985;44(5):704–706
29. Hedgpeth PL, Thurmond AS, Fry R, Schmidgall JR, Rosch J. Radiographic fallopian tube recanalization: absorbed ovarian radiation dose. Radiology 1991;180(1):121–122
30. Thurmond AS. Use of hydrophilic guide wires in the fallopian tubes: effect on sperm survival and mouse embryo development. Radiology 1993;188(1):276
31. Thurmond AS, Brandt KR, Gorrill MJ. Tubal obstruction after ligation reversal surgery: results of catheter recanalization. Radiology 1999;210(3):747–750
32. Thurmond AS, Rosch J. Fallopian tubes: improved technique for catheterization. Radiology 1990;174(2):572–573
33. Sulak PJ, Letterie GS, Coddington CC, Hayslip CC, Woodward JE, Klein TA. Histology of proximal tubal occlusion. Fertil Steril 1987;48(3):437–440
34. Papaioannou S. A hypothesis for the pathogenesis and natural history of proximal tubal blockage. Hum Reprod 2004;19(3):481–485
35. Halme J, Hammond MG, Hulka JF, Raj SG, Talbert LM. Retrograde menstruation in healthy women and in patients with endometriosis. Obstet Gynecol 1984;64(2):151–154
36. Kosseim M, Brunham RC. Fallopian tube obstruction as a sequela to *Chlamydia trachomatis* infection. Eur J Clin Microbiol 1986;5(5):584–590
37. Critoph FN, Dennis KJ. Ciliary activity in the human oviduct. Br J Obstet Gynaecol 1977;84(3):216–218
38. Lyons RA, Djahanbakhch O, Mahmood T, et al. Fallopian tube ciliary beat frequency in relation to the stage of menstrual cycle and anatomical site. Hum Reprod 2002;17(3):584–588
39. Kerin JF, Surrey ES, Williams DB, Daykhovsky L, Grundfest WS. Falloposcopic observations of endotubal isthmic plugs as a cause of reversible obstruction and their histological characterization. J Laparoendosc Surg 1991;1(2):103–110
40. Lang EK. Organic vs functional obstruction of the fallopian tubes: differentiation with prostaglandin antagonist- and beta 2-agonist-mediated hysterosalpingography and selective ostial salpingography. AJR Am J Roentgenol 1991;157(1):77–80
41. World Health Organization. Comparative trial of tubal insufflation, hysterosalpingography, and laparoscopy with dye hydrotubation for assessment of tubal patency. World Health Organization. Fertil Steril 1986;46(6):1101–1107
42. Perquin DA, Dorr PJ, de Craen AJ, Helmerhorst FM. Routine use of hysterosalpingography prior to laparoscopy in the fertility workup: a multicentre randomized controlled trial. Hum Reprod 2006;21(5):1227–1231
43. Lang EK, Dunaway HH. Recanalization of obstructed fallopian tube by selective salpingography and transvaginal bougie dilatation: outcome and cost analysis. Fertil Steril 1996;66(2):210–215
44. Confino E, Tur-Kaspa I, De Cherney A, et al. Transcervical balloon tuboplasty: A multicenter study. JAMA 1990;264:2079–2082
45. Papaioannou S, Afnan M, Girling AJ, et al. The effect on pregnancy rates of tubal perfusion pressure reductions achieved by guide-wire tubal catheterization. Hum Reprod 2002;17(8):2174–2179

45. Karande CV, Pratt ED, Gleicher N. The assessment of tubal functional status by tubal perfusion pressure measurements. Hum Reprod Update 1996;2(5):429–433
46. Hilgers TW, Yeung P. Intratubal pressure before and after transcervical catheterization of the fallopian tubes. Fertil Steril 1999;72(1):174–178
47. Gleicher N, Parrilli M, Redding L, Pratt D, Karande V. Standardization of hysterosalpingography and selective salpingography: a valuable adjunct to simple opacification studies. Fertil Steril 1992;58(6):1136–1141
48. Schmitz-Rode T, Neulen J, Gunther RW. Fluoroscopically guided fallopian tube recanalization with a simplified set of instruments. Rofo 2004;176(10):1506–1509
49. Pinto AB, Hovsepian DM, Wattanakumtornkul S, Pilgram TK. Pregnancy outcomes after fallopian tube recanalization: oil-based versus water-soluble contrast agents. J Vasc Interv Radiol 2003;14(1):69–74
50. Thurmond AS. Selective salpingography and fallopian tube recanalization. AJR Am J Roentgenol 1991;156(1):33–38
51. Lang EK, Dunaway HH. Transcervical recanalization of strictures in the postoperative fallopian tube. Radiology 1994;191(2):507–512
52. Houston JG, Anderson D, Mills J, Harrold A. Fluoroscopically guided transcervical fallopian tube recanalization of post-sterilization reversal mid-tubal obstructions. Cardiovasc Intervent Radiol 2000;23(3):173–176
53. Thurmond AS, Machan LS, Maubon AJ, et al. A review of selective salpingography and fallopian tube catheterization. Radiographics 2000;20(6):1759–1768
54. Thurmond AS. Pregnancies after selective salpingography and tubal recanalization. Radiology 1994;190(1):11–13
55. Sweeney W. The interstitial portion of the uterine tube - its gross anatomy, course, and length. Obstet Gynecol 1962;19:3–8
56. Hayashi N, Kimoto T, Sakai T, et al. Fallopian tube disease: limited value of treatment with fallopian tube catheterization. Radiology 1994;190(1):141–143
57. Houston JG, Machan LS. Salpingitis isthmica nodosa: technical success and outcome of fluoroscopic transcervical fallopian tube recanalization. Cardiovasc Intervent Radiol 1998;21(1):31–35
58. Thurmond AS, Burry KA, Novy MJ. Salpingitis isthmica nodosa: results of transcervical fluoroscopic catheter recanalization. Fertil Steril 1995;63(4):715–722

13 Fallopian Tube Occlusion

Hugh McSwain and Mark F. Brodie

Permanent sterilization, which includes bilateral tubal sterilization (BTS) and vasectomy, is a widely used method of birth control because of its proven safety and effectiveness. An estimated 220 million people worldwide use permanent sterilization for birth control.[1] Approximately 10.7 million and 4.2 million American women currently rely on BTS and vasectomy for contraception, which represents 27.7% and 10.9%, respectively, of all contraceptive users in the United States.[2] BTS is the most common birth control method in the United States with over 700,000 procedures performed annually. With 500,000 vasectomy patients per year, the estimated annual market in the United States for permanent sterilization is 1.2 million patients.

Although both methods of permanent sterilization are effectively equivalent, BTS is more popular despite having greater morbidity.[3,4] Over the past 40 years, vasectomy has dropped in popularity relative to BTS; this is possibly due to the increasing safety of tubal ligation.[3] A recent development in female sterilization decreases the morbidity of BTS by accessing the fallopian tubes transcervically, thus eliminating the need for laparoscopy and the inherent risks of general anesthesia and the procedure itself.[5,6] In November 2002, the U.S. Food and Drug Administration (FDA) granted approval for transcervical hysteroscopic placement of the Essure device (Conceptus Inc., Mountain View, CA) for permanent birth control. Fluoroscopic placement of the device is possible and currently performed as an off-label use of the product.[7]

Background

The first known description of a method for fallopian tube occlusion was written by Blundell and published in 1828.[8] The method described bilateral partial salpingectomy with the theoretical result of permanent sterility, but no known attempts by Blundell to perform this procedure were published. Friorep followed in 1849 with his transcervical technique for tubal sterilization.[9] This is the earliest documented record of a transcervical method for tubal sterilization (TTS). His method used an application of silver nitrate solution into the proximal fallopian tubes to induce tubal occlusion. Pantaleoni built on the early work of Bozzini and used hysteroscopy as a diagnostic tool in 1869.[10] In 1934, Schroeder used hysteroscopy with electrocoagulation on two patients for TTS.[11] However, both patients had tubal patency when studied with a follow-up hysterosalpingogram (HSG). Hysteroscopic electrocoagulation for TTS was used in the 1970s with Quinones et al reporting a bilateral tubal occlusion rate of 80%.[12] Subsequent work did not reproduce this success and the method fell into disfavor.

Concurrent development of female sterilization via abdominal access proceeded in the early 20th century.[10] Laparotomy was most commonly used to access the fallopian tubes. Laparoscopic tubal sterilization using electrocoagulation was reported by Boesch in 1936.[13] Frangenheim first applied the method of bipolar electrocoagulation for tubal sterilization in 1972;[14] today, it is the most common method in the United States for laparoscopic tubal sterilization.[15] Other techniques use mechanical devices (e.g., Filshie clip, Falope ring, Hulka clip) to occlude the fallopian tube, which cause less destruction of the fallopian tube and pose no risk of electrical burns. Preserving the maximal amount of tube should always be considered given the possibility that a fallopian tube reconstruction procedure may be desired in the future. Reconstruction procedures are performed when a patient desires to regain her fertility after previous tubal sterilization.

Many methods for TTS have been reported in the literature. Though these methods vary greatly in design, the common endpoint is tubal occlusion. This is mediated via mechanical occlusion,[16–21] inflammation,[22–28] or a combination of the two.[5,6,29–34] Thurmond et al performed the initial evaluation of the Essure device in rabbits using hysteroscopy and fluoroscopy during the placement procedure.[35] This success led to FDA clinical trials of the device with subsequent approval for permanent birth control.

Patient Selection

Indications

Tubal sterilization is indicated when a woman does not want or cannot tolerate a pregnancy. This includes multiparous women not yet at menopause and women whose medical conditions are aggravated by or whose lives may be at risk during a pregnancy. The typical patient is a woman older than 30 years of age with two or more children and no plans for future childbearing. A patient should be screened carefully to determine if permanent sterilization is the correct form of birth control for her particular situation. For example, if she is concerned about protection against sexually transmitted disease and human immunodeficiency virus or regulating her menstrual cycle, permanent tubal sterilization may not be the best choice for her.

Contraindications

The foremost contraindications to tubal sterilization are a desire to maintain childbearing potential and concerns about permanent sterility. Other contraindications include pregnancy or a recent or current pelvic infection given the possibility of infecting the implanted device. Specific contraindications for the Essure device include patients who have had prior tubal ligation, termination of a pregnancy or child delivery <6 weeks prior to placement, the limitation of one coil for placement in the patient (i.e., uterine anomaly with single fallopian tube or proximal tubal occlusion on the contralateral side), immunosuppression, and menorrhagia/menometrorrhagia without a diagnosis.[36] Additional contraindications, which are annotated in the package insert for this device, are a known allergy to iodinated contrast media and a known hypersensitivity to nickel confirmed by a skin test.

A contrast allergy can be addressed by premedicating the patient using prednisone and diphenhydramine. Nickel hypersensitivity with intravascular stents and orthopedic prostheses has been addressed in the literature.[37–39] The possibility of early restenosis with nitinol intravascular stents in patients who exhibit nickel hypersensitivity has been debated.[38,39] Although no work has been published concerning hypersensitivity with nitinol in the fallopian tubes, nickel allergy is likely to remain a relative contraindication given the unknown long-term effects that may result from this condition.

■ Equipment

The optimal setup for performing fluoroscopy-guided transcervical tubal sterilization includes an all-purpose fluoroscopy room with a rotating C-arm. The use of lithotomy stirrups is highly recommended. A kit for sterilely preparing the perineum and vagina is needed; draping the legs and abdomen is also necessary. Either a metal speculum that can be resterilized after use or a disposable plastic speculum can be used to access the vaginal vault and visualize the cervix. A transcervical catheter is needed for uterine cavity access; we use a 12F catheter with a 5F catheter inner diameter and a side arm (Cook Medical Inc., Bloomington, IN) for injecting contrast and saline. A sterile cervical tenaculum for traction and sterile set of disposable cervical dilators (Cook Medical) should be available for every case, but may not be needed necessarily. Long-handle sponge forceps are useful to keep the vaginal vault dry during and after the procedure. Iodinated contrast (Visipaque 320; Amersham Health, Princeton, NJ) is used to perform the initial hysterosalpingogram (HSG) with selective salpingograms, if necessary. A 40 cm angled-tip 4F catheter (Cook Medical) is preferred for the selective salpingograms.

Because only the Essure device (Conceptus) is FDA-approved for transcervical BTS, all further references to the coil(s) will refer to this device (**Fig. 13.1**). The coil measures 4 cm in length with a maximum diameter of 2 mm when fully expanded (**Fig. 13.2**). An outer Nitinol coil surrounds a flexible stainless steel core wire containing polyethylene terephthalate fibers (Dacron; Invista Inc., Wichita, KS). The Dacron causes an inflammatory reaction in the fallopian tubes with resultant fibrosis limiting the possibility for tubal recanalization. The fibrotic in-growth occluding the tube at 3 months postprocedure has been well documented histologically.[40]

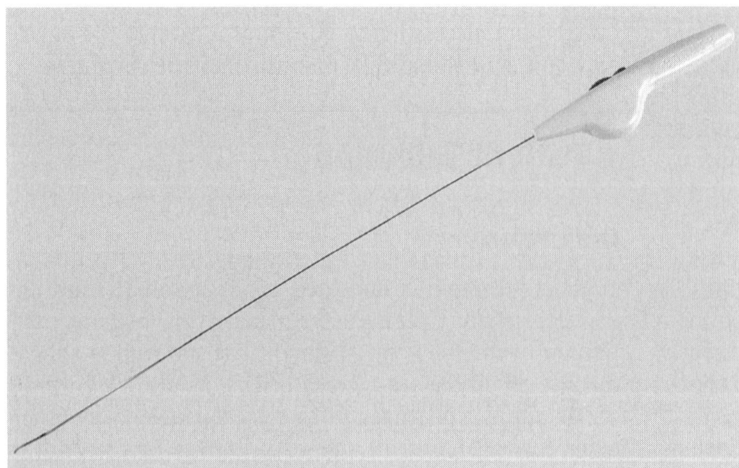

Fig. 13.1 The Essure device. The device contains the coil in its constrained configuration with a 10-degree angled tip to aid in selecting out the tubal ostium for placement. The outer diameter of the device shaft is 4.3F.

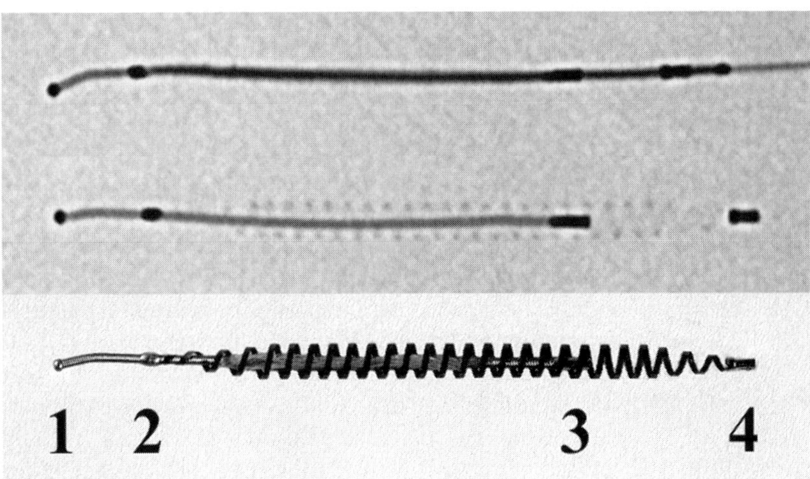

Fig. 13.2 From top to bottom, fluoroscopic images of the Essure device and a deployed coil with a photograph of a deployed coil. The radiopaque markers are labeled 1 to 4. The third marker is ideally placed at the tubal ostium.

■ Technique

Anatomy and Approach

The fallopian tube provides a conduit from the ovary to the uterus and consists primarily of circular and longitudinal smooth muscle fibers with multiple epithelial folds. The smooth muscle layers become thinner as the tube tracks from the uterus to the ovary; the diameter of the tube also increases correspondingly. The average fallopian tube measures 11 cm in length (range 7 to 16 cm) and is divided into four segments (**Fig. 13.3**): intramural (interstitial), isthmic, ampullary, and infundibular. The intramural segment is contained in the wall of the uterus beginning at the uterotubal ostium and ending at the uterotubal junction (UTJ). It measures 1.5 to 2.5 cm in length with a lumen of 0.8 to 1.4 mm in diameter in in vivo specimens.[41] The narrowest point of the fallopian tube is at the UTJ. The isthmus begins at the UTJ and ends at the ampullary–isthmic junction. Its length ranges from 2 to 3 cm with a diameter of 1 to 2 mm, making it the narrowest extrauterine segment. The ampullary segment is the most variable; it ranges from 5 to 8 cm in length with a diameter of 1.5 mm at the ampullary–isthmic junction to 10 mm at the ampullary–infundibular junction. The infundibular segment contains the fimbria and the opening to the peritoneal cavity.

The preprocedure workup prior to fallopian tube occlusion includes documentation of a recent pelvic examination with a normal Pap smear and negative gonorrhea and *Chlamydia* cultures. Fallopian tube embolization should be performed in the follicular phase (day 7 to 14) of the patient's menstrual cycle to limit the chance of a luteal phase

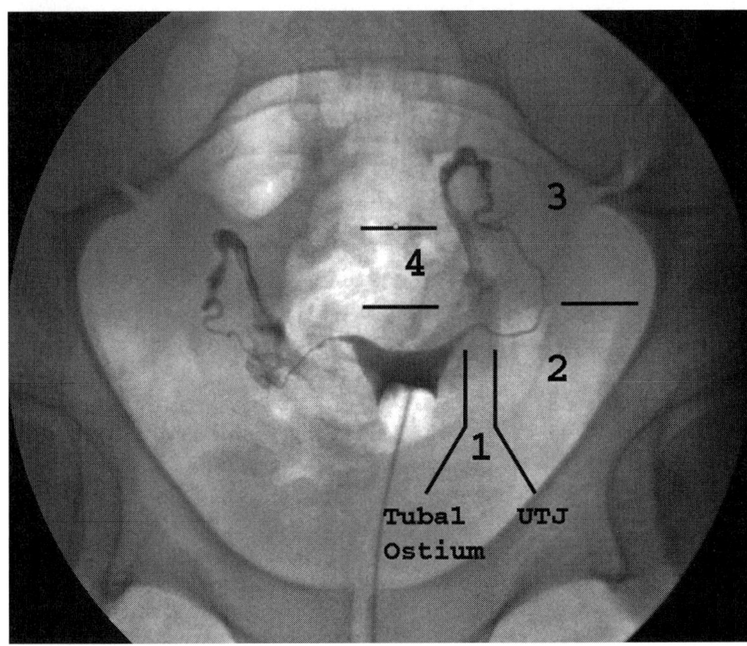

Fig. 13.3 Hysterosalpingogram demonstrates the relevant uterotubal anatomy. The labeled segments of the fallopian tube include (1) intramural (interstitial), (2) isthmic, (3) ampullary, and (4) infundibular. Note the uterotubal junction (UTJ) is the narrowest portion of the fallopian tube. The UTJ should be spanned with the coil to effectively occlude the tube.

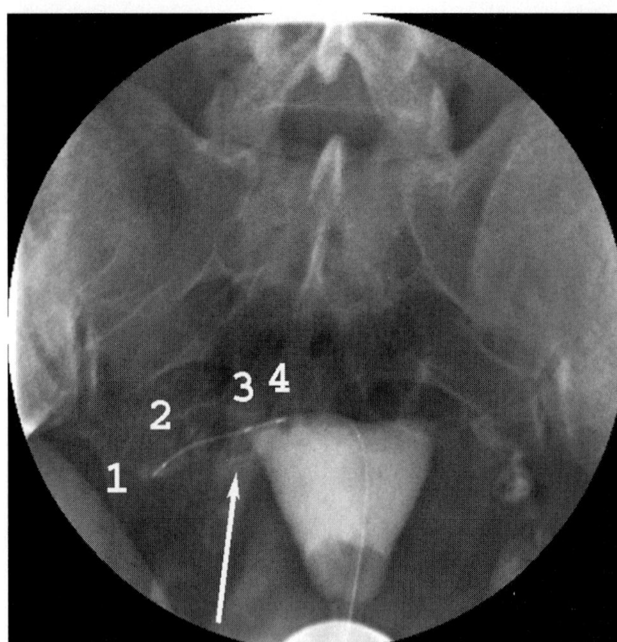

Fig. 13.4 Placement of the Essure device into the right fallopian tube with radiopaque markers labeled 1 to 4. The device has been advanced to place the third marker at the tubal ostium (*white arrow*). After satisfactory positioning, the coil is deployed.

pregnancy. A qualitative urine human chorionic gonadotropin (HCG) test is performed on the day of the procedure and the negative result documented before the start of the procedure. Preprocedure medications include 30 mg of ketorolac and 1 g of ceftriaxone intravenously. Ketorolac, a nonsteroidal antiinflammatory drug (NSAID), is helpful for postprocedure pain and cramping and may help with tubal spasm. With radiologic procedures such as HSGs and fallopian tube recanalizations (FTR), periprocedural administration of antibiotics (i.e., doxycycline) is widely practiced, but not universally. At our institution, we administer antibiotics for all gynecologic interventions. No preoperative antibiotics were given during the Essure pivotal trial with 507 attempted hysteroscopic device placement procedures and there were no reported cases of infection.[6]

This procedure can be performed under intravenous conscious sedation (i.e. midazolam and fentanyl) or with local anesthetic utilizing paracervical block anesthesia. If a paracervical block without intravenous conscious sedation is used for pain control during placement, several anatomic factors should be considered. The uterovaginal plexus lies predominantly lateral and posterior to the junction of the uterus and cervix. The cardinal ligaments transmit uterine nerves at the 3 and 9 o'clock positions and similarly, the uterosacral ligaments transmit nerves at the 5 and 7 o'clock positions. Injections of 1% lidocaine at the 3, 5, 7, and 9 o'clock positions at the cervicovaginal junction place the local anesthetic adjacent to the appropriate nerves; however, the injections at the 3 and 9 o'clock positions along the cervix risk entering the uterine arteries or veins that are present in the neurovascular bundles. Lidocaine injections with 3 to 5 mL at the 4 and 8 o'clock or 5 and 7 o'clock positions are recommended to maximize anesthesia and minimize risk to adjacent vessels.

The procedure begins with the patient in the lithotomy stirrups on the angiography table. The vulvar and perineal areas are sterilely prepared with an iodine-based solution followed by the placement of sterile drapes over the legs and the abdomen. A sterile speculum is placed in the vaginal vault and the cervix identified. Both the vaginal vault and cervix are prepared with the iodine solution. A 12F balloon cannula is used to access the uterine cavity transcervically. The internal balloon is inflated to seal against contrast leakage. A cervical tenaculum can be used if needed for traction on the uterus. An HSG is performed with an injection of contrast through the cannula sidearm. If neither or only one of the fallopian tubes is identified on the HSG, a 4F angled-tip catheter is used for selective salpingogram(s). Both fallopian tubes should be clearly seen in their entirety before beginning the placement of the device. After identification of the fallopian tubes, the tube that appears to offer more of a challenge to correct device placement should be selected for initial placement. This is based on Conceptus' recommendation: if bilateral microcoils cannot be placed, the procedure should be aborted.[36] Several factors that correlate with a more difficult device placement have been identified including a smaller caliber tube, a more tortuous tube, and a more acute angle at the UTJ.

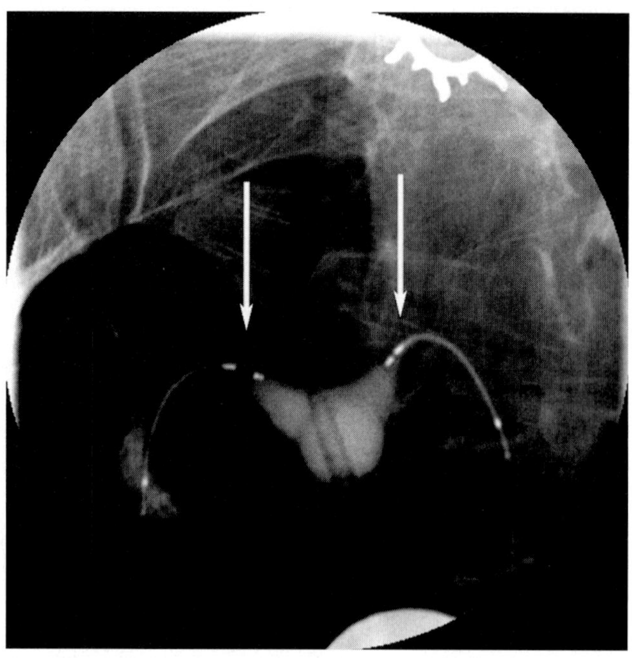

Fig. 13.5 Postbilateral coil placement in a different patient. Note the approximation of the third radiopaque markers to the tubal ostia (*white arrows*).

The Essure device has a 4.3F catheter outer diameter; it is placed through the 5F catheter working port of the cervical cannula. Using fluoroscopy, the device is engaged into the tubal ostium. The device is then advanced into the fallopian tube until the third radiopaque marker is at the level of the tubal ostium (**Fig. 13.4**). The coil is deployed and the placement process is then repeated with another Essure device to occlude the contralateral fallopian tube (**Fig. 13.5**). The internal balloon is deflated and the cervical cannula is then removed from the patient. The long-handle sponge forceps are used if needed to clean the vaginal vault of contrast and/or blood. The patient is taken to a holding or observation area for recovery and monitoring by a nurse postprocedure.

The patient and her significant other are instructed to use another form of contraception until correct coil position and tubal occlusion can be documented by HSG at a 3-month follow-up appointment. Alternate forms of birth control do not include a condom alone (it must be used in combination with another method) or an intrauterine method (i.e., an intrauterine device or intrauterine system – these may cause problems with the coils).

The HSG at the 3-month follow-up appointment is performed in a fashion similar to the FTE procedure previously described in the technique section with the following exceptions: no conscious sedation or local anesthesia is used with the 3F balloon transcervical catheter that can be used for uterine cavity access. The prescribed protocol for the 3-month HSG includes a minimum of six images: scout, minimal fill of the uterine cavity, partial fill of the uterine cavity, total fill of the uterine cavity, and bilateral oblique magnification views of the uterine cornua (**Fig. 13.6**). The

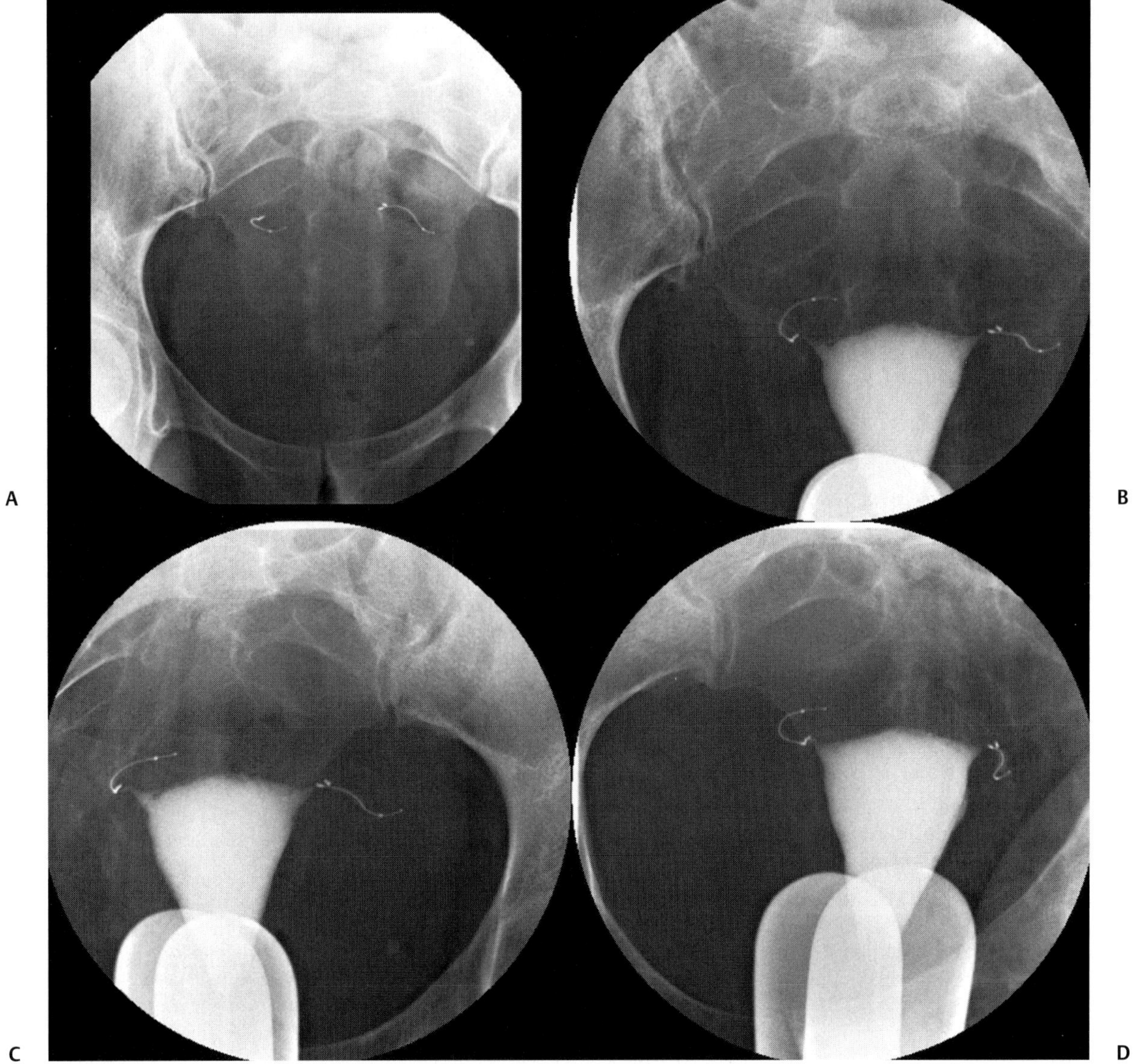

Fig. 13.6 Three-month follow-up hysterosalpingogram with **(A)** scout, **(B)** total fill of the uterine cavity, **(C)** oblique of the left cornua, and **(D)** oblique of the right cornua. The minimal fill and partial fill views are not shown.

Table 13.1 Hysterosalpingogram (HSG) Criteria for Grading Coil Placement and Tubal Occlusion

Grade	Coil Placement	Tubal Occlusion
I	Expulsion of coil or >50% of the coil inner length trails into uterine cavity	Tube is occluded at the cornua
II	Less than 50% of the inner coil length trails into uterine cavity or proximal end of inner coil is <30 mm into the tube from the tubal ostium	Contrast within the tube but not past any portion of the coil
III	Coil inner length proximal end is >30 mm distal to the tubal ostium or the coil is within the peritoneal cavity	Contrast past the coil or in the peritoneal cavity

To rely on the coils for sole method of birth control, the coil placement must be grade II and tubal occlusion must be grade I or II (gray shaded area). The coil inner length is defined as the coil between the first (distal end) and the third (proximal end) radiopaque markers.

coil placement and degree of tubal occlusion are assessed and graded (**Table 13.1**).

Technical Aspects

Although the procedure is not technically difficult in most cases, there are situations that can be challenging. In the case of a flexed uterus, the device can have problems tracking into the tubal ostium. Use of a cervical tenaculum to straighten the angles of the cervix and uterus is invaluable in this scenario to allow the device tip to engage the tubal ostium. Once the device has engaged the tubal ostium, there is a high likelihood that the device will track across the UTJ without difficulty. It is possible that the device tip can engage the tubal ostium and advance into the intramural tube segment, but then not progress significantly past the UTJ. In this case, a selective tubal ostium injection of 100 µg of nitroglycerin in a normal saline may allow the device to be advanced distally past the UTJ for successful device deployment. In the intramural and isthmic segments, the largest portion of the tubal wall consists of smooth muscle cells. Ekerhovd and Norström[42] documented the effects of nitric oxide donors on the contractility of the isthmic segment of human fallopian tubes. Nitroglycerin had a concentration-dependent inhibition of the smooth muscle contraction of fallopian tubes. Although our evidence is anecdotal, we feel the use of intratubal nitroglycerin has a physiologic basis for use during the procedure to relieve tubal spasm with few inherent risks.

■ Controversies

It is important to remember that a patient undergoing this procedure receives exposure to radiation using fluoroscopic guidance that she would not have experienced had she elected for hysteroscopic placement. The radiation dose for the follow-up HSG is equivalent for both placement methods. Hedgpeth et al reported their dose for fallopian tube recanalization patients as an estimated mean ovarian dose of 8.5 mGy.[43] We reported our initial results for device placement with a similar estimated dose of 8.5 mGy based on the fluoroscopy time and spot radiographs.[7] This dose is felt to represent a minimal risk to the ovaries.

The 3-month follow-up HSG is mandated by the FDA, but this requirement is not desirable for most patients. Other methods to assess coil location at 3 months postprocedure include pelvic radiographs or ultrasound, both of which have been described in the literature and are in clinical use in Europe and Australia.[44,45] Follow-up with radiographs is limited to patients in whom the initial placement was judged as satisfactory by the physician performing the procedure. A pelvic x-ray is obtained 3-months postprocedure and bilateral coil retention and location are confirmed. In the absence of abnormal positioning of the coils, tubal occlusion is assumed. HSG is only performed if the placement is felt to be suboptimal or there is an abnormality on the radiograph at 3 months. Heredia et al followed a series of 78 patients using the guidelines described above from October 2001 to early 2004.[44] Sixty-five patients (83%) underwent only pelvic radiograph followup; 17% underwent HSG due to perceived suboptimal placement at the time of the procedure. No pregnancies were reported in this patient population. This algorithm is used to limit the patients' discomfort, radiation exposure, added cost and inconvenience from an HSG. Ultrasound is used in a similar fashion, with or without contrast media to detect tubal patency; the coils are highly echogenic and easily visible on ultrasound (**Fig. 13.7**).[45] Although these methods may eventually replace the postprocedure HSG, they are not currently approved by the FDA and should not be considered as alternatives to the HSG in the United States.

Other transcervical sterilization devices (e.g., Adiana Complete [Cytyc Corp., Marlborough, MA], Ovion Eclipse [American Medical Systems, Minnetonka, MN], Invectus Intratubal Ligation Device [Invectus Biomedical, Salt Lake City, UT]) are not currently available in the United States for clinical application. The Adiana system uses a polymer matrix combined with a radiofrequency ablation limited exclusively to the UTJ.[46] Because the Essure coil has a uterine cavity component, the issue of future endometrial ablation

A

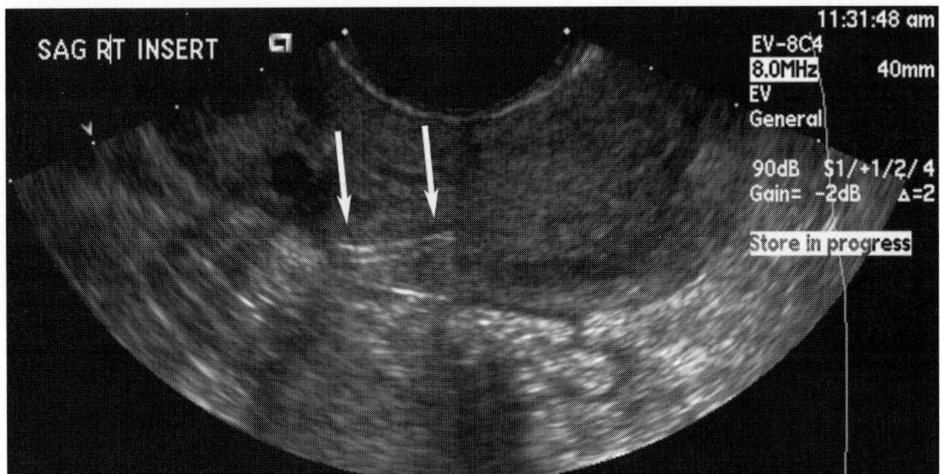

B

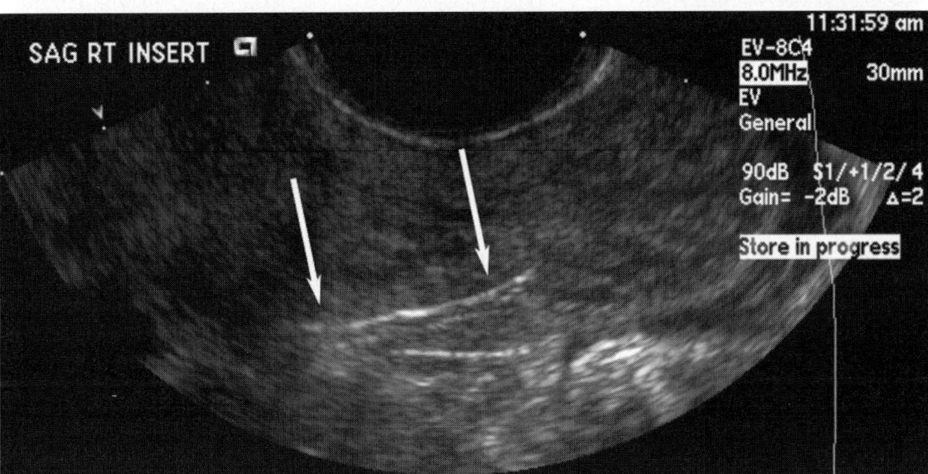

Fig. 13.7 (A,B) Endovaginal ultrasound. Note the echogenic outer nitinol coil (*white arrows*) easily distinguishable from the surrounding uterus and fallopian tube.

for Essure patients has been raised. Although the overall significance of this issue is unclear at this point, future technologies may have an advantage in this subset of patients.

■ Results

Data from the Essure phase II ($n = 227$) and pivotal trials using hysteroscopic placement ($n = 518$) included attempted placements in 745 patients;[5,6] the bilateral placement rates after two procedures were 88% (phase II) and 92% (pivotal). The reliance rate, which is defined as [(the number of women who are able to rely on the coils for birth control) divided by (the number of women with bilateral coil placement)] times 100, was 97% for both trials. The efficacy rate for the device in preventing pregnancy is 99.8%, effectively equal to BTL and vasectomy.

■ Complications

In the pivotal trial for the Essure device, the most common complications for hysteroscopic placement included coil expulsion (2.9%) and perforation (1.1%).[6] Cramping and/or pain and vaginal spotting occurred in the majority of patients and should be considered expected events postcoil placement.

No method of birth control is 100% effective. The possibility of pregnancy, including a high risk for an ectopic location, exists after a patient begins to rely on the coils for her primary birth control. For all methods of tubal sterilization, the probability of pregnancy after 10 years with tubal sterilization is 1.3% with 32.9% of these pregnancies occurring in ectopic locations.[47] To date, there have been 220,000 hysteroscopic Essure placements worldwide.[48] The most common cause (57%) of pregnancy in these patients is noncompliance with postplacement procedure protocol (physicians and patients). This includes failure to undergo the follow-up HSG and failure to prescribe alternative contraception following device placement. Also contributing to these pregnancies were probable pregnancy before coil placement (16%) and failure to adequately interpret the follow-up HSG (16%).

■ Postprocedure and Follow-up Care

After the coil placement procedure, virtually all patients are immediately ambulatory. Patients can expect vaginal spotting and abdominal and/or pelvic cramping. These are expected events and the cramping can be treated with NSAIDS. The patient is instructed to use an alternate form of birth control for 3 months after the coil placement, until the follow-up HSG is performed. After the follow-up HSG, the patient is informed of her results and whether or not she should rely solely on the coils for birth control. If she cannot rely on the coils at that time, the options and ramifications are discussed with her. All patients are instructed to take a home pregnancy test for any missed menses. If a home test result is positive, the patient should be seen expeditiously to evaluate for pregnancy, with special concern for an ectopic location.

Patients who have had coil placement or their referring physicians have expressed concerns regarding the safety of magnetic resonance imaging (MRI) after the procedure. The Essure coils have been reported as safe for both 1.5 and 3 Tesla MRI[49]; however, Muehler recently questioned this assertion.[50] He stated that "the publication refers to an examination of the interaction of biomedical implants with a 3-T static magnetic field, yielding no harmful deflection or torque for the Essure device. Nevertheless, determination of whether a device is MR safe goes beyond the interaction with the static magnetic field." The MR safety of the Essure coil at 1.5 T is not in question. The MR artifacts produced by the coil at 1.5 T in an ex vivo environment are relatively low. Unless the coil is exactly in the area of interest on the MR, the artifact should not be a limiting factor. On gradient echo sequences at 1.5 T or on sequences at 3 T, the metal artifact will be exaggerated; it is likely even under these circumstances, diagnostic quality images will be obtained.[51]

■ Conclusions

Transcervical fallopian tube occlusion for permanent birth control has been proven safe and effective when performed hysteroscopically; preliminary results for fluoroscopic placement are encouraging. The interventional radiologist should be familiar with expected outcomes and complication rates with this procedure; the patient should understand placement using fluoroscopic guidance is an off-label use of an FDA-approved medical device. Patient follow-up at 3 months after the initial placement procedure for an HSG is essential. Continued research in this area will be necessary to validate the fluoroscopic approach against hysteropic placement in hopes of approval by the FDA for this method.

References

1. Engender Health. Contraceptive sterilization: global issues and trends. New York: Engender Health; 2002
2. Piccinino LJ, Mosher WD. Trends in contraceptive use in the United States: 1982–1995. Fam Plann Perspect 1998;30:4–10
3. Chandra A. Surgical sterilization in the United States: prevalence and characteristics, 1965–95. Vital Health Stat 23 1998;20:1–33
4. Hendrix NW, Chauhan SP, Morrison JC. Sterilization and its consequences. Obstet Gynecol Surv 1999;54:766–777
5. Kerin JF, Cooper JM, Price T, et al. Hysteroscopic sterilization using a micro-insert device: results of a multicentre Phase II study. Hum Reprod 2003;18:1223–1230
6. Cooper JM, Carignan CS, Cher D, Kerin JF. Microinsert nonincisional hysteroscopic sterilization. Obstet Gynecol 2003;102:59–67
7. McSwain H, Shaw C, Hall LD. Placement of the Essure permanent birth control device with fluoroscopic guidance: a novel method for tubal sterilization. J Vasc Interv Radiol 2005;16:1007–1012
8. Blundell J. Lectures on the theory and practice of midwifery: a standard pelvis. Lancet 1828;8:65
9. Friorep R. Zur vorbeugung der notwendigkeit des kaiserschnitts und der perforation. Notiz Geburtshilfe Natur Und Heilkunde 1849;221:9–10
10. Magos A, Chapman L. Hysteroscopic tubal sterilization. Obstet Gynecol Clin North Am 2004;31:705–719
11. Schroeder C. Uber den avsbau und die leistungen der hysteroskopie. Arch Gynecol Obstet 1934;156:407
12. Quinones R, Alvarado A, Lev E. Hysteroscopic sterilization. Int J Gynaecol Obstet 1976;14(1):27–34
13. Boesch PF. Laproskopie. Schweiz Z Krankenh Anstaltw 1936;6:62.
14. Frangenheim H. Laparoscopy and culdoscopy in gynaecology. London: Butterworth; 1972.
15. Clinical Management Guidelines for Obstetrician-Gynecologists. ACOG Practice Bulletin No. 46. Benefits and Risks of Sterilization. Obstet Gynecol 2003;102:647–658
16. Schmitz-Rode T, Ross PL, Timmermans H, Thurmond AS, Gunther RW, Rosch J. Experimental nonsurgical female sterilization: transcervical implantation of microspindles in fallopian tubes. J Vasc Interv Radiol 1994;5:905–910
17. Ross PL, Thurmond AS, Uchida BT, Jones MK, Scanlan RM, Kessel E. Transcatheter tubal sterilization in rabbits: technique and results. Invest Radiol 1994;29:570–573
18. Maubon AJ, Thurmond AS, Laurent A, et al. Tubal sterilization by means of selective catheterization: comparison of a hydrogel and a collagen glue. J Vasc Interv Radiol 1996;7:733–736
19. Reed TP, Erb R. Hysteroscopic tubal occlusion with silicone rubber. Obstet Gynecol 1983;61:388–392
20. Ligt-Veneman NGP, Tinga DJ, Kragt H, Brandsma G, van der Leij G. The efficacy of the intratubal silicone in the Ovabloc hysteroscopic method of sterilization. Acta Obstet Gynecol Scand 1999;78:824–825
21. Hart R, Scott P, Ruach M, Magos A. Development of a novel method of female sterilization. Retention of tubal screws in patients undergoing simultaneous laparoscopic sterilization. J Laparoendosc Adv Surg Tech A 2002;12:435–439
22. Zipper J, Cole LP, Goldsmith A, et al. Quinacrine hydrochloride pellets: preliminary data on a nonsurgical method of female sterilization. Int J Gynaecol Obstet 1980;18:275–279

23. Mullick B, Mumford SD, Kessel E. Studies of quinacrine and of tetracycline for nonsurgical female sterilization. Adv Contracept 1987;3:245–254
24. Hieu DT, Tan TT, Tan DN, Nguyet PT, Than P, Vinh DQ. 31,781 cases of non-surgical female sterilization with quinacrine pellets in Vietnam. Lancet 1993;342:213–217
25. Tang GW, Kwan M. Non-surgical sterilization using phenol-mucilage: acceptability versus efficacy. Contraception 1988;37:599–606
26. Brumsted JR, Shirk G, Soderling MJ, Reed T. Attempted transcervical occlusion of the fallopian tube with the Nd:YAG laser. Obstet Gynecol 1991;77:327–328
27. Kukreja LM. In vitro occlusion of human fallopian tubes with the Nd: YAG laser. Natl Med J India 1998;11:122–124
28. Hurst BS, Thomsen S, Lawes K, Ryan T. Controlled radiofrequency endotubal sterilization. Adv Contracept 1998;14:147–152
29. Kerin JF, Carignan CS, Cher D. The safety and effectiveness of a new hysteroscopic method for permanent birth control: results of the first Essure PBC clinical study. Aust N Z J Obstet Gynaecol 2001;41:364–370
30. Maubon AJ, Thurmond AS, Laurent A, Honiger JE, Scanlan RM, Rouanet JP. Selective tubal sterilization in rabbits: experience with a hydrogel combined with a sclerosing agent. Radiology 1994;193:721–723
31. Berkey GS, Nelson R, Zuckerman AM, Delehey D, Cope C. Sterilization with methylcyano-acrylate induced fallopian tube occlusion and a nonsurgical transvaginal approach in rabbits. J Vasc Interv Radiol 1995;6:669–674
32. Pelage JP, Herbreteau D, Paillon JF, Murray JM, Rymer R, Garance P. Selective salpingography and fallopian tubal occlusion with n-butyl-2-cyanoacrylate: report of two cases. Radiology 1998;207:809–812
33. Abdala N, Levitin A, Dawson A, et al. Use of ethylene vinyl alcohol copolymer for tubal sterilization by selective catheterization in rabbits. J Vasc Interv Radiol 2001;12:979–984
34. Post JH, Cardella JF, Wilson RP, et al. Experimental nonsurgical transcervical sterilization with a custom-designed platinum microcoil. J Vasc Interv Radiol 1997;8:113–118
35. Thurmond AS, Nikolchev J, Khera A, et al. Nonsurgical sterilization using the Essure device in fallopian tubes: results in rabbits. J Women's Imaging 2004;6:75–80
36. Conceptus. Physician training manual. Mountain View, CA: Conceptus Inc; 2003
37. Hallab N, Merritt K, Jacobs JJ. Metal sensitivity in patients with orthopaedic implants. J Bone Joint Surg Am 2001;83:428–436
38. Koster R, Vieluf D, Kiehn M, et al. Nickel and molybdenum contact allergies in patients with coronary in-stent restenosis. Lancet 2000;356:1895–1897
39. Hillen U, Haude M, Erbel R, et al. Evaluation of metal allergies in patients with coronary stents. Contact Dermatitis 2002;47:353–356
40. Valle RF, Carignan CS, Wright TC. Tissue response to the STOP microcoil transcervical permanent contraceptive device: results from a prehysterectomy study. Fertil Steril 2001;76:974–980
41. Kerin JF. New methods for transcervical cannulation of the fallopian tube. Int J Gynaecol Obstet 1995;51(Suppl. 1):S29–S39
42. Ekerhovd E, Norström A. Involvement of a nitric oxide-cyclic guanosine monophosphate pathway in control of fallopian tube contractility. Gynecol Endocrinol 2004;19(5):239–246
43. Hedgpeth PL, Thurmond AS, Fry R, et al. Radiographic fallopian tube recanalization: absorbed ovarian dose. Radiology 1991;180:121–122
44. Heredia F, Cos R, Moros S, et al. Radiological control of Essure placements. Gynecol Surg 2004;1(3):201–203
45. Kerin JF, Levy BS. Ultrasound: an effective method for localization of the echogenic Essure sterilization micro-insert: correlation with radiologic evaluations. J Minim Invasive Gynecol 2005;12(1):50–54
46. Johns DA. Advances in hysteroscopic sterilization: report on 600 patients enrolled in the Adiana EASE pivotal trial. Paper presented at: the Global Meeting of the American Association of Gynecological Laparoscopy; November 9–12, 2005; Chicago, IL
47. Peterson HB, Xia Z, Hughes JM, et al. The risk of ectopic pregnancy after tubal sterilization. N Engl J Med 1997;336:762–767
48. Kerin JF. Hysteroscopic sterilization: long-term safety and efficacy. Paper presented at: the Global Meeting of the American Association of Gynecological Laparoscopy; November 9–12, 2005; Chicago, IL
49. Shellock FG, Crues JVMR. Procedures: biologic effects, safety, and patient care. Radiology 2004;232:635–652
50. Muhler MR. Can intrauterine devices actually be considered safe at 3-T MR imaging? Radiology 2005;235:709
51. Wittmer MH, Brown DL, Hartman RP, et al. Sonography, CT, and MRI appearance of the Essure microinsert permanent birth control device. AJR Am J Roentgenol 2006;187:959–964

14 Clinical Perspective: Interventional Radiology and Patient Fertility

Robert L. Worthington-Kirsch

Interventional radiologists have become increasingly involved with women's health issues over the last few decades. This has led to increased participation in the care of patients presenting with symptomatic uterine fibroids, pain due to pelvic congestion syndrome, or infertility due to fallopian tube pathology. In any of these cases, fertility issues become a significant consideration during the course of managing these patients. Fertility issues are important when considering any procedure performed on women of childbearing age, but are especially critical when contemplating procedures treating the genitourinary system. Radiation safety concerns are paramount in this population as outlined in an earlier chapter. However, there also should always be an awareness of what direct effects a particular procedure will have on fertility. This chapter will provide an overview of fertility issues surrounding the treatment of fibroids and fallopian tube interventions.

Before any discussion of the clinical issues surrounding treatment, one has to address the importance of building a team to address these issues. There must be clear and continuous channels of communication between the interventional radiologist and both the primary gynecologist and the reproductive endocrinologist providing care for each patient. This ensures that each patient is provided with a plan for care that is thorough and coherent. In my practice, there is a steady stream of correspondence between all three of these physicians, as well as frequent personal communications by phone and e-mail, regarding each patient.

In addition, it is important for the interventional radiologist to develop a true physician–patient relationship with each patient. All women should be seen for an office consultation before any elective invasive procedure. This allows the interventional radiologist to become familiar with the patient's medical history and current situation. It also is invaluable for setting a woman at ease regarding a physician who is going to be providing medical care in an area of life (and anatomy) that may have tremendous emotional repercussions. To gain that trust, an open discussion that includes the potential risks as well as the potential benefits of any procedure being considered must be held with the patient. This relationship continues after any procedure because the interventional radiologist is responsible for postprocedure and recovery issues, follow-up, and management of any complications that may occur. The importance of this is that physicians who do not have training in interventional radiology (IR) including the gynecologist, primary care physician, or local emergency room [ER] staff will likely be unfamiliar with issues that arise after IR procedures and therefore may not be able to manage them appropriately.

■ Fibroid Interventions

Fibroid disease is extremely common and is one of the most frequently encountered diseases of the uterus; as many as 40% of all women will experience fibroid-related symptoms during the reproductive phase.[1,2] Fibroids most commonly cause symptoms of abnormally heavy menstrual bleeding (menorrhagia and/or menometrorrhagia) and/or bulk or pressure symptoms such as urinary frequency or urgency (occasionally bladder outlet obstruction), sensation of a pelvic/abdominal mass, and dyspareunia. Fibroid disease can also contribute to subfertility. The exact relationship between fibroids and subfertility is unclear in many cases. It is generally accepted that submucosal fibroids can interfere with progression of a pregnancy by distorting the uterine cavity, which can contribute to increasing the risk of miscarriage.[3] If fibroids grow in the vicinity of the uterine cornua, they can occlude or distort the fallopian tubes. Although some have suggested other mechanisms for fibroids to impact fertility, these are less well understood.

When it comes to fertility issues, in my experience there are two types of fibroid patients. The majority of women presenting for treatment of uterine fibroids are seeking relief from fibroid-related abnormal bleeding and/or pressure. Most of these women have completed childbearing or have no interest in future fertility. In some of these women, preservation of fertility may be a consideration, but is usually of secondary importance. Many of these patients have no immediate plans to have children or additional children, but are not yet ready to abandon that possibility. However, a small number of women who present to an interventional radiologist for fibroid therapy have fibroid-related subfertility as their primary concern and may or may not have fibroid-related symptoms as well.

The most common therapy offered to women with fibroid-related subfertility is myomectomy. In women who have small numbers of small to moderate-sized fibroids that are easily accessible, myomectomy provides excellent results for preserving or improving fertility, especially if a hysteroscopic approach can be utilized.[4] However, as the fibroid burden increases (number and/or size of fibroids) there may be a greater likelihood of surgical complications or poor fertility outcomes.[2] There is also a significant incidence of fibroid recurrence after myomectomy, and fertility outcomes after repeat procedures are generally poor.[5] Women who have large fibroid burdens may also run an unacceptably high risk of conversion of an attempted myomectomy to hysterectomy due to intraoperative bleeding.

As outlined in earlier chapters, uterine fibroid embolization (UFE or uterine artery embolization, UAE) has recently emerged as a definitive therapy for fibroids given its durable success at controlling most fibroid-related symptoms.[6–8] UFE may also be a valuable option for some women who desire to maintain fertility after treatment of their fibroids, especially in light of emerging evidence suggesting that fertility after UFE is probably similar to fertility after multiple myomectomy.[9] When discussing treatment options with these patients, it is important that the interventional radiologist and the patient have a realistic understanding of the patient's likelihood of fertility and available alternatives.

In women with a limited fibroid burden and a strong desire for future fertility, myomectomy may well be the procedure of choice. This may offer the patient control of her symptoms with minimal risk of negative impact on her chance for fertility. If a woman opts for myomectomy, it would be appropriate for the interventional radiologist to establish UFE as an option if fibroid symptoms are not adequately controlled, or recur in the future. There are also women who are good candidates for myomectomy, but prefer to undergo UFE given the less invasive nature of this treatment. In my experience, this scenario requires that an extensive discussion take place between the physician and the patient that reviews the various available treatment options and their respective risks and benefits. In my practice, if a patient then decides that she wishes to avoid surgical management if at all possible, UFE will then be offered as an option. Finally, women with larger fibroid burdens (multiple fibroids, large uteri) are likely poor candidates for myomectomy. Because of the extent of their fibroid disease, the chance of preserving fertility may be relatively low with either myomectomy or UFE. In these women, UFE may well be the only uterine-sparing therapy available. The author has seen at least one successful pregnancy in a patient who has multiple fibroids resulting in a uterine size greater than 20 weeks before embolization. This patient had been told by an experienced fertility surgeon that there was little likelihood that she would preserve her uterus if myomectomy were attempted, and that even after a successful myomectomy she would not be able to carry a pregnancy to term. Therefore, UFE was an option that should have been and was offered to her.

In summary, it is important to have a logical framework when evaluating a patient for fibroid therapy who wishes to preserve fertility. The answers to the following questions should guide the discussion and recommendations made to the patient:

1. Does the patient desire treatment of her fibroids primarily for fertility issues or is fertility a secondary concern to relief of her fibroid symptoms?
2. How realistic are the patient's desires and plans for future fertility (fibroid burden, patient age, life situation, etc.)?
3. Would this patient be better served by myomectomy (opinion of reproductive endocrinologist and/or fertility surgeon)?

One should also consider the issue of adenomyosis before leaving the topic of embolotherapy. There have been mixed results published about the outcome of embolization to treat adenomyosis;[10,11] therefore, I do not offer embolotherapy to most women who prove to have adenomyosis on preprocedure magnetic resonance imaging (MRI). Unfortunately the only definitive therapy currently available for adenomyosis is hysterectomy, which is clearly not a good option for a patient desiring future fertility. Hence, I do offer embolization to those women for whom preservation of a chance at fertility is a high priority, even given the incidence of symptom recurrence in patients with adenomyosis.[12]

■ Fallopian Tube Interventions

Diagnostic hysterosalpingography (HSG) is the foundation for interventions in the fallopian tubes. In most facilities, hysterosalpingograms are performed on a cooperative basis between gynecology and radiology. In this setting, the gynecologist placing the catheter and injecting contrast while a diagnostic radiologist (typically whoever is doing gastrointestinal [GI] studies that day) does the fluoroscopy and provides the interpretation for the examination. In my practice, the fertility surgeon used to do this, but had chronic problems of coordinating the clinic and operating schedule with the fluoroscopy schedule within radiology. Several years ago, this was changed and I now perform hysterosalpingograms in interventional radiology. The cases are scheduled as outpatients and fit easily into the daily schedule of interventional radiology, without disrupting the fertility surgeon's patient schedule and the fluoroscopy schedule within radiology.

The major advantage of a diagnostic hysterosalpingogram being completely performed within interventional radiology is that appropriate patients can potentially be diagnosed and treated at the same time. Previously, if the hysterosalpingogram performed by the gynecologist revealed proximal occlusion of the fallopian tubes, the patient would need to be scheduled for another appointment in interventional radiology for fallopian tube recanalization (FTR). Now the patient is scheduled for diagnostic hysterosalpingogram with a possible fallopian tube recanalization to follow if indicated. This markedly simplifies the schedule and the lives of all involved. Most importantly, the patient is pleased to have everything taken care of at one time, without having to rearrange her life for a second procedure.

Fallopian tube recanalization to treat a proximal occlusion of the fallopian tube was first reported in 1987 by Amy Thurmond and colleagues[13] with more recent results reviewed in a previous chapter. This procedure is fairly straightforward and can be performed by any physician with an appropriate degree of image-guided catheterization skills. It has been associated with a high technical success rate (70 to 90%), a low risk of complications, and reasonable clinical success. Successful pregnancies are seen in ~30% of women who undergo a successful fallopian tube recanalization procedure.[14]

For most interventional radiologists, it is a small step to move from the fallopian tube recanalization procedure, which reestablishes fallopian tube patency, to other procedures that are performed with the goal of occluding the fallopian tube for purposes of permanent contraception. Both procedures are similar in their skill sets and both fall well within the typical procedures performed within interventional radiology. A variety of procedures and devices for the purpose of causing fallopian tube occlusion have been evaluated over time.[15] As discussed in an earlier chapter, the ESSURE fallopian tube micro-insert system (Conceptus Inc., Mountain View, CA) has been approved by the FDA for permanent birth control since 2002. The device was designed to be placed hysteroscopically and has been approved with that mode of delivery in mind. However, the device can also be easily inserted under fluoroscopic control, especially in a woman with a normal uterine cavity.[16] Given the large number of patients being seen and treated for symptomatic uterine fibroids in my practice, a desire to offer comprehensive services to this patient population is a logical next step for practice growth. In the case of a practice performing UFE procedures, procedures such as fallopian tube occlusion in addition to procedures to treat varicose veins (such as saphenous vein ablation, sclerotherapy, and ambulatory phlebectomy) go a long way toward achieving this goal of offering additional services to this population. In my experience, placement of the ESSURE device is an outpatient procedure that can typically take 5 to 10 minutes to perform within any facility performing interventional radiology procedures. This procedure can be performed in women who have had a UFE, although catheterizing the fallopian tubes in a cavity distorted by fibroids can be quite challenging. Despite this potential obstacle, I have found that the addition of fallopian tube occlusion procedures to a practice can help interventional radiologists offer a comprehensive range of services to a population of patients seeking minimally invasive solutions to problems that have traditionally had surgical solutions.

References

1. Schwartz SM. Epidemiology of uterine leiomyomata. Clin Obstet Gynecol 2001;44:316–326
2. Myers ER, Barber MD, Couchman GM, et al. Evidence Report: Management of Uterine Fibroids (Contract No. 290–97–0014, Task Order 4). Rockville, MD: Agency for Healthcare Research and Quality; 2000
3. Parker WH. Etiology, symptomatology, and diagnosis of uterine myomas. Fertil Steril 2007;87:725–736
4. Shokeir TA. Hysteroscopic management in submucous fibroids to improve fertility. Arch Gynecol Obstet 2005;273:50–54
5. Frederick J, Hardie M, Reid M, Fletcher H, Wynter S, Frederick C. Operative morbidity and reproductive outcome in secondary myomectomy: a prospective cohort study. Hum Reprod 2002;17:2967–2971
6. Razavi MK, Hwang G, Jahed A, Modanloo S, Chen B. Abdominal myomectomy versus uterine fibroid embolization in the treatment of symptomatic uterine leiomyomas. AJR Am J Roentgenol 2003;180:1571–1575
7. Edwards RD, Moss JG, Lumsden MA, et al. Uterine artery embolization versus surgery for symptomatic uterine fibroids. N Engl J Med 2007;356:360–370
8. Spies JB, Bruno J, Czeyda-Pommershein F, Magee ST, Ascher SA, Jha RC. Long-term outcome of uterine artery embolization of leiomyomata. Obstet Gynecol 2005;106:933–939
9. Domenico L, Siskin GP. Uterine artery embolization and infertility. Tech Vasc Interv Radiol 2006;9:7–11
10. Kim MD, Kim S, Kim NK, et al. Long-term results of uterine artery embolization for symptomatic adenomyosis. AJR Am J Roentgenol 2007;188:176–181
11. Pelage JP, Jacob D, Fazel A, et al. Midterm results of uterine artery embolization for symptomatic adenomyosis: initial experience. Radiology 2005;234:948–953
12. Goldberg J. Uterine artery embolization for adenomyosis: looking at the glass half full. Radiology 2005;236:1111–1112
13. Thurmond AS, Novy M, Uchida BT, Rösch J. Fallopian tube obstruction: selective salpingography and recanalization. work in progress. Radiology 1987;163:511–514
14. Thurmond AS, Machan LS, Maubon AJ, et al. A review of selective salpingography and fallopian tube catheterization. Radiographics 2000;20:1759–1768
15. Maubon AJ, Thurmond AS, Laurent A, et al. Tubal sterilization by means of selective catheterization: comparison of a hydrogel and a collagen glue. J Vasc Interv Radiol 1996;7:733–736
16. McSwain H, Shaw C, Hall LD. Placement of the Essure permanent birth control device with fluoroscopic guidance: a novel method for tubal sterilization. J Vasc Interv Radiol 2005;16:1007–1012

IV Ovarian Interventions

15 Clinical Review: Pelvic Pain

Jafar Golzarian, Fadi Youness, and Colleen M. Kennedy

The definition of chronic pelvic pain is noncyclic pain of 6 or more months duration that localizes to the anatomic pelvis, abdominal wall at or below the umbilicus, lumbosacral back, or the buttocks and is of sufficient severity to cause functional disability or lead to medical care.[1] Pelvic pain may further be categorized as acute (typically less than 3 months in duration), or chronic (pain lasting longer than 6 months in duration). Estimates suggest that 15 to 20% of women in the United States between the ages of 18 and 50 years have experienced chronic pelvic pain.[2] Although chronic pelvic pain accounts for 10 to 40% of all outpatient gynecologic visits,[3] it is important to note that the most frequent disorders associated with chronic pelvic pain are often nongynecologic, including irritable bowel syndrome, painful bladder syndrome, and musculoskeletal disorders.[4] Patients younger than 35 years and white women are at higher risk of developing this condition. Chronic pelvic pain is responsible for 35% of diagnostic laparoscopies and 15% of all hysterectomies performed in the United States. Finally, this condition is associated with a substantial economic impact as manifested by work absenteeism and health care cost. It is estimated that the cost of care for women with chronic pelvic pain approaches $39 billion per year in the United States.[1]

Acute pelvic pain often warrants investigation, including laboratory and radiologic studies, to determine whether or not the etiology of pain necessitates an immediate intervention such as with appendicitis or a ruptured ectopic pregnancy. Although, patients with an acute surgical abdomen will often have a rapid onset of symptoms, patients with bowel obstruction necessitating emergent surgery may present with weeks of vague abdominal pain, followed by a sudden deterioration. The list of disorders causing pelvic pain is exhaustive; common etiologies of acute pelvic pain are noted in **Table 15.1**.[5]

In contrast to patients presenting with acute pelvic pain, women presenting for an evaluation of chronic pelvic pain have typically already undergone an extensive evaluation, which may or may not have revealed an etiology for their pain. They may have been seen by a variety of different medical specialists given the many nongynecologic conditions associated with chronic pelvic pain. However, up to 20% of patients remain symptomatic after undergoing multiple diagnostic and therapeutic procedures. This is a source of frustration and anxiety for patients with chronic pelvic pain. It is also increases the importance for any practitioner evaluating these patients to understand the extensive differential diagnosis that must be applied to these patients. Common conditions that may exacerbate or cause chronic pelvic pain are noted in **Table 15.2**.[1]

Evaluating a Patient with Chronic Pelvic Pain

When a patient with pelvic pain is being evaluated, it is often tempting to attribute this to gynecologic causes, especially in the context of an interventional radiology practice evaluating patients prior to procedure such as uterine fibroid embolization (UFE) or ovarian vein embolization. However, it is important to remember that these patients

Table 15.1 Common Causes of Acute Pelvic Pain

Gynecologic
Ruptured ectopic pregnancy (rule out first!)
Endometriosis
Endometritis
Pelvic inflammatory disease
Leiomyomas (degeneration, infarction, torsion)
Ovarian cysts or masses with bleeding, torsion, or rupture
Gastrointestinal
Appendicitis
Diverticulitis
Colitis/ Ileitis (viral, bacterial, other)
Peritonitis
Bowel obstruction
Urologic
Bladder outlet obstruction
Cystitis
Renal lithiasis
Pyelonephritis
Vascular
Mesenteric ischemia/ infarction
Dissecting or ruptured aortic aneurysm
Bowel wall hematoma
Sickle cell disease

Table 15.2 Common Conditions That May Cause or Exacerbate Chronic Pelvic Pain

Condition
Gynecologic
Endometriosis
Pelvic congestion syndrome
Pelvic inflammatory disease
Ovarian retention syndrome
Ovarian remnant syndrome
Leiomyomas
Adenomyosis
Adhesions
Cervical stenosis
Pudendal nerve entrapment
Vulvodynia
Gastrointestinal
Colon cancer
Constipation
Inflammatory bowel disease
Irritable bowel syndrome
Urologic
Bladder cancer
Interstitial cystitis
Radiation cystitis
Urethral syndrome
Musculoskeletal
Abdominal wall myofascial pain
Chronic coccygeal or back pain
Fibromyalgia
Pelvic floor myalgia
Other
Depression
Hyperalgesia
Somatization disorder
Celiac disease
Porphyria
Shingles

may suffer from one of a large number of etiologies including gastrointestinal (GI), urologic, musculoskeletal, neurologic, psychologic, and vascular disorders among others. Therefore, a comprehensive history and physical examination are critically important parts of the evaluation of a patient with chronic pelvic pain.

When obtaining a history from these patients, their obstetric, surgical, psychosocial, and sexual history must be covered. In addition, the characteristics of their pain (e.g., location, severity, quality, timing, and exacerbating and relieving factors) must be reviewed because they may point toward an etiology for their pain.[7] If the patient has undergone previous therapy, the effect that these treatments have had on the pain must be reviewed. A complete review of systems is important due to the multifactorial etiology that is often present in patients with chronic pelvic pain. The goal of a physical examination is to detect the exact anatomic location of tenderness and to then correlate these findings with the location of the patient's pain. The evaluation must cover the reproductive tract, in addition to the musculoskeletal, GI, urinary, and neurologic systems.[8]

Imaging studies will likely make up the next component of the evaluation of patients with chronic pelvic pain. The imaging tests ordered will be based on the most highly suspected etiology for the patient's pain based on the above history and physical examination. Laparoscopy remains an important part of the diagnostic evaluation of these patients; more than one-third of diagnostic laparoscopies are done in this setting. Although conditions such as endometriosis and adhesions are often diagnosed with laparoscopy, it is important to remember that up to one-third of laparoscopic studies in women with chronic pelvic pain have normal findings. This, however, does not mean that a woman has no physical basis for her pain.[7] In addition, pathology identified at laparoscopy may not be responsible for the patient's pain.[9–11]

After a typically extensive evaluation has taken place, treatment options will be discussed with the patient. Some of the conditions that can potentially be addressed by interventional radiologists are reviewed in this chapter and others within this text. Other conditions highlighted in this chapter, though not likely to be treated by interventional radiologists, are ones that will likely already have been discussed with patients and will therefore come up during their evaluations of patients with chronic pelvic pain.

■ Differential Diagnosis

Endometriosis

The most common gynecologic diagnosis among women with chronic pelvic pain is endometriosis.[12] Although 30% of women evaluated for chronic pain in the general population are found to have endometriosis, over 70% of women were given a diagnosis of endometriosis when seen in a gynecology specialty practice.[12] Despite the fact that interventional radiologists may not themselves be directly involved in treating these patients, it is important to be aware of this condition when evaluating patients with chronic pelvic pain for procedures such as ovarian vein embolization or uterine artery embolization.

Endometriosis is classically described as the presence of endometrial-like tissue (glands and stroma) outside the uterine cavity and musculature.[13] The etiology of this remains unknown, but theories do exist including coelomic metaplasia, lymphatic or hematologic spread, or implantation of cells carried in retrograde menstrual flow. Retrograde menstruation can seed the peritoneal cavity with endometrial cells, which leads to stimulated angiogenesis and lesion development.[13,14] This can lead to an intraperitoneal cascade of cytokines and other factors that result in the pain associated with endometriosis.[15,16] However, because retrograde menstruation can occur in up to 90% of normal patients, it is clear that other factors are involved in the pathogenesis of endometriosis.[17]

A history including pelvic pain, dysmenorrhea, dyspareunia, and infertility is suggestive of endometriosis. The pain associated with endometriosis is generally cyclical, although it may become continuous as the disease worsens.[18,19] Lesions involving the bladder or rectum can cause pain during urination or defecation.[18,20] Endometriosis is also associated with infertility, especially when there is advanced disease due to the distortion of normal pelvic anatomy and impairment of tuboovarian function.[21,22] Finally, endometriosis tends to be associated with a negative impact on quality due to the symptoms of pelvic pain and infertility as well as from the effects of treatment.[23] Given the nonspecific nature of many of these symptoms, endometriosis is often difficult to diagnose.

Findings on physical examination may include increased tenderness during a bimanual pelvic examination, a fixed retroverted uterus, lateral displacement of the cervix, decreased uterine mobility, uterosacral ligament nodularity, and enlarged adnexa (suggestive of an endometrioma). Most women with endometriosis will have a normal pelvic examination.[24] There have been no laboratory findings strongly associated with endometriosis, although some have reported that increased CA-125 levels may be associated with severe disease; CA-125 is of limited value in women with minimal or mild disease.[25]

Imaging studies are of mixed value in diagnosing endometriosis, but are helpful in identifying associated findings that have endometriosis as an underlying etiology, including simple ovarian cysts, endometriomas, complex ovarian cysts, and ovarian torsion. Ultrasonography is commonly included in the evaluation of women with chronic pelvic pain and may identify adnexal findings consistent with an endometrioma. The appearance of endometriomas on ultrasound (preferably transvaginal) is described as homogeneous hypoechoic "tissue" of low level echoes, mostly multifocal, within the ovaries (**Fig. 15.1**).[26] There should be absence of particular neoplastic features in these lesions.[27] On color Doppler sonography (CDS), the lesions show poor or no vascularization.[28] However, some reports indicate that CDS does not improve the diagnostic accuracy of transvaginal ultrasound alone in the diagnosis of endometriomas.[29] Magnetic resonance imaging (MRI) is an excellent means for detection of macroscopic endometrial implants in the pelvis (particularly the posterior cul-de-sac and uterosacral ligaments) as areas of variable high signal intensity on T1-weighted images and low signal intensity on T2-weighted images.[30] Other sequences, such as fat-suppressed imaging, are also useful for diagnosis (**Fig. 15.2**).

Although a presumptive clinical diagnosis is commonly assigned, the diagnosis is pathologic and typically con-

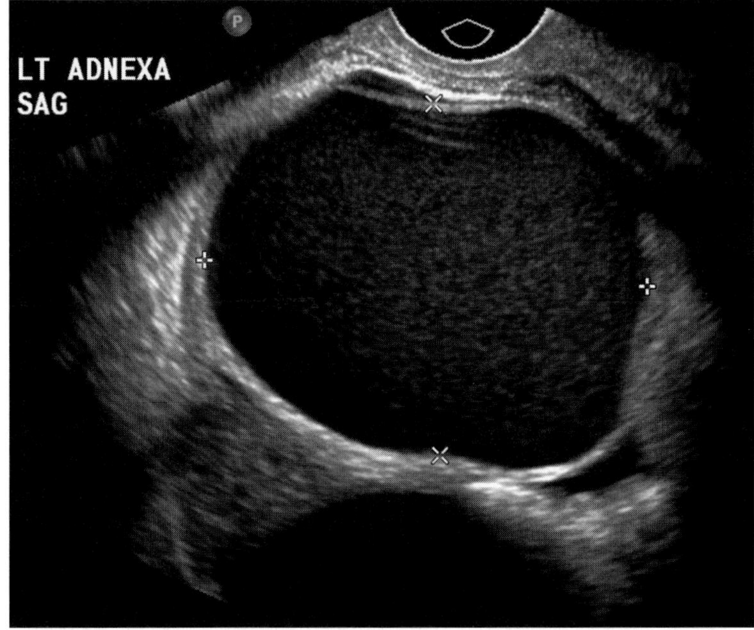

Fig. 15.1 Longitudinal image from a transvaginal ultrasound examination of the left adnexa region. This demonstrates a hypoechoic cystic structure containing low-level echoes seen in association with an endometrioma.

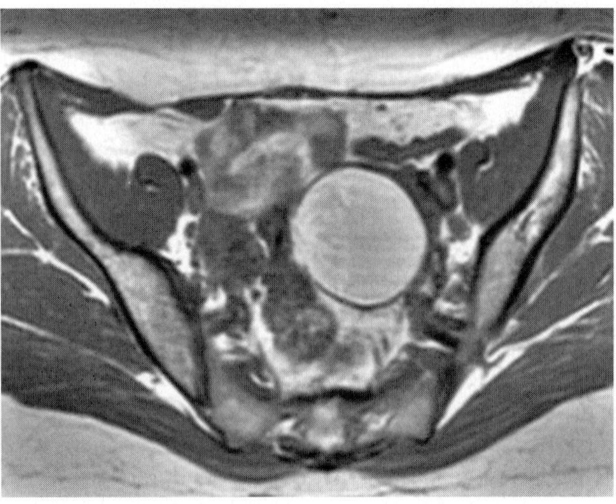

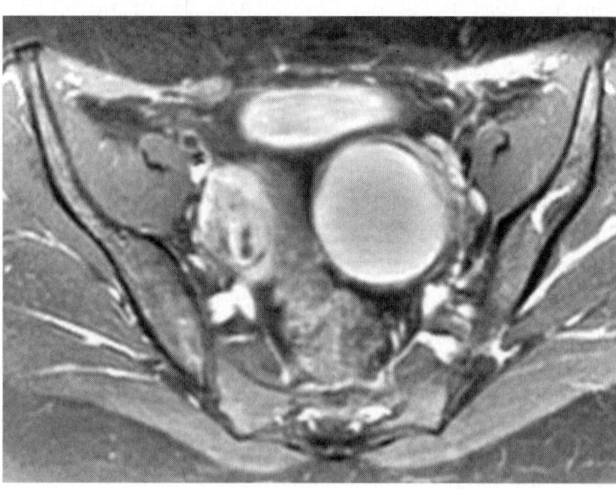

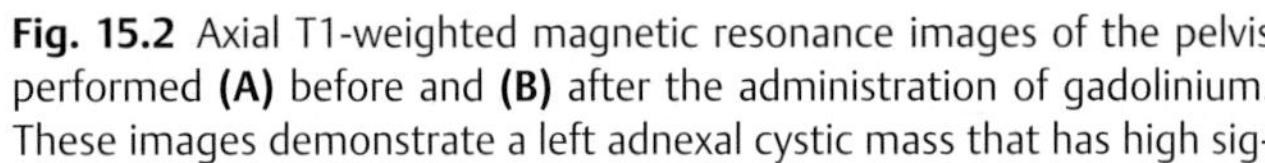
Fig. 15.2 Axial T1-weighted magnetic resonance images of the pelvis performed **(A)** before and **(B)** after the administration of gadolinium. These images demonstrate a left adnexal cystic mass that has high signal on T1-weighted images and does not enhance with contrast, which is characteristic of an endometrioma.

firmed with laparoscopy. Most physicians accept visualization of apparent lesions as enough to make a diagnosis of endometriosis.[31] This approach, however, may lead to errors in diagnosis. Following a clinical diagnosis of endometriosis, laparoscopy has been found to confirm visible endometriosis in 70 to 90% of patients.[12] However, the positive predictive value of visual findings compared with histologic findings varies from 14 to 65% based on the anatomic site of the lesion and from 0 to 76% based on the type of lesion present.[32] For example, the positive predictive value is high in the posterior cul-de-sac, but low in unusual sites such as the psoas muscle. Overall, the positive predictive value for laparoscopic visualization is 43 to 45%.[32,33] On laparoscopy, a variety of lesions can be confused visually with endometriosis implants including endosalpingiosis, mesothelial hyperplasia, hemosiderin deposition (rather than hemosiderin-laden macrophages), hemangiomas, adrenal rests, residual carbon from previous ablation procedures, reactions to oil-based radiographic dyes, inflammatory changes, and splenosis.[13] In general, infiltrating lesions are most likely associated with pain symptoms, whereas superficial lesions are less likely to cause pain and may be found incidentally in asymptomatic women.[34] The findings at laparoscopy, however, do not necessarily correlate with symptom severity.[35]

If the diagnostic impression is most consistent with endometriosis, medical therapy can be considered empirically without surgical (pathologic) confirmation.[36] The primary goals of medical treatment are to address the symptoms associated with endometriosis and to possibly induce atrophy of the abnormal tissue.[19,37,38] Because endometriotic tissue is known to be hormonally sensitive, and because the symptoms of endometriosis usually improve during pregnancy or after menopause, medical therapy is designed to induce or mimic states including menopause (GnRH analogues), amenorrhea (danazol), or pregnancy (oral contraceptives or progestins).[18,23] The initial medical treatment options are noted in **Table 15.3**. Oral contraceptives are the drug of choice among many gynecologists in managing women with endometriosis and are therefore considered the first line of therapy.[13] They are comparably effective to medroxyprogesterone acetate or GnRH analogues in addressing dysmenorrhea.[39] Pathologically, it is known that long-term exposure to progestins leads to decidualization and atrophy of the endometriotic lesions.[13] Other medications that are helpful with these patients include danazol, which is an androgen that suppresses pituitary secretion of gonadotropins and inhibits ovulation, and GnRH analogues, which lead to a hypoestrogenic state.[13]

When it comes to the surgical options for endometriosis, there are both radical and conservative options. The most radical option is a total hysterectomy and bilateral oophorectomy, but even this is associated with a 5 to 10% rate of recurrence.[40,41] Conservative options are typically performed from a laparoscopic approach and include excision or ablation of lesions; ablation techniques include vaporization, cauterization, or desiccation. Reports have been

Table 15.3 Medical Therapeutic Options for the Management of Endometriosis and Chronic Pelvic Pain

Nonsteroidal antiinflammatory medications
Oral contraceptive pills
Continuous progestin treatment, oral or intrauterine (IUS)
Danazol (androgen agonist)
Aromatase inhibitors
Gonadotropin-releasing hormone agonist analogue (GnRH)

published concerning the failure rate after laparoscopic treatment with some claiming a 51% rate of recurrent symptoms within 1 year and others claiming a 40 to 50% rate of symptom recurrence after 5 years.[15,42,43] Adjunctive laparoscopic options include presacral neurectomy or uterosacral nerve ablation, both of which may have a potential role in relieving pain associated with endometriosis.[44] Potential complications of these laparoscopic procedures include vascular, ureteral, and bowel injuries.[45]

Fibroids

Uterine fibroids (leiomyomata) are the most common pelvic tumors in women. They represent the most frequent indication for hysterectomy in premenopausal women; 600,000 hysterectomies are performed annually in the United States, with uterine fibroids listed as the indication in one-third of them. Although many patients with fibroids will present with abnormal bleeding, others will present with pelvic pain or back pain. In addition, large fibroids exert mass effect on surrounding organs, leading to urinary, GI, and neurologic symptoms. The surgical options for fibroids, including hysterectomy and myomectomy, are effective at addressing the symptoms associated with fibroids. As described in earlier chapters in this text, UFE is also effective at treating the pain and other symptoms associated with fibroids.

Adenomyosis

Adenomyosis is another condition that is associated with chronic pelvic pain, in addition to dysmenorrhea, menorrhagia, and infertility. It is characterized by the presence of endometrial glands and stroma within the myometrium (at least 2.5 cm below the endometrial–myometrial junction) with adjacent myometrial hyperplasia.[46] It occurs with a frequency that has been reported as high as 30%.[47] The dysmenorrhea associated with adenomyosis is due to the myometrial contractions that are caused by prostaglandins produced by adenomyosis tissue.[48] Up to 35% of patients with adenomyosis may be symptom free.[49] In addition to dysmenorrhea and menorrhagia, patients with adenomyosis can present with bulk-related symptoms due to uterine enlargement. Given this complex of symptoms, these patients are often thought to have fibroids until definitive testing is completed.

Adenomyosis can be focal, which is also known as an adenomyoma, mimicking a uterine fibroid in ultrasound. In these cases, ultrasound shows an ill-defined echogenic mass within the myometrium. On color Doppler ultrasound (CDS), the lesion shows penetrating vessels within the mass. Adenomyosis can also be diffuse with endometrial glands distributed throughout the myometrium. Ultrasound shows a heterogeneous and asymmetric myometrium. In up to 50% of cases, myometrial cysts are seen that are highly specific of this condition.[50] However, magnetic resonance imaging (MRI) is considered the modality of choice for diagnosis of adenomyosis. T2-weighted images show foci of increased signal within the myometrium corresponding with endometrial glands or subendometrial (myometrial) cysts. The thickening of junctional zone of more than 12 mm is another characteristic MRI finding (**Fig. 15.3**). Focal adenomyosis is presented as a low signal intensity and ill-defined mass inside the myometrium.[31]

Hysterectomy is considered as the definitive treatment for adenomyosis. Hormonal treatment (e.g., progestins,

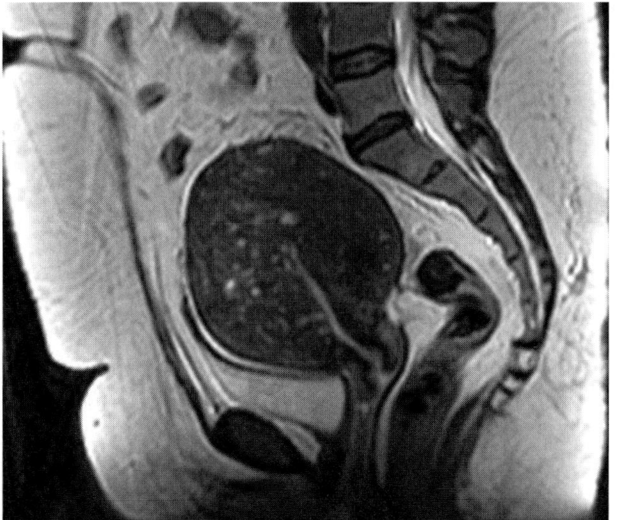

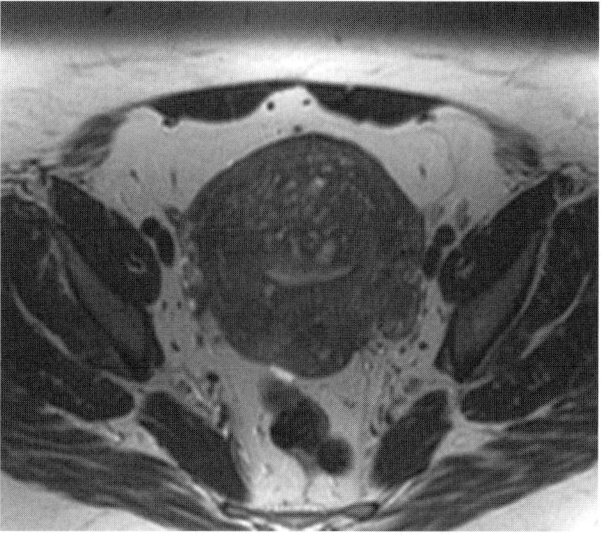

Fig. 15.3 **(A)** Sagittal and **(B)** axial T2-weighted magnetic resonance images of the pelvis in a patient with diffuse adenomyosis. These images demonstrate a thickened junctional zone containing multiple foci of high signal consistent with subendometrial cysts.

gonadotropin-releasing hormone agonists, danazol) to reduce the symptoms and junctional zone thickening is effective, but temporary and often not effective in the acute setting. Other surgical modalities include endometrial ablation and myometrial excision.[46] Uterine artery embolization (UAE) has been reported to be a potential treatment option in this patient population, as discussed in Chapter 5.[51–53] Although the results are not as good when compared with embolization performed for uterine fibroids, it can save more than 50% of patients from undergoing a hysterectomy by addressing their most significant symptoms.[54]

Postoperative Adhesions

Adhesions are defined as the abnormal attachment of tissue surfaces that occur due to tissue trauma (e.g., injury, infection, radiation, ischemia, foreign body reactions, etc.).[55] After trauma, vasoactive substances are released that increase vascular permeability, leading to the formation of fibrin deposits.[56] Adhesions can have significant consequences, including infertility, bowel obstruction, and abdominal or pelvic pain. Pain occurs due to the fact that adhesions impair organ mobility.[57] However, there has been no relationship between the extent of adhesions and the severity of pain experienced by a patient. In addition, a randomized trial observed no difference in pain relief among patients who underwent laparoscopic lysis of adhesions or sham surgery.[58] Therefore, lysis of adhesions may result in little or no improvement in abdominal and pelvic pain.[55]

Interstitial Cystitis

Interstitial cystitis is a chronic inflammatory disease of the bladder that is another potential cause for chronic pelvic pain in women. It is a condition that often goes unrecognized, and patients therefore experience symptoms for a long time and see many different physicians before a diagnosis is made.[59] These patients can present with pelvic pain and dyspareunia in addition to a history of frequency, urgency, nocturia, and frequent culture-negative urinary tract infections.[60] Some patients will have pelvic pain in the absence of urinary symptoms. Most cases are mild to moderate in severity, with symptoms that tend to occur in cycles of flares and remissions.[61] In some women, flares occur during or after sexual activity and during the week before the onset of menses.[62] All patients with suspected interstitial cystitis should have a urinalysis and urine culture performed to rule out microscopic hematuria and infections. Patients with hematuria should have a cystoscopy performed to rule out a bladder neoplasm.[63] Cystoscopic findings associated with interstitial cystitis include glomerulations, submucosal hemorrhages, ulcers, and a reduced bladder capacity to <400 cc.[60,63] The potassium chloride (KCl) sensitivity test can be used for interstitial cystitis because it is positive (increased intravesical sensitivity) in 66 to 75% of patients; false-positive results can occur with detrusor instability, radiation cystitis, and urinary tract infections.[63–65]

Medical therapy is designed to address the pathophysiologic processes that have been identified in this condition.[7,66–68] This includes pentosan polysulfate sodium (PPS) and/or intravesical heparin for dysfunctional epithelium. PPS is the only U.S. Food and Drug Administration (FDA)-approved medication for interstitial cystitis, which works by repairing the altered permeability of the bladder surface.[67] Approximately 30% of patients will have improvement with this therapy. Other therapies include hydroxyzine for mast cell activation and allergies and tricyclic antidepressants for neural upregulation and sleeping difficulties. Procedures such as hydrodistention of the bladder, laser destruction of the vesicoureteric plexus, sacral nerve stimulation, and even cystectomy with urinary diversion have been reported as well.[66,69,70]

Irritable Bowel Syndrome

Irritable bowel syndrome (IBS) can lead to alternating constipation and diarrhea, abdominal distension, mucus from the rectum, improvement in pain after a bowel movement, and the sensation of incomplete evacuation after defecation.[71] The age at onset varies, but the incidence appears to increase during adolescence and peaks in the third and fourth decades of life.[72] As the number of women being diagnosed with IBS has increased, it has become apparent that this condition can be found in as many as 80% of women with chronic pelvic pain.[7,23] Dyspareunia has been reported in association with IBS.[73] Various mechanisms for this disorder have been described, including abnormalities of gastrointestinal sensation, motility, autonomic function, bacterial flora, the mucosal immune system, and serotonin pathways.[74]

Medical treatment is used to address the symptoms of IBS. Antispasmodic medications such as dicyclomine hydrochloride and hyoscyamine can be used to address abdominal pain, gas, and bloating symptoms because they relax the smooth muscle of the gut and reduce its contractility.[7,72,75] Stool softeners and laxatives can be used when constipation is the predominant symptom; loperamide can be used when diarrhea is predominant.[7] Psychologic treatment with tricyclic antidepressants improves the clinical response above that seen with medical treatment alone.[76,77] Dietary treatment is important for these patients as well including elimination of lactose, sorbitol, fructose, and caffeine.[7] Fiber supplementation is effective for the constipation symptoms of IBS, but not for pain and diarrhea.[70]

Pelvic Venous Incompetence

Pelvic venous incompetence (PVI), also referred to as pelvic congestion syndrome, is defined as pelvic (typically ovarian) varicosities associated with chronic pelvic pain.[78,79] First described in 1857 by Richet, it was not before the middle of the last century that this entity has been recognized. However, there is still controversy related to pelvic congestion syndrome and it remains an underdiagnosed disease. In many patients with chronic pelvic pain, it is usually considered as a diagnosis of exclusion.

The pain associated with pelvic congestion syndrome is described as heaviness or deep and prolonged pelvic pain with varying severity. The pain is exacerbated by position change (with pain typically worse in the upright position), abdominal pressure, and at the end of the day. It is associated with dyspareunia and dysmenorrhea. Approximately 150,000 to 200,000 women in the United States have pelvic varicosities, of which only a portion will present with the clinical picture of chronic pelvic pain.[80] The risk factors for pelvic congestion syndrome include hormonal factors, heredity, history of varicose veins (lower extremities), and multiple pregnancies.

Many different imaging studies, including Doppler ultrasound (transabdominal or transvaginal), computed tomography (CT), and MRI can potentially demonstrate pelvic varicosities.[81–83] It is known, however, that MRI can underestimate venous pathology because it is typically performed in the supine position. New MRI technology is being developed that allows imaging of patients in the standing position. Ultrasonography can be performed in both supine and upright positions. Another way to demonstrate ovarian varices is with vulvar phlebography (injection of contrast into vulvar varices after surgical exposure of vein or percutaneous venous puncture) and transuterine venography (a needle is placed into myometrium) with pelvic images taken.[84] Once varicosities have been identified in a patient with chronic pelvic pain, consideration can be given toward embolizing the abnormal veins responsible for the reflux of blood into the varices, including the ovarian and/or internal iliac veins.[80,85] This technique is outlined in Chapter 16.

■ Conclusions

Chronic pelvic pain is frequent and disabling in most patients. The knowledge of different causes and their treatment is of utmost importance to help these patients. Although the differential diagnosis for chronic pelvic pain is extensive, interventional radiology is playing an increasing role in the management of these patients, primarily due to its role in the treatment of conditions such as uterine fibroids, adenomyosis, and pelvic congestion syndrome.

References

1. ACOG Committee on Practice Bulletin – Gynecology. Chronic pelvic pain. Obstet Gynecol 2004;103:589–605
2. Mathias SD, Kuppermann M, Ziberman RF, Lipschutz RC, Steege JF. Chronic pelvic pain: prevelance, health related quality of life and economic correlates. Obstet Gynecol 1996;87:321–327
3. Zondervan KT, Yudkin PL, Vessey MP, et al. Chronic pelvic pain in the community: symptoms, investigations, and diagnoses. Am J Obstet Gynecol 2001;184:1149–1155
4. Parker JD, Leondires M, Sinaii N, Premkumar A, Nieman LK, Stratton P. Persistence of dysmenorrhea and nonmenstrual pain after optimal endometriosis surgery may indicate adenomosis. Fertil Steril 2006;86:711–715
5. Fishman MB, Aronson MD. Differential diagnosis of abdominal pain in adults. UpToDate. Available at: http://www.uptodate.com. Accessed December 1, 2006
6. Howard F, Barbieri RL. Chronic pelvic pain in women. UpToDate. Available at: http://www.uptodate.com. Accessed November 16, 2006
7. Howard FM. Chronic pelvic pain. Obstet Gynecol 2003;101:594–611
8. Howard FM. Physical examination. In: Howard FM, Carter JE, Perry CP, El-Minawi AM, eds. Pelvic pain: Diagnosis and management. Philadelphia: Lippincott, Williams, and Wilkins, 2000:26–42
9. Kresch AJ, Seifer D, Sachs L, et al. Laparoscopy in 100 women with chronic pelvic pain. Obstet Gynecol 1984;64:672–674
10. Rawson JMR. Prevalence of endometriosis in asymptomatic women. J Reprod Med 1991;36:513–515
11. Moen MH. Is mild endometriosis a disease? Why do women develop endometriosis and why is it diagnosed? Hum Reprod 1995;10:8–11
12. Scialli AR. Evaluating chronic pelvic pain: a consensus recommendation. Pelvic Pain Expert Working Group. J Reprod Med 1999;44:945–952
13. Winkel CA. Evaluation and management of women with endometriosis. Obstet Gynecol 2003;102:397–408
14. Ramey JW, Archer D. Peritoneal fluid: its relevance to the development of endometriosis. Fertil Steril 1993;60:1–14
15. Hornung D, Ryan IP, Chao VA, Vigne JL, Schriock ED, Taylor RN. Immunolocalization and regulation of the chemokine RANTES in human endometrial and endometriosis tissues and cells. J Clin Endocrinol Metab 1997;82:1621–1628
16. Piva M, Horowitz GM, Sharpe-Timms KL. Interleukin-6 differentially stimulates haptoglobin production by peritoneal and endometriotic cells in vitro: a model for endometrial-peritoneal interaction in endometriosis. J Clin Endocrinol Metab 2001;86:2553–2561
17. Gazvani R, Templeton A. Peritoneal environment, cytokines and angiogenesis in the pathophysiology of endometriosis. Reproduction 2002;123:217–226
18. Child TJ, Tan SL. Endometriosis: aetiology, pathogenesis and treatment. Drugs 2001;61:1735–1750
19. Chwalisz K, Garg R, Brenner RM, Schubert G, Elger W. Selective progesterone receptor modulators (SPRMs): a novel therapeutic concept in endometriosis. Ann N Y Acad Sci 2002;955:373–388
20. Milingos S, Protopapas A, Drakakis P, et al. Laparoscopic management of patients with endometriosis and chronic pelvic pain. Ann N Y Acad Sci 2003;997:269–273
21. D'Hooghe TM, Debrock S, Hill JA, Meuleman C. Endometriosis and subfertility: is the relationship resolved? Semin Reprod Med 2003;21:243–253
22. Gianetto-Berrutti A, Feyles V. Endometriosis related to infertility. Minerva Ginecol 2003;55:407–416
23. Crosignani P, Olive D, Bergqvist A, Luciano A. Advances in the management of endometriosis: an update for clinicians. Hum Reprod Update 2006;12:179–189
24. Vercellini P, Trespidid L, De Giorgi O, Cortesi I, Parazzini F, Crosignani PG. Endometriosis and pelvic pain: Relation to disease stage and localization. Fertil Steril 1996;65:299–304
25. Mol BW, Mayram N, Lijmer JG, et al. The performance of CA 125 measurement in the detection of endometriosis: a meta-analysis. Fertil Steril 1998;70:1101–1108

26. Guerriero S, Mais V, Ajossa S, et al. The role of endovaginal ultrasound in differentiating endometriomas from other ovarian cysts. Clin Exp Obstet Gynecol 1995;22(1):20–22
27. Patel MD, Feldstein VA, Chen DC, Lipson SD, Filly RA. Endometriomas: diagnostic performance of US. Radiology 1999;210:739–745
28. Guerriero S, Ajossa S, Mais V, et al. The diagnosis of endometiomas using color Doppler energy imaging. Hum Reprod 1998;13:1691–1695
29. Alcazar JL, Laparte C, Jurado M, Lopez-Garcia G. The role of transvaginal ultrasonography combined with color velocity imaging and pulsed Doppler in the diagnosis of endometrioma. Fertil Steril 1997;67:487–491
30. Kinkel K, Chapron C, Balleyguier C, Fritel X, Dubuisson JB, Moreau JF. Magnetic resonance imaging characteristics of deep endometriosis. Hum Reprod 1999;14:1080–1086
31. Ascher SM, Arnold LL, Patt RH, et al. Adenomyosis: prospective comparison of MRI and transvaginal sonography. Radiology 1994;190:803–806
32. Walter AJ, Hentz JG, Magtibay PM, Cornella JL, Magrina JF. Endometriosis: correlation between histologic and visual findings at laparoscopy. Am J Obstet Gynecol 2001;184:1407–1413
33. Stratton P, Winkel CA, Sinaii N, Merino MJ, Zimmer C, Nieman LK. Location, color, size, depth, and volume may predict endometriosis in lesions resected at surgery. Fertil Steril 2002;78:743–749
34. Koninckx PR, Meuleman C, Demeyere S, Lesaffre E, Cornillie FJ. Suggestive evidence that pelvic endometriosis is a progressive disease, whereas deeply infiltrating endometriosis is associated with pelvic pain. Fertil Steril 1991;55:759–765
35. Fedele L, Parazzini F, Bianchi S, Arcaini L, Candiani G. Stage and localization of pelvic endometriosis and pain. Fertil Steril 1990;53:155–158
36. Ling FW. Randomized controlled trial of depot leuprolide in patients with chronic pelvic pain and clinically suspected endometriosis. Pelvic Pain Study Group. Obstet Gynecol 1999;93:51–58
37. Rice VM. Conventional medical therapies for endometriosis. Ann N Y Acad Sci 2002;955:343–352
38. Valle RF, Sciarra JJ. Endometriosis: treatment strategies. Ann N Y Acad Sci 2003;997:229–239
39. Winkel CA, Scialli AR. Medical and surgical therapies for pain associated with endometriosis. J Womens Health Gend Based Med 2001;10:137–162
40. Clayton RD, Hawe JA, Love JC, Wilkinson N, Garry R. Recurrent pain after hysterectomy and bilateral salpingooophorectomy for endometriosis: evaluation of laparoscopic excision of residual endometriosis. Br J Obstet Gynaecol 1999;106:740–744
41. Namnoum AB, Hickman TM, Goodman SB, Gehlbach DL, Rock JA. Incidence of symptom recurrence after hysterectomy for endometriosis. Fertil Steril 1995;64:898–902
42. Abbott J, Hawe J, Hunter D, Holmes M, Finn P, Garry R. Laparoscopic excision of endometriosis: a randomized, placebo-controlled trial. Fertil Steril 2004;82:878–884
43. Hornstein MD, Hemmings R, Yuzpe AA, Heinrichs WL. Use of nafarelin versus placebo after reductive laparoscopic surgery for endometriosis. Fertil Steril 1997;68:860–864
44. Proctor ML, Farquhar CM, Sinclair OJ, Johnson NP. Surgical interruption of pelvic nerve pathways for primary and secondary dysmenorrhoea. Cochrane Database Review 2003; (2):CD001896
45. Feste JR, Winkel CA. Is the standard of care what we think it is? JSLS 1999;3:331–334
46. Levgur M. Therapeutic options for adenomyosis: a review. Arch Gynecol Obstet 2007;276:1–15
47. Benson RC, Sneeden VD. Adenomyosis: a reappraisal of symptomatology. Am J Obstet Gynecol 1958;76:11044–11061
48. Hoike H, Ikerone T, Mori N. Relationship between dysmenorrhea severity and prostaglandin production in women with adenomyosis (Abstract P-21). Abstract presented at: Fifth World Congress on Endometriosis; October 21–24 1996; Yokohama, Japan
49. Adenomyosis AR. current perspectives. Obstet Gynecol Clin North Am 1989;16:221–235
50. Fedele L, Bianchi S, Dorta M, et al. Transvaginal ultrasonography in the diagnosis of diffuse adenomyosis. Fertil Steril 1992;58:94–97
51. Lohle PN, De Vries J, Klazen CA, et al. Uterine artery embolization for symptomatic adenomyosis with or without uterine leiomyomas with the use of calibrated tris-acryl gelatin microspheres: midterm clinical and MR imaging follow-up. J Vasc Interv Radiol 2007;18:835–841
52. Kim MD, Kim S, Kim NK, et al. Long-term results of uterine artery embolization for symptomatic adenomyosis. AJR Am J Roentgenol 2007;188:176–181
53. Pelage JP, Jacob D, Fazel A, et al. Midterm results of uterine artery embolization for symptomatic adenomyosis: initial experience. Radiology 2005;234:948–953
54. Goldberg J. Uterine artery embolization for adenomyosis: looking at the glass half full. Radiology 2005;236:1111–1112
55. The Practice Committee of the American Society for Reproductive Medicine. Control and prevention of peritoneal adhesions in gynecologic surgery. Fertil Steril 2006;86(Suppl 4):S1–S5
56. Diamond MP, El-Mowafi DM. Pelvic adhesions. Surg Technol Int 1998;VII:273–283
57. Kresch AJ, Seifer DB, Sachs LB, Barrese I. Laparoscopy in 100 women with chronic pelvic pain. Obstet Gynecol 1984;64:672–674
58. Swank DJ, Swank-Bordewijk SC, Hop WC, et al. Laparoscopic adhesiolysis in patients with chronic abdominal pain: a blinded randomized controlled multi-centre trial. Lancet 2003;361:1247–1251
59. Metts JF. Interstitial cystitis: urgency and frequency syndrome. Am Fam Physician 2001;64:1199–1214
60. Gunter J. Chronic pelvic pain: an integrated approach to diagnosis and treatment. Obstet Gynecol Surv 2003;58:615–623
61. Evans RJ, Grannum RS. Current diagnosis of interstitial cystitis: an evolving paradigm. Urology 2007;69(Suppl 4A):64–72
62. Hand JR. Interstitial cystitis: report of 223 cases (204 women and 19 men). J Urol 1949;61:291–310
63. Sant GR, Hanno PM. Interstitial cystitis: current issues and controversies in diagnosis. Urology 2001;57(suppl 6A):82–88
64. Parsons CL, Greenberger M, Gabal L, et al. The role of urinary potassium in the pathogenesis and diagnosis of interstitial cystitis. J Urol 1998;159:1862–1866
65. Chambers GK, Fenster HN, Cripps S, et al. An assessment of the use of intravesical potassium in the diagnosis of interstitial cystitis. J Urol 1999;162:699–701
66. Moldwin RM, Evans RJ, Stanford EJ, Rosenberg MT. Rational approaches to the treatment of patients with interstitial cystitis. Urology 2007;69(Suppl 4A):73–81
67. Moldwin RM, Sant GR. Interstitial cystitis: a pathophysiology and treatment update. Clin Obstet Gynecol 2002;45:259–272
68. Oberpenning F, van Ophpven A, Hertle L. Interstitial cystitis: an update. Curr Opin Urol 2002;12:321–332
69. Messing EM. Interstitial cystitis and related syndromes. In: Walsh PC, Gittes RF, Perlmutter AD, et al, eds. Campbell's Urology. 5th ed. Philadelphia: WB Saunders; 1986:1070–1092
70. Gillespie L. Destruction of the vesicoureteric plexus for the treatment of hypersensitive bladder disorders. Br J Urol 1994;74:40–43
71. Manning AP, Tompson WG, Heaton KW, et al. Towards a positive diagnosis of the irritable bowel. BMJ 1978;2:653–654
72. Mertz HR. Irritable bowel syndrome. N Engl J Med 2003;349:2136–2146
73. Whitehead WE, Palsson O, Jones KR. Systematic review of the comorbidity of irritable bowel syndrome with other disorders: what are the causes and implications? Gastroenterology 2002;122:1140–1156
74. Spiller R, Aziz Q, Creed F, et al. The British Society of Gastroenterology. Guidelines on the Irritable Bowel Syndrome: Mechanisms and Practical Management. Gut 2007;56(12):1770–1798
75. Horwitz BJ, Fisher RS. The irritable bowel syndrome. N Engl J Med 2001;344:1846–1850
76. Guthrie E, Creed F, Dawson D, Tomenson B. A controlled trial of psychological treatment for the irritable bowel syndrome. Gastroenterology 1991;100:450–457

77. Svedlund J, Ottosson JO, Sjodin I, Dotevall G. Controlled study of psychotherapy in irritable bowel syndrome. Lancet 1983;2(8350):589–591
78. Edlundh KO. Pelvic varicocities in women: a preliminary report. Acta Obstet Gynecol Scand 1964;43:399–407
79. Beard RW, Belsey EM, Lieberman BA, Wilkinson JC. Pelvic pain in women. Am J Obstet Gynecol 1977;128:566–570
80. Machan L, Vogelzang R. Interventional radiologic diagnosis and embolization of ovarian varicoceles in the treatment of chronic pelvic pain. Female Patient 1997;22:25–28
81. Liu SZ, Chou CP, Lion WS, Huang JS, Pan HB. Pelvic congestion syndrome–findings on multi-detector row computerized tomography: a case report. Kaohsiung J Med Sci 2003;19:569–573
82. Nascimento AB, Mitchell DG, Holland G. Ovarian veins: magnetic resonance imaging findings in an asymptomatic population. J Magn Reson Imaging 2002;15:551–556
83. Park SJ, Lim JW, Ko YT, et al. Diagnosis of pelvic congestion syndrome using transabdominal and transvaginal sonography. AJR Am J Roentgenol 2004;182:683–688
84. Beard RW, Highman JH, Pearce S, Reginald PW. Diagnosis of pelvic varicosities in women with chronic pelvic pain. Lancet 1984;2:946–949
85. Vembrux AC, Chang AH, Kim HS, et al. Pelvic congestion syndrome (pelvic venous incompetence): impact of ovarian and internal iliac vein embolotherapy on menstrual cycle and chronic pelvic pain. J Vasc Interv Radiol 2002;13:171–178

16 Pelvic Congestion Syndrome and Ovarian Vein Embolization

Anthony Andrew Nicholson

Pelvic congestion syndrome (PCS) was first described in 1857 and was associated with chronic pelvic pain in 1949.[1,2] Despite this history, PCS is a condition that is often not considered during the evaluation of a patient with chronic pelvic pain. Even when it is considered, PCS is a condition that is difficult to diagnose. This does not diminish its importance, however, because PCS is a condition that causes distress to a significant number of women. There are many options for treating PCS; some are more successful than others, but none are completely successful. In this respect, embolotherapy is no different but the results of endovascular treatment are at least equivalent to those of surgery and better than conventional medical therapy.

Chronic pelvic pain accounts for up to 40% of female patients attending gynecology outpatient clinics and is said to occur in 15% of all women between the ages of 18 and 50 years.[3] Fifteen percent of all hysterectomies and 35% of diagnostic laparoscopies are performed to diagnose and treat patients with chronic pelvic pain.[4] Many of these patients will undergo clinical and ultrasound examinations that are normal and will ultimately get better without any intervention.[3] However, approximately one-third of these patients will have endometriosis and another third will have some other structural abnormality of the fallopian tubes, bowel, or bladder. It is important that these significant pathologies are excluded before a diagnosis of PCS is considered. The diagnosis of PCS should be on every gynecologist's list of causes of chronic pelvic pain, but unfortunately often it is not.

■ Etiology

Pelvic congestion syndrome has a mixed etiology. The demands made on venous return by the constant hormonal changes associated with pregnancy leads to variable increases in intraluminal pressure. This can ultimately result in weakening of the ovarian vein walls and valvular incompetence. In some patients, there is a congenital absence of valves in the ovarian veins. These conditions can all result in reflux of blood down the ovarian vein into the tributaries of the internal iliac veins within the pelvis. This occurs more frequently on the left than the right because of the anatomic configuration of these veins.

The left ovarian vein drains into the left renal vein, which then takes a roughly perpendicular course to drain into the inferior vena cava. The right ovarian vein usually drains directly into the inferior vena cava, just below the right renal vein. The resulting congestion of the infundibulopelvic and broad ligaments leads to swelling and engorgement, which, in part, leads to the pain experienced by the patient. However, it is not just the physical blood volume and back pressure that causes the pain: venous ischemia, both in the vessel wall and the end organ also plays a role and most interestingly the stretching and shear stress on the inner surface of the ovarian vein distorts both the endothelial and the smooth muscle cells that respond by releasing vasodilator substances. These include neuropeptide transmitters such as substance P and the neurokinins A and B.[5] The nutcracker syndrome has a different etiology and implications and is discussed separately.

■ Patient Presentation

One of the reasons why a diagnosis of PCS is often not considered is because it can present with a variety of symptoms (**Table 16.1**). These findings tend to be nonspecific and are therefore potentially indicative of several of the conditions that can cause chronic pelvic pain. PCS occurs most often in women who are multigravida and in their 20s and 30s. It classically presents with pelvic pain or a

Table 16.1 Symptoms Associated with Pelvic Congestion Syndrome

Symptoms
Pain brought on by an increase in intraabdominal pressure
Pain relieved by lying down
May be unilateral or bilateral
Dull aching pain
Dysfunctional bleeding and dysmenorrhea common
Low back pain
Postcoital ache that may last for hours or days
Acute episodes of pain common
Menstrual disorders
Bladder irritability (24 to 45% of patients)
Functional gastrointestinal symptoms
Family history of varicose veins and associated with vulval varicosities

postcoital ache that is worse on the left side, may last for hours or days, and may be relived by lying down. The pelvic fullness experienced by these patients can be acute and severe or chronic and dull. It can be unilateral or bilateral. These symptoms, when combined with ovarian point tenderness, are said to be 94% sensitive and 77% specific for pelvic congestion syndrome.[6] Such specificity and sensitivity figures indicate that women do have a variety of other symptoms including pain brought on by increased intraabdominal pressure, bladder irritability (which occurs in 24 to 45% of all patients), functional gastrointestinal (GI) symptoms (such as constipation), and low back pain. A history of varicose veins and associated vulval varicosities is often present in patients with PCS. Other features on physical examination that may point to the diagnosis include cervical motion tenderness and an engorged blue-looking cervix.

Women with PCS are often described as being depressed and anxious. This is partly due to the fact that they have very real symptoms, which are chronic and potentially debilitating. In addition, they have often gone through an extensive diagnostic workup and in many cases, the cause for their discomfort is difficult to find. There are also good pharmacologic and physiologic reasons why these patients might be suffering from psychological stress. Substance P and the neurokinins A and B, released in response to stretching by endothelial and smooth muscle cells described earlier, play a key role in the regulation of emotions and are an integral part of central nervous system pathways involved in psychological stress.

■ Imaging

Following the performance of a detailed history and physical examination, most patients presenting with chronic pelvic pain will undergo some type of imaging evaluation. This most commonly includes an ultrasound examination and laparoscopy. Sonographic findings of pelvic congestion syndrome include a dilated left ovarian vein with reversed caudal flow, dilated arcuate veins crossing the uterine myometrium, polycystic changes of the ovary, and variable duplex waveform during a Valsalva maneuver.[7] Computed tomography (CT), magnetic resonance imaging (MRI), and magnetic resonance angiography (MRA) (**Fig. 16.1**) can all aid in the diagnosis of PCS, but in all of these investigations the patient is likely to be supine. Therefore, although all of these studies may demonstrate venous engorgement in the pelvis in severe cases, in less severe cases this same venous engorgement might not be seen, which will result in a false-negative examination.[8]

Cross-sectional imaging studies remain important because they may reveal associated abnormalities that suggest a diagnosis of PCS. For instance, polycystic ovaries

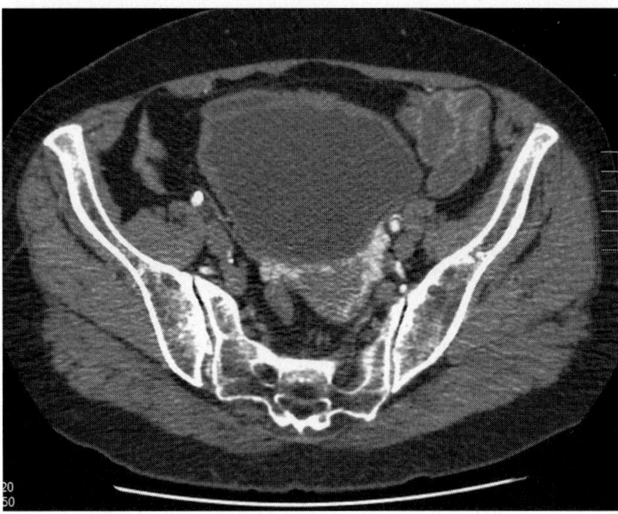

Fig. 16.1 Contrast-enhanced computed tomography scan of the pelvis in a woman with chronic pelvic pain demonstrates multiple enlarged varicosities around the uterus. She responded well to endovascular treatment.

may be found on ultrasound and these are associated with pelvic congestion syndrome in 56% of patients. Similarly, imaging may reveal an increase in uterine cross-sectional area and an endometrial thickness, which is marginally greater than normal. On CT, these findings may cause confusion with adenomyosis. None of these imaging modalities, however, should be considered as a primary tool for diagnosing PCS.

Presently, ovarian venography remains the definitive modality for evaluating patients for PCS (**Fig. 16.2**). Ideally, a percutaneous venogram should be performed on a tilting table so that the patient is partially upright during the examination. This will maximize the ability of venography to detect reflux and perhaps address the false-negative cases seen on cross-sectional imaging or laparoscopy performed in the supine position. Ovarian venography can be performed from a jugular or femoral vein approach. The jugular vein is often preferred because the angles favor selective catheterization of the ovarian veins from this approach. In addition, it is preferred by many if embolization is being considered at the same sitting for the same reason. Selective catheterization of the left renal vein (LRV) can usually be performed with 4 French cobra or multipurpose catheters. The same catheters can be used to catheterize the right ovarian vein (ROV), though a sidewinder is often required if the study is being performed via femoral vein access. The LRV should be catheterized first because it is typically more straightforward and often has the greatest yield for a positive finding.

Once the LRV is catheterized, a venogram should be performed with the patient in a semiupright position or while the patient is performing a Valsalva maneuver (if a

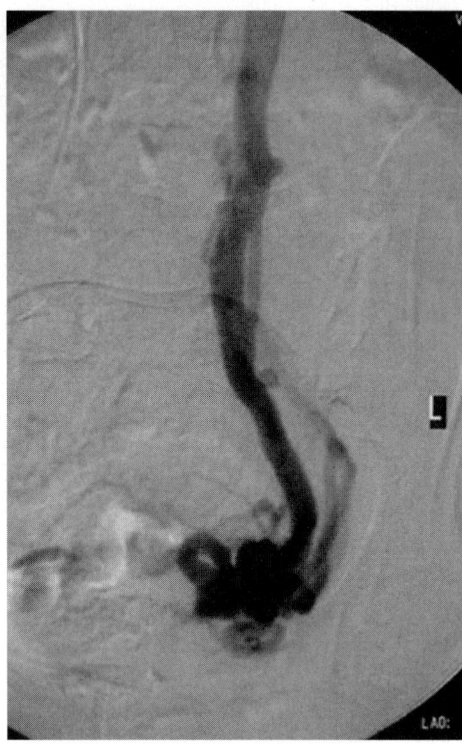

Fig. 16.2 Contrast injection into the left renal vein during Valsalva maneuver caused gross reflux of contrast down the left ovarian vein in a woman with a long history of chronic pelvic pain.

tilting table is not available). This can be achieved using an old-fashioned sphygmomanometer. With this technique, the patient is asked to blow into the rubber tubing and to hold the mercury at ~20 mm. The venogram should be performed prior to catheterization of the LOV for two reasons.

First, it is important not to miss the diagnosis of nutcracker syndrome (see below). Second, if significant reflux is present, an injection of contrast into the LRV (under the above-described conditions) will immediately determine whether or not the patient has reflux down the ovarian vein. If no reflux is seen then it is highly unlikely that the patient has PCS. An attempt can be made at this point to catheterize the ROV, but if this is also not seen or is not quickly catheterized, it is probable that it is small and not refluxing. The examination can be terminated at this point. The diagnostic criteria for PCS on venography include a minimum ovarian diameter of 8 to 10 mm, uterine venous engorgement, congestion of the ovarian plexus, filling of the pelvic veins across the midline, and/or filling of vulvovaginal and thigh varicosities.[9,10]

The LOV can be catheterized with a hydrophilic guide wire and the chosen catheter. Great care should be taken in performing this selective catheterization because in its distended state, the ovarian vein is fragile and can easily be ruptured. In addition, it can go into spasm very quickly if it is overly irritated and this can prevent treatment and occasionally prevent the removal of the catheter until it relaxes. The guide wire and catheter should be carefully advanced further into the ovarian vein until it is positioned just above the pelvic brim. At that point, additional contrast should be injected to confirm reflux into the pelvic veins. In addition, this injection can demonstrate cross filling to the right side of the pelvis (if present) and reflux into any vulvar or thigh varicosities that may be present.

■ Nutcracker Syndrome

The so-called nutcracker syndrome is caused by LRV compression between the superior mesenteric artery and the aorta (**Fig. 16.3**), with associated retrograde hypertension within the LRV (and its tributaries).[11,12] The renal venous

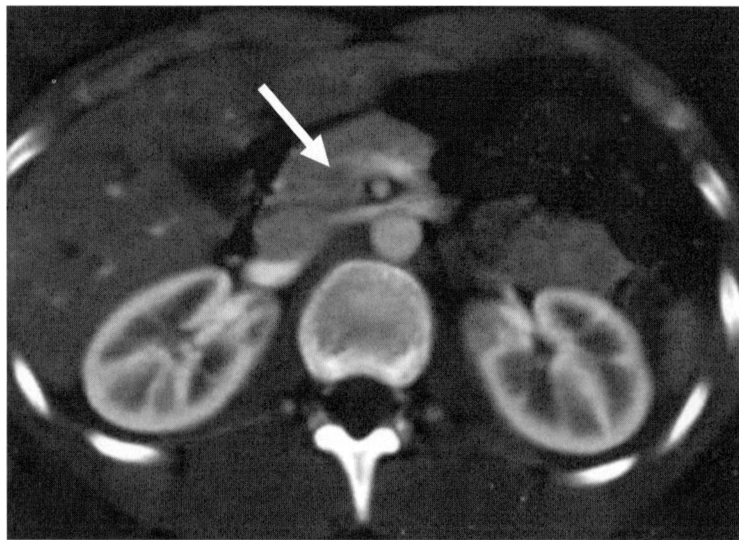

Fig. 16.3 Contrast-enhanced computed tomography scan demonstrating compression of the left renal vein by the superior mesenteric artery (*arrow*) causing the nutcracker syndrome.

hypertension found in patients with nutcracker syndrome leads to the development of collaterals around the renal pelvis that may cause hematuria and retrograde flow in the LOV.[13] This can result in the symptoms of PCS.

There are two peaks of incidence at young and middle age, which correspond to two different pathophysiological stages of the nutcracker syndrome. At an early stage, LRV compression leads to LRV hypertension and the development of venous collaterals around the renal capsule. Because incompetence of the LOV veins has presumably not yet occurred, no reflux is seen in these vessels at this stage; furthermore, high pressure in the LRV potentially leads to the development of direct communications between the dilated veins and adjacent calyces with consequent hematuria and flank pain.[14,15]

At a later stage, the persistence of LRV hypertension causes valvular incompetence and massive reflux of blood into ovarian or lumbar veins leading to pelvic or vulvar varices with the symptomatology of PCS. This is mainly encountered in middle-age women.[16,17] The diagnosis of nutcracker syndrome is based on an association of symptoms of hematuria, left-sided flank pain, pelvic congestion, pelvic and vulvar varices, and imaging findings of LRV compression on cross-sectional imaging confirmed by venography and documentation of a pressure gradient of more than 3 mm Hg between the LRV and IVC.[18]

A variety of surgical procedures, including LRV bypass with polytetrafluoroethylene (PTFE) graft interposition, and autotransplantation of the left kidney into the left iliac fossa have been described to alleviate the LRV compression associated with the nutcracker syndrome.[19] Recent reports describe endovascular procedures such as renal venous stenting from a femoral vein approach (**Fig. 16.4**).[20–22] Follow-up in these series, which total nine patients only, ranges from 4 to 54 months. These few case reports and series are encouraging, especially in light of the fact that venous stenting is proving successful in the short treatment of venous diseases such as vena cava syndromes and Budd–Chiari syndrome. However, it is my experience that venous stenting is successful only for a short time in patients with nutcracker syndrome. Studies require much longer follow-up if intravascular stenting is to become a treatment option.

■ Treatment

There are few medical options to treat patients with PCS, all of which revolve around addressing the pain associated with this syndrome. Nonsteroidal antiinflammatory drugs may help with pain relief in the short term, but they are not a long-term solution to this problem. Medroxyprogesterone acetate has been shown to relieve symptoms in ~40% of patients and a combination of this and psychotherapy may be effective in ~60% of patients. However, Farquhar et al[23] performed a study in which patients were assigned to psychotherapy alone, medroxyprogesterone acetate alone, these two in combination, or placebo and found that placebo use was effective at one year in 50% of patients. Analgesia is a good first line treatment, but patients symptoms

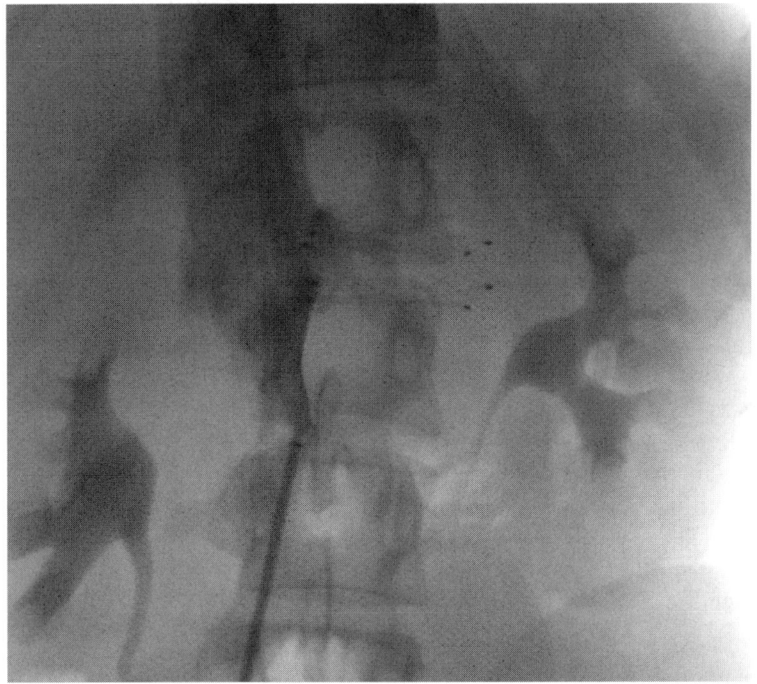

Fig. 16.4 Left renal vein stenting has been suggested as a treatment option in nutcracker syndrome as in this case where a 10 mm self-expanding stent has been inserted successfully. However, longer-term studies are required to evaluate the real efficacy of this treatment.

should not be ignored if it is not completely effective or pain recurs when it is stopped.

Surgical treatment utilizing hysterectomy and bilateral oophorectomy with hormone replacement is said to effectively cure, or at least bring symptomatic improvement in two-thirds of patients.[4] Despite the definitive nature of a hysterectomy, it does not appear to be as effective as simply ligating the ovarian vein, which is reported as having a 73% cure rate with 78% of patients demonstrating symptomatic improvement.[24] Ligation of the ovarian vein(s) can be done using an open or laparoscopic approach. However, ligation of the ovarian vein can also result in transaction to nerves of the pelvis and still leaves open the possibility of establishing collateral channels leading to symptomatic recurrence. Surgery is rarely used because endovascular treatments are more effective and less invasive.

Since Edwards et al[25] reported the first case in 1993, embolization used to treat ovarian varices has become an effective treatment option for these patients. Unlike ovarian vein ligation, embolization of the ovarian vein leaves the nerves that accompany the vein intact. Though it does potentially allow for the establishment of collaterals, these are limited by occlusion of collaterals that drain into the high ovarian vein. Embolization is reported to have a 73 to 78% rate of symptomatic improvement or cure.[26] There is still controversy among interventional radiologists regarding the best technique to use and it is clear from the literature that the technique is still evolving. Specific questions that remain unanswered include the following:

- Should only refluxing veins be embolized (usually the left)?
- Should both ovarian veins be embolized regardless of whether they are both refluxing?
- Should both ovarian veins and the internal iliac veins be embolized?
- If the latter, should this be done all at once or should treatment be staged?
- What embolization material should be used – coils, sclerosants, glue, or Gelfoam (Pfizer, Inc., New York, NY)?

Initially, patients were treated with unilateral ovarian vein embolization. This was invariably the left ovarian vein given the anatomic predisposition of this vessel toward causing PCS.[27–29] In this early experience, coils were the main embolization material used. Results were variable, with significant relief being described in ~66% of all patients. It is not always clear in these articles how "significant relief" was defined. Approximately 33% of patients were described as having partial or no relief.

Although these figures are slightly disappointing, they are at least as good as those described for surgical treatment. By the late 1990s, bilateral ovarian vein embolization was becoming the standard of care for this patient population. Many operators were embolizing the refluxing left ovarian vein and the right ovarian vein whether it was refluxing or not. This is not always as easy as it sounds. Occasionally, the right ovarian vein cannot be found or is extremely small and therefore difficult to catheterize.[30] In these circumstances only the left ovarian vein is embolized because it is reasonable to conclude that a small vein that is difficult to catheterize may not be responsible for significant reflux and symptoms.

The use of foam sclerotherapy has also been applied to the ovarian veins when treating patients with PCS. A total dose of 3 to 6 cc of 3% sodium tetradecyl sulfate (STD), mixed with either air or Gelfoam and then passed rapidly back and forth across a three-way stopcock between two syringes, can be injected into the ovarian vein below the level of the pelvic brim (**Fig. 16.5**) to treat PCS. This can then be followed by coil embolization to within one centimeter of the vein origin (**Fig. 16.6**).[30] In addition, the internal iliac

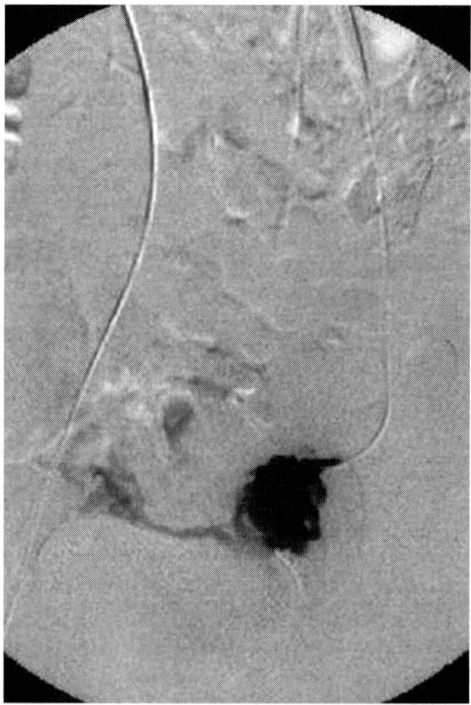

Fig. 16.5 A catheter in the left ovarian vein has been advanced to the pelvic brim in this patient with classical pelvic congestion syndrome. Venography reveals multiple large varicosities with cross filling to the right. Following injection of 3 cc of 3% sodium tetradecyl sulfate and Gelfoam (Pfizer, Inc., New York, NY), mixed into a foam between two syringes there is stasis in the varicosities. This was followed by coil embolization of the left and right ovarian veins.

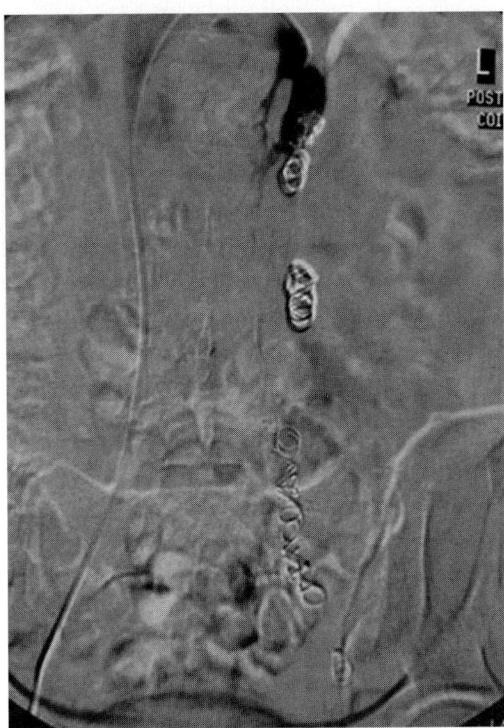

Fig. 16.6 Coils inserted to within a centimeter of the left ovarian origin from the left renal vein following Gelfoam (Pfizer, Inc., New York, NY) sodium tetradecyl sulfate sclerotherapy to pelvic varicosities.

veins can be embolized with either coils or sclerosant. Results using this approach seemed to improve, though it is difficult to determine objectively how this improvement was being measured.

The largest series to date describes 127 patients, 106 of whom underwent bilateral ovarian vein sclerotherapy followed by coil embolization.[30] The remaining patients underwent unilateral embolization and sclerotherapy. All patients underwent a venogram of the internal iliac veins 4 to 6 weeks after ovarian vein embolization. The internal iliac veins were then occluded proximally with a balloon and contrast was injected into the internal iliac vein to determine if and when contrast refluxed into the contralateral internal iliac vein. If residual varices were seen, the same volume of sclerosant/Gelfoam slurry was then injected. After 5 minutes, the balloon was deflated and the procedure was repeated in the opposite internal iliac vein. One hundred eight of the 127 patients in this study underwent bilateral internal iliac vein embolization in this way. A visual analogue score similar to that used for pain relief in cancer was used to assess outcome in this study. Eighty three percent of patients demonstrated relief of symptoms, 13% were no better, and 4% were worse. It would seem from these results that there can be a significant improvement in the success rate of embolization by embolizing the internal iliac veins.

My approach is to embolize the incompetent left ovarian vein by using a slurry of Gelfoam and a sclerosing agent together with coils. The same approach can then be utilized on the right if there is obvious reflux or to just use coil embolization if the reflux is not obvious (assuming that the vessel can be easily catheterized). Patients are seen 6 weeks later in the outpatient setting, and if they are still complaining of significant symptoms, the internal iliac veins are embolized in the manner described by Kim et al.[30]

■ Complications

Significant pulmonary embolic disease does not appear to be a complication of ovarian or internal iliac vein embolization. The use of coils in the internal iliac veins in some patients can lead to coil displacement with migration into the lungs; this can potentially require retrieval of these coils. This problem, however, has not been reported in association with the use of a Gelfoam/sclerosant slurry. Occasionally a patient's symptoms can be made worse by embolization, but this is exceptional, occurring in only 4% of patients.[30] Spasm and occasional rupture of the thin-walled ovarian vein can occur, but this rarely leads to any sequelae and can be treated with simple analgesia. There have not been significant changes in basal follicle-stimulating hormone, luteinizing hormone, or estradiol levels associated with this procedure.[30]

■ Conclusions

Patients with pelvic congestion syndrome are generally unhappy and have often been through a plethora of investigations to exclude other causes of pelvic pain. Pelvic venography performed in an upright or semiupright position, should be the procedure of choice when evaluating these patients because other investigations can misdiagnose subtle pelvic congestion syndrome. If pelvic congestion is caused by the nutcracker syndrome it can be treated by embolization and renal vein stenting, but this may fail in the medium to long term. In classic pelvic congestion syndrome, embolization, if done carefully, is not a difficult or time-consuming procedure, especially if performed from the jugular approach. The evolution of the embolization technique would now dictate that both ovarian veins are embolized if the right ovarian vein can be found and easily catheterized. Gelfoam sclerosant slurry is very effective for this purpose, followed by coil embolization. The internal iliac veins can be embolized as described if the patient's symptoms persist. Finally, it is very important not to build the patient's expectations too high as treatment may fail to relieve symptoms on a long-term basis.

References

1. Richet MA. Traite Pratique d'Anatomie Medico-Chirugicale. Paris: E. Chamerot Libraire Editeur;1857
2. Taylor HC. Vascular congestion and hyperemia; their effects on structure and function in the female reproductive system. Am J Obstet Gynecol 1949;57:637–653
3. Harris RD, Holtzman SR, Poppe AM. Clinical outcome in female patients with pelvic pain and normal pelvic ultrasound findings. Radiology 2000;216:440–443
4. Association of Professors of Gynecology and Obstetrics (APGO). APGO Educational Series on Women's Health Issues. Chronic Pelvic Pain: An Integrated Approach. Washington, DC: APGO; 2000
5. Stones RW, Beard RW, Burnstock G. Pharmacology of the human ovarian vein: responses to putative neurotransmitters and endothelin-1. Br J Obstet Gynaecol 1994;101:701–706
6. Beard RW, Reginald PW, Wadsworth J. Clinical features of women with chronic lower abdominal pain and pelvic congestion. Br J Obstet Gynaecol 1988;95:153–161
7. Park SJ, Lim JW, Ko YT, et al. Diagnosis of pelvic congestion syndrome using transabdominal and transvaginal sonography. AJR Am J Roentgenol 2004;182:683–688
8. Venbrux AC, Chang AH, Kim HS, et al. Pelvic congestion syndrome (pelvic venous incompetence): impact of ovarian and internal iliac vein embolotherapy on menstrual cycle and chronic pelvic pain. J Vasc Interv Radiol 2002;13:171–178
9. Kennedy A, Hemmingway A. Radiology of ovarian varices. Br J Hosp Med 1990;44:38–43
10. Giacchetto C, Cotroneo GB, Marincolo F, Cammisuli F, Caruso G, Catizone F. Ovarian varicocele: ultrasonic and phlebographic evaluation. J Clin Ultrasound 1990;18:551–555
11. Rudloff U, Holmes RJ, Prem JT, Faust GR, Moldwin R, Siegel D. Mesoaortic compression of the left renal vein (nutcracker syndrome): case reports and review of the literature. Ann Vasc Surg 2006;20:120–129
12. El Sadr AR, Mina A. Anatomical and surgical aspects of the operative management of varicoceles. Urol Cutaneous Rev 1950;54:257–262
13. Nicholson T, Basile A. Pelvic congestion syndrome: who should we treat and how? Tech Vasc Interv Radiol 2006;9:19–23
14. MacMahon HE, Latorraca R. Essential renal hematuria. J Urol 1954;71:667–676
15. Pytel A. Renal fornical hemorrhages: their pathogenesis and treatment. J Urol 1960;83:783–789
16. Scultetus AH, Villavicencio JL, Gillespie DL. The nutcracker syndrome: its role in the pelvic venous disorders. J Vasc Surg 2001;34:812–819
17. Wendel RG, Crawford ED, Hehman KN. The "nutcracker" phenomenon: an unusual cause for renal varicosities with hematuria. J Urol 1980;123:761–763
18. Ahmed K, Sampath R, Khan MS. Current trends in the diagnosis and management of renal nutcracker syndrome: a review. Eur J Vasc Endovasc Surg 2006;31:410–416
19. Segawa N, Azuma H, Iwamoto Y, et al. Expandable metallic stent placement for nutcracker phenomenon. Urology 1999;53:631–633
20. Kim SJ, Kim CW, Kim S, et al. Long-term follow-up after endovascular stent placement for treatment of nutcracker syndrome. J Vasc Interv Radiol 2005;16:428–431
21. Van der Laan L, Vos JA, de Boer E, et al. The central-venous compression syndrome: rare, but adequately treatable with endovascular stenting. Ned Tijdschr Geneeskd 2004;148:433–437
22. Hartung O, Grisoli D, Boufi M, et al. Endovascular stenting in the treatment of pelvic vein congestion caused by nutcracker syndrome: lessons learned from the first five cases. J Vasc Surg 2005;42: 275–280
23. Farquhar CM, Rogers V, Franks S, et al. The value of medroxyprogesterone acetate (MPA) and of psychotherapy in the treatment pelvic congestion. Br J Obstet Gynaecol 1989;96:1153–1162
24. Rundqvist E, Sandholm LE, Larsson G. Treatment of pelvic varicosities causing lower abdominal pain with extraperitoneal resection of the left ovarian vein. Ann Chir Gynaecol 1984;73:339–341
25. Edwards RD, Robertson JR, MacLean AB, Hemingway AP. Case report: pelvic pain syndrome – successful treatment of a case by ovarian vein embolization. Clin Radiol 1993;47:429–431
26. Machan L. Embolization in the female pelvis. In Dyet JD, Ettles D, Nicholson AA, et al, eds. Textbook of Endovascular Procedures. Philadelphia, PA: Churchill-Livingstone;2000:367
27. Tarazov PG, Prozorovskij KV, Ryzhkov VK. Pelvic pain syndrome caused by ovarian varices: treatment by transcatheter embolization. Acta Radiol 1997;38:1023–1025
28. Capasso P, Simons C, Trotteur G, et al. Treatment of symptomatic pelvic varices by ovarian vein embolization. Cardiovasc Intervent Radiol 1997;20(2):107–111
29. Cordts PR, Eclavea A, Buckley PJ, et al. Pelvic congestion syndrome: early clinical results after transcatheter ovarian vein embolization. J Vasc Surg 1998;28:862–868
30. Kim HS, Malhotra AD, Rowe PC, et al. Embolotherapy for pelvic congestion syndrome: long-term results. J Vasc Interv Radiol 2006;17:289–297

17 Ovarian Drainage: Cyst Aspiration

Gary P. Siskin

In recent years, the frequency of diagnosing ovarian cysts in pre- and postmenopausal patients has increased. This can most likely be attributed to improvements in ultrasound technology and increased utilization of ultrasound in female patients.[1] Most of these cysts are diagnosed as benign or functional based on their ultrasound characteristics (**Fig. 17.1**).[2–4] In fact, Granberg et al[5] observed that increased accuracy of ultrasound has allowed benign cysts to be identified reliably on ultrasound with only a 0.5% risk of malignancy. However, just because the ability of ultrasound to characterize an ovarian cyst has improved over the years, it must still be acknowledged that a benign cyst can still cause problems for patients. In the late 1980s, ovarian cysts were the fourth most common gynecologic cause of hospital admission in the United States.[6] Most ovarian cysts are asymptomatic, but a small number of patients may present with pelvic pain. In many of these patients, the presence of a cyst can lead to significant anxiety about the possibility of malignancy, despite the fact many of these patients have sonographically benign cysts.[3] For these reasons, treatment is often pursued for these patients. Even though many of these patients undergo laparoscopic or surgical resection of the cyst or the involved ovary, it has been suggested that this is overtreatment with considerable cost to patients and society and the risks often outweighing the benefits.[1,7] Therefore, it is helpful and important to be able to offer a less invasive option for these patients, which is why some interventionalists have turned to ultrasound-guided aspiration of ovarian cysts.

■ Ovarian Cyst Aspiration

Before a patient with an ovarian cyst is considered for an ultrasound-guided aspiration, interventionalists must evaluate the patient thoroughly and exclude a malignancy prior to the procedure.[8] In addition, the success of ultrasound-guided cyst aspiration depends on the criteria used for patient selection, which often include a combination of the patient's symptoms, laboratory results (tumor markers such as CA-125 and CA 19/9), and imaging findings.[5,8,9] The imaging evaluation prior to aspiration typically includes a pelvic ultrasound. Benign cysts tend to be unilocular and homogeneously anechoic with a uniformly thin wall; these

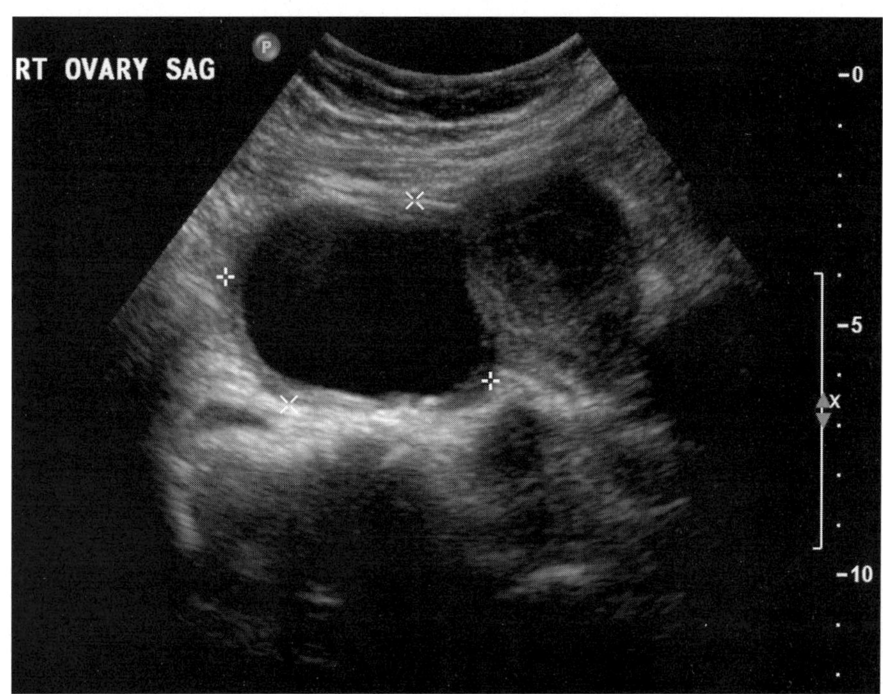

Fig. 17.1 Longitudinal ultrasound image of the pelvis demonstrating a simple ovarian cyst (with uniformly hypoechoic cyst contents, no internal septations, and no mural nodules).

are the cysts that can be considered for aspiration. Complex cysts may be multilocular and have wall thickening, septations, mural nodules, or internal echoes within the cyst cavity. Even though these cysts may be benign, there may still be too many questions regarding the etiology of the cyst to consider aspiration as primary treatment.[10] Clinically, patients who are not ideal candidates for surgery, such as obese patients, those with a history of previous pelvic surgery, and those at high risk for anesthesia, may also be considered suitable candidates for ultrasound-guided aspiration.[7]

There have been several published studies evaluating the role of both transabdominal and transvaginal ultrasound-guided aspiration in the treatment of ovarian cysts (**Fig. 17.2**). One can review this data and interpret it to either support or dispute its use in this population of patients, depending on one's individual perspective. For those that support the use of this procedure, there is data demonstrating symptomatic improvement and resolution of the cyst after aspiration. Those who do not recommend the use of this procedure cite the high rates of cyst recurrence after aspiration. Caspi et al[11] evaluated ultrasound-guided simple ovarian cyst aspiration in 107 patients who were followed for a mean of 2.7 years. In 42 patients, cyst aspiration was definitive and in another 27 patients, the cyst recurred but was followed due to a size <5 cm. Therefore, 69 patients (65%) were able to avoid surgery after aspiration. Duke et al[7] reported their results in 24 patients. Using conscious sedation, a 20 g needle was used to aspirate the cysts under transvaginal ultrasound guidance. In this population, there was a 75% recurrence rate with a mean follow-up of 39.5 months (which was longer than seen in other studies). Additional studies have reported recurrence rates ranging from 11.1 to 27.5%,[12–15] but the maximum follow-up in all of these studies was 24 months. This data supports the observation that the likelihood of finding a recurrent cyst aspiration will increase with time. Both Duke et al and Weinrub et al found a higher incidence of recurrence when the cysts were left-sided, possibly due to the differences in venous drainage between the right and left ovaries.[7,16] Bret et al[10] reported their experience with transvaginal ultrasound aspiration of ovarian cysts in 48 patients. They found that some large cysts can cause acute symptoms due to their size. In these patients, aspiration was able to provide immediate symptomatic relief. This was also found by Caspi

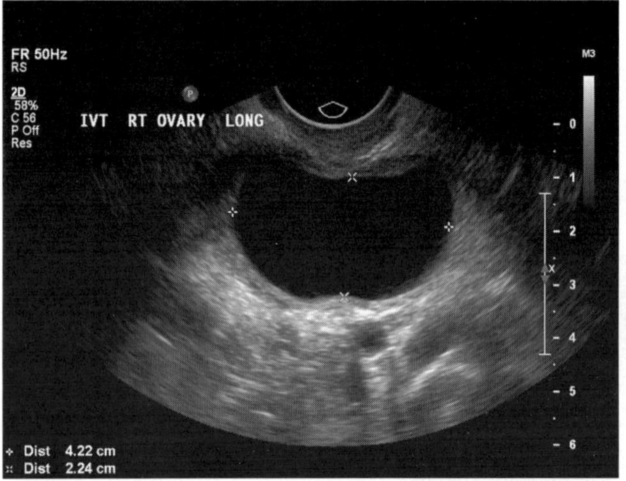

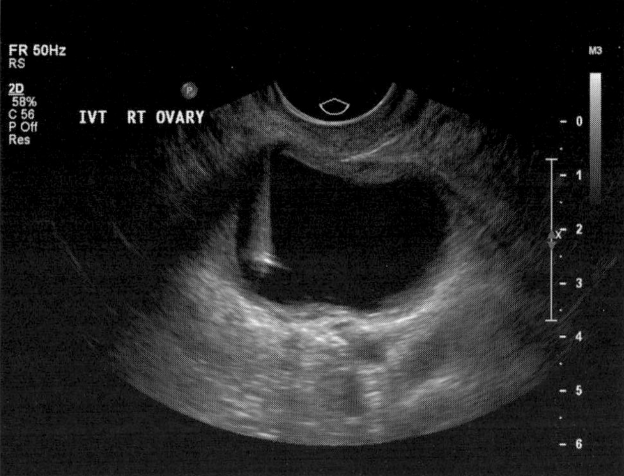

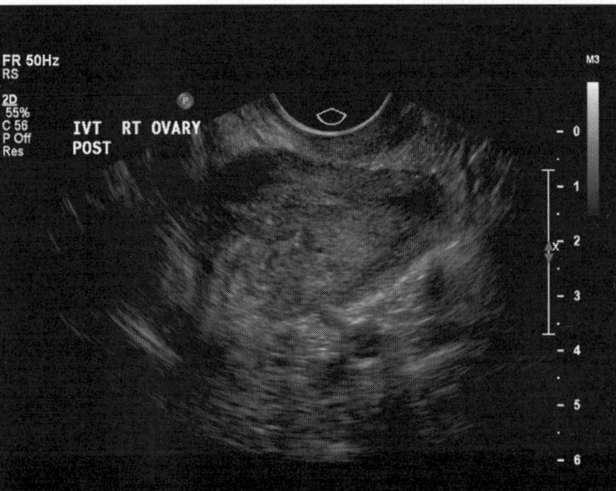

Fig. 17.2 Longitudinal images of a right ovarian cyst before **(A)**, during **(B)**, and after **(C)** transvaginal aspiration of this cyst. **B** demonstrates the needle within the cyst from a transvaginal approach.

et al[17] who found that there was immediate relief of pain in 18 patients with symptomatic ovarian cysts after aspiration. Balat et al found that 73% of patients remain free of symptoms during the follow-up period.[15]

Despite these results, the management of ovarian cysts within the gynecology community remains debatable with the potential benefits of aspiration challenged by other studies. Zanetta et al[18] performed a prospective randomized trial on 278 patients with 143 assigned to simple observation and 135 patients assigned to ultrasound-guided aspiration. In this study, it was found that there was no superiority of aspiration over simple observation. In fact, spontaneous cyst resolution occurred in 45% of patients treated conservatively.[18] Therefore, time alone may be enough to address the cysts in these patients, but unfortunately, this does not address the often acute need for treatment and the anxiety associated with this diagnosis.

Once aspiration is performed, it is mandatory to perform an evaluation of the cyst fluid to determine if a malignancy is present.[8] An initial characterization of the fluid is important to make at the time of the aspiration. Patients need to be counseled that laparoscopy or exploratory laparotomy will be recommended if there is an abnormality of the cyst fluid, including the presence of mucus or blood within the aspirate.[8,19,20] Following this initial gross evaluation of the fluid, samples must be sent for cytologic analysis. However, it has been established that cytology has a relative poor predictive value and low sensitivity for the diagnosis of an ovarian malignancy.[7,18,21,22] This, together with the fear and risk of preoperative spill of malignant cells and its negative impact on survival,[7,23] are the reasons why ultrasound-guided cyst aspiration remains controversial within the gynecology community.

Certainly, one possible solution to the problem of recurrence after aspiration is the injection of material into the cavity of the cyst. Different studies have been performed to evaluate several different agents to use in this setting. Mesogitis et al[1] utilized methotrexate, which is a folate antagonist mentioned earlier in this text in the context of treating a cervical ectopic pregnancy. Methotrexate was felt to represent a good choice of material to inject because cells within endometriomas show a high mitotic index and may be addressed with the methotrexate.[1] Thirty milligrams of methotrexate, diluted in 3 cc of normal saline, were injected into 122 patients with either a simple cyst or an endometrioma after transabdominal aspiration. Using this technique, resolution was seen in 84.6% of patients with a simple cyst and 83.6% of patients with an endometrioma.

Another possible solution for treating patients with endometriomas was described by Fisch and Sher in 2004.[24] In this study, 32 infertile women with ovarian endometriomas were treated by sclerotherapy with tetracycline. Using a transvaginal approach, an 18 g needle was used to aspirate the endometrioma and the cyst cavity was flushed with normal saline until the aspirated fluid was clear. At this point, tetracycline 5% was injected into the cyst. The volume used was slightly less than the approximate volume of the endometrioma. Following injection of the tetracycline, sterile saline (100 to 300 cc) was injected into the cul-de-sac to minimize the potential for peritoneal irritation secondary to the tetracycline. In 75% of patients, the endometriomas were completely resolved at the 6-week follow-up. Eight patients had a residual simple cyst that required repeat aspiration. Two patients required an additional course of sclerotherapy.

Noma and Yoshida reported their experience with ethanol sclerotherapy of endometriomas.[25] They treated 74 patients who were then followed for at least 6 months. The endometrioma was aspirated with a 16 g needle introduced via a transvaginal approach. Following this, pure ethanol having a volume equal to 80% of the aspirated volume with a maximum of 80 cc was injected. Using this technique, the recurrence rate was found to be 14.9%. They recommended that only patients with one cyst should be treated and that the duration of ethanol instillation should be >10 minutes. Adequate washing of the cyst following sclerotherapy was recommended to reduce alcohol intoxication. Messalli et al[26] also evaluated the role of ethanol sclerotherapy in 10 patients. They instilled ethanol into the cyst cavity after aspiration. The volume of ethanol utilized was 50% of the volume of fluid aspirated initially from the cyst. The ethanol was left in place within the cyst for 10 to 20 minutes. In 90% of patients, there was no recurrence after a mean follow-up period of 21 months.

Ultrasound-guided cyst aspiration is an option for patients with symptomatic ovarian cysts who are either not candidates for surgery or who have a laboratory and imaging evaluation suggesting a benign etiology for the cyst. In these patients, aspiration can lead to symptomatic improvement. Concerns with recurrence and the possibility of intraperitoneal spill of malignant fluid have led some to discourage the use of this procedure. However, an appropriate evaluation prior to aspiration and the potential applicability of sclerotherapy is likely to support an increased role for this procedure in suitable patients.

■ Tuboovarian Abscess Drainage

Pelvic inflammatory disease (PID) is a significant problem among reproductive-aged women. It is responsible for more hospitalizations in this population than conditions such as ovarian cysts, menstrual disorders, and uterine fibroids.[27] Despite the fact that admissions for PID have been declining since outpatient treatment has become more common, patients with a tuboovarian abscess complicating PID are usually hospitalized.[28] It has been shown that ~100,000 women in the United States are annually hospitalized with a tuboovarian abscess.[29] A tuboovarian abscess occurs in 15% of cases of PID; it most commonly occurs in the third and fourth decades of life.[30,31] If left untreated, a tuboovarian abscess can lead to complications including adhesion formation, reduced fertility, and chronic pelvic pain.[31] Antibiotic therapy can result in a clinical response rate of 35 to 87%.[32] If the patient does not respond to antibiotic therapy within 2 to 3 days, surgical treatment ranging from colpotomy to total abdominal hysterectomy and bilateral salpingo-oophorectomy is typically recommended.[33] Although definitive treatment with hysterectomy and bilateral salpingo-oophorectomy is inarguably effective, it comes at a cost to the premenopausal patients typically affected by PID. Given the age of this patient population, the primary aim of management is to be as conservative as possible. That is why many physicians have turned to image-guided aspiration of a tuboovarian abscess for treatment. The decision to use percutaneous drainage as opposed to surgery depends on local expertise and preference.[34]

At the present time, percutaneous drainage of tuboovarian abscess can be successful in 95% of patients.[35] Various approaches have been described for percutaneous drainage of a tuboovarian abscess: transabdominal,[36,37] transgluteal,[38,39] transrectal,[40,41] and transvaginal.[34,42–48] A computed tomography (CT) scan of the upper abdomen and pelvis is recommended before draining a tuboovarian abscess to better assess the anatomy and to determine if there are collections elsewhere in the abdomen, which may have been missed on a pelvic ultrasound (**Fig. 17.3**).[49]

The transvaginal approach often provides the most direct route from the vagina into the cul-de-sac or adnexal region where the tuboovarian abscesses are typically located,[31,50] although some feel that transvaginal drainage provides a less effective drainage of large abscesses compared with laparoscopy.[51] In addition, this procedure may not be appropriate for young, prepubertal, or sexually inactive patients; in these patients, a transabdominal or transgluteal approach may be more suitable.[31] That said, transvaginal aspiration has been well studied and has been the subject of several articles demonstrating its success. The largest of these studies is by Gjelland et al who performed 449 transvaginal aspirations on 302 women.[48] Technically, this procedure was performed under ultrasound guidance. Once fluid was aspirated from the abscess, the cavity was irrigated with saline to make aspiration easier. Saline irrigation was used when the abscess contents were particularly viscous and when multiple loculations were seen on ultrasound; 93.4% of patients were successfully treated for transvaginal aspiration of purulent fluid together with antibiotic therapy. The remaining patients underwent surgery due to diagnostic or therapeutic uncertainty after aspiration based on persistent pain or signs of residual infection. It appeared in this study that the success rate of the transvaginal procedure was not affected by the size of the abscess or the multilocularity of the abscess. Similar success rates have been reported by numerous authors in association with transvaginal drainage of a tuboovarian abscess.[42–44,52–55]

There are several variations in technique that have been described for drainage, ranging from simple needle aspiration to catheter placement using trocar technique or an over-the-wire technique with serial dilatation prior to catheter placement. The use of needle aspiration alone versus catheter drainage for a tuboovarian abscess is not universally agreed upon. The advantages of needle aspiration are that the treatment is completed in one session, it can be performed on an outpatient basis and it avoids the

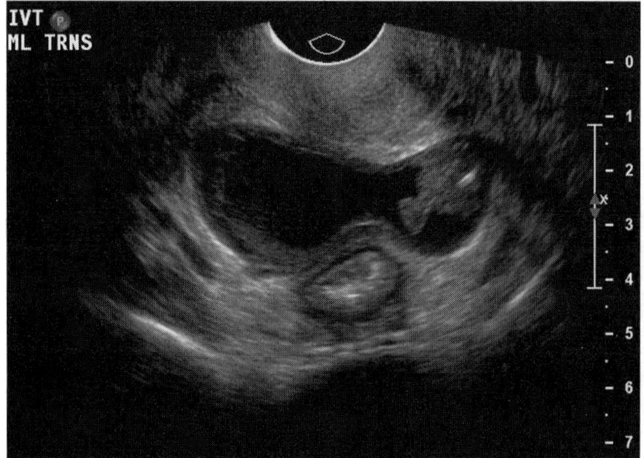

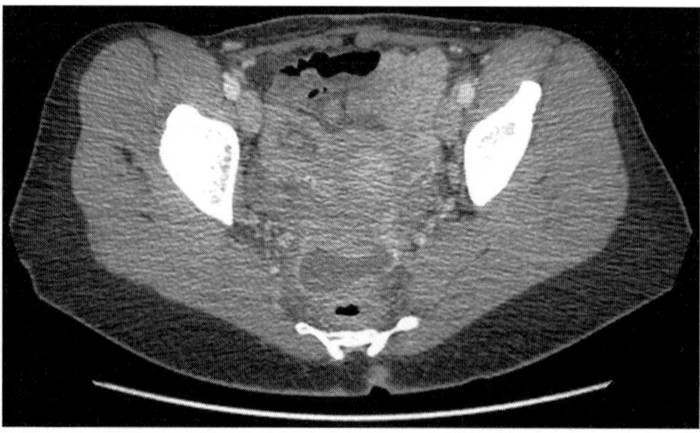

Fig. 17.3 (A) Transvaginal ultrasound image in a 27-year-old patient presenting with pelvic pain and fever. This demonstrates a thick-walled fluid collection suspicious for an abscess. **(B)** The pelvic computed tomography scan in this patient demonstrated the posterior fluid collection with a thickened and enhancing wall consistent with an abscess.

inconvenience of the patient needing an indwelling catheter.[44] One drawback of needle aspiration without catheter placement is the potential need for repeated punctures to fully aspirate a complex abscess. In addition, an extended period of antibiotic coverage is typically required to control residual infection after a simple aspiration.[34,41,42] A catheter may be indicated when the abscess material is too viscous for drainage or if the collection is multiloculated.[34,42] Catheter placement has the benefit of permitting repeat flushing of large abscesses to help break down loculi and lower the viscosity of the abscess contents.[31] When the output is >100 cc/day, a sinogram can be performed through a catheter to determine if an underlying fistula is present.[37] Catheters are generally removed when there is improvement in a patient's condition as demonstrated by a normal temperature, a normal white blood cell (WBC) count, and a reduction in catheter output to <20 cc over 24 hours.[34]

Lee et al[31] reported a success rate of 86% in 22 patients when using the trocar technique via a transvaginal approach. The wall of the vaginal vault consists of thick muscular tissue that is often difficult to puncture and difficult for subsequent passage of dilators due to patient discomfort. The pain and discomfort occurs secondary to the inflammation of the vaginal wall that often accompanies PID and abscess formation.[34] Using the trocar technique, there is one stick and no need for repeated catheter exchanges and dilatation.

Nelson et al[56] reported success using a transrectal approach to treat tuboovarian abscesses that are too posterior to be amenable to transvaginal aspiration. In many of their patients, it was not necessary to place a drainage catheter; needle aspiration was enough. Their sense was that the transrectal approach was better tolerated than the transvaginal approach because manipulation around a tender cervix and uterus can be intrinsically more uncomfortable for women with salpingitis.

Possible complications of transvaginal drainage include bleeding, infection, underlying organ damage, and vaginal fistula formation.[43] Introduction of infection into the pelvis or dissemination of the infection within the pelvis as a direct result of transvaginal drainage has not been reported.[34] Catheter dislodgement when using the transvaginal approach can be a problem as well. This can be addressed using a locking pigtail catheter and by attaching the catheter to the anterior thigh using adhesive tape.[34]

References

1. Mesogitis S, Daskalakis G, Pilalis A, et al. Management of ovarian cysts with aspiration and methotrexate injection. Radiology 2005;235:668–673
2. Schwartz PE. The role of tumor markers in the preoperative diagnosis of ovarian cysts. Clin Obstet Gynecol 1993;36:384–394
3. Bhan V, Amso N, Whitehead MI, et al. Characteristics of persistent ovarian masses in asymptomatic women. Br J Obstet Gynaecol 1989;96:1384–1391
4. Modesitt SC, Pavlik E, Ueland F, et al. Risk of malignancy in unilocular ovarian cystic tumors less than 10 centimeters in diameter. Obstet Gynecol 2003;102:594–599
5. Granberg S, Wikland M, Jansson I. Macroscopic characterization of ovarian cancer and relation to the histological diagnosis: criteria to be used for ultrasound evaluation. Gynecol Oncol 1989;35:139–144
6. Grimes DA, Hughes JM. Use of multiphasic oral contraceptives and hospitalization of women with functional ovarian cysts in the United States. Obstet Gynecol 1989;73:1037–1039
7. Duke D, Colville J, Keeling A, et al. Transvaginal aspiration of ovarian cysts: long-term follow-up. Cardiovasc Intervent Radiol 2006;29:401–405
8. Mathevet P, Dargent D. Role of ultrasound guided puncture in the management of ovarian cysts. J Gynecol Obstet Biol Reprod (Paris) 2001; 30(1, Suppl)S53–S58
9. Troiano RN, Quendens-Case C, Taylor KJW. Correlation of findings on transvaginal sonography with serum CA125 levels. AJR Am J Roentgenol 1997;168:1587–1590
10. Bret PM, Guibaud L, Atri M, et al. Transvaginal US-guided aspiration of ovarian cysts and solid pelvic masses. Radiology 1992;185:377–380
11. Caspi B, Goldchmit R, Zalel Y, Appelman Z, Insler V. Sonographically guided aspiration of ovarian cyst with simple appearance. J Ultrasound Med 1996;15:297–300
12. Lee CL, Lai YM, Chang SY, et al. The management of ovarian cysts by sono-guided transvaginal cyst aspiration. J Clin Ultrasound 1993;21:511–514
13. Troiano RN, Taylor KJ. Sonographically guided therapeutic aspiration of benign appearing ovarian cysts and endometriomas. AJR Am J Roentgenol 1998;171:1601–1605
14. Bonilla-Musoles F, Ballester MJ, Simon C, et al. Is the avoidance of surgery possible in patients with perimenopausal ovarian tumours using transvaginal ultrasound and duplex color Doppler sonography? J Ultrasound Med 1993;12:33–39
15. Balat O, Sarac K, Sonmez S. Ultrasound guided aspiration of benign ovarian cysts: an alternative to surgery. Eur J Radiol 1996;22:136–137
16. Weinraub Z, Avrech O, Fuchs C, et al. Transvaginal aspiration of ovarian cysts: prognosis based on outcome over a 12-month period. J Ultrasound Med 1994;13:275–279
17. Caspi B, Zalel Y, Lurie S, Elchlal U, Katz Z. Ultrasound-guided aspiration for relief of pain generated by simple ovarian cysts. Gynecol Obstet Invest 1993;35:121–122
18. Zanetta G, Lissoni A, Torri V, et al. Role of puncture and aspiration in expectant management of simple ovarian cysts: a randomised study. BMJ 1996;313:1110–1113
19. Dordoni D, Zaglio S, Zucca S, Favalli G. The role of sonographically guided aspiration in the clinical management of ovarian cysts. J Ultrasound Med 1993;12:27–31
20. Khaw KT, Walker WJ. Ultrasound guided fine needle aspiration of ovarian cysts: diagnosis and treatment in pregnant and non-pregnant women. Clin Radiol 1990;41:105–108
21. Moran O, Menczer J, Ben-Baruch G, et al. Cytological examination of ovarian cyst fluid for the distinction between benign and malignant tumors. Obstet Gynecol 1993;82:444–446
22. Diernaes E, Rasmussen J, Soerensen T, Hasch E. Ovarian cysts: management by puncture? Lancet 1987;1(8541):1084
23. Sainz de la Cuesta R, Goff BA, Fuller AF, et al. Prognostic importance of intraoperative rupture of malignant ovarian epithelial neoplasms. Obstet Gynecol 1994;84:1–7
24. Fisch JD, Sher G. Sclerotherapy with 5% tetracycline is a simple alternative to potentially complex surgical treatment of ovarian endometriomas before in vitro fertilization. Fertil Steril 2004;82:437–441
25. Noma J, Yoshida N. Efficacy of ethanol sclerotherapy for ovarian endometriomas. Int J Gynaecol Obstet 2001;72:35–39
26. Messalli EM, Cobellis G, Pecori E, et al. Alcohol sclerosis of endometriomas after ultrasound-guided aspiration. Minerva Ginecol 2003;55:359–362

27. Velebil P, Wingo PA, Xia Z, Wilcox LS, Peterson HB. Rate of hospitalization for gynecologic disorders among reproductive-age women in the United States. Obstet Gynecol 1995;86:764–769
28. Rein DB, Kassler WJ, Irwin KL, Rabiee L. Direct medical cost of pelvic inflammatory disease and its sequelae: decreasing, but still substantial. Obstet Gynecol 2000;95:397–402
29. Wiesenfeld HC, Sweet RL. Progress in the management of tuboovarian abscesses. Clin Obstet Gynecol 1993;36:433–444
30. Franklin EW, 3rd, Hevron JE Jr, Thompson JD. Management of the pelvic abscess. Clin Obstet Gynecol 1973;16:66–79
31. Lee BC, McGahan JP, Bijan B. Single-step transvaginal aspiration and drainage for suspected pelvic abscesses refractory to antibiotic therapy. J Ultrasound Med 2002;21:731–738
32. McNeeley SG, Hendrix SL, Mazzoni MM, Kmak DC, Ransom SB. Medically sound, cost-effective treatment for pelvic inflammatory disease and tuboovarian abscess. Am J Obstet Gynecol 1998;178:1272–1278
33. Fabiszewski NL, Sumkin JH, Johns CM. Contemporary radiologic percutaneous abscess drainage in the pelvis. Clin Obstet Gynecol 1993;36:445–456
34. Varghese JC, O'Neill MJ, Gervais DA, Boland GW, Mueller PR. Transvaginal catheter drainage of tuboovarian abscess using the trocar method: technique and literature review. AJR Am J Roentgenol 2001;177:139–144
35. Worthen NJ, Gunning JE. Percutaneous drainage of pelvic abscesses: management of the tuboovarian abscess. J Ultrasound Med 1986;5: 551–556
36. Shulman A, Maymon R, Shapiro A, Bahary C. Percutaneous catheter drainage of tuboovarian abscesses. Obstet Gynecol 1992;80:555–557
37. Casola G, van Sonnenberg E, D'Agnostino HB, et al. Percutaneous drainage of tuboovarian abscess. Radiology 1992;182:399–402
38. Butch RJ, Mueller PR, Ferrucci JT, et al. Drainage of pelvic abscesses through the greater sciatic foramen. Radiology 1986;158:487–491
39. Harisinghani MG, Gervais DA, Maher MM, et al. Transgluteal approach for percutaneous drainage of deep pelvic abscesses: 154 cases. Radiology 2003;228:701–705
40. Alexander AA, Eschelman DJ, Nazarian LN, Bonn J. Transrectal sonographically guided drainage of deep pelvic abscesses. AJR Am J Roentgenol 1994;162:1227–1232
41. Kuligowska E, Keller E, Ferrucci JT. Treatment of pelvic abscesses: value of one-step sonographically guided transrectal needle aspiration and lavage. AJR Am J Roentgenol 1995;164:201–206
42. Nelson AL, Sinow RM, Renslo R, Renslo MJ, Atamded F. Endovaginal ultrasonographically guided transvaginal drainage for treatment of pelvic abscesses. Am J Obstet Gynecol 1995;172:1926–1932
43. Feld R, Eschelman DJ, Sagerman JE, et al. Treatment of pelvic abscesses and other fluid collections: efficacy of transvaginal sonographically guided aspiration and drainage. AJR Am J Roentgenol 1994;163:1141–1145
44. Aboulghar MA, Mansur RT, Serour GI. Ultrasonographically guided transvaginal aspiration of tuboovarian abscesses and pyosalpinges: an optional treatment for acute pelvic inflammatory disease. Am J Obstet Gynecol 1995;172:1501–1503
45. McGahan JP, Brown B, Jones CD, Stein M. Pelvic abscesses: transvaginal US-guided drainage with the trocar method. Radiology 1996;200:579–581
46. vanSonnenberg E, D'Agostino HB, Casola G, et al. US-guided transvaginal drainage of pelvic abscesses and fluid collections. Radiology 1991;181:53–56
47. Corsi PJ, Johnson SC, Gonik B, et al. Transvaginal ultrasound-guided aspiration of pelvic abscesses. Infect Dis Obstet Gynecol 1999;7:216–221
48. Gjelland K, Ekerhovd E, Granberg S. Transvaginal ultrasound-guided aspiration for treatment of tubo-ovarian abscess: a study of 302 cases. Am J Obstet Gynecol 2005;193:1323–1330
49. Maher MM, Gervais DA, Kalra MK, et al. The inaccessible or undrainable abscess: how to drain it. Radiographics 2004;24:717–735
50. Abbitt PL, Goldwag S, Urbanski S. Endovaginal sonography for guidance in draining pelvic fluid collections. AJR Am J Roentgenol 1990;154:849–850
51. Raiga J, Canis M, Le Bouedec G, et al. Laparoscopic management of adnexal abscesses: consequences for fertility. Fertil Steril 1996;66:712–717
52. Teisala K, Heinonen PK, Punnonen R. Transvaginal ultrasound in the diagnosis and treatment of tuboovarian abscess. Br J Obstet Gynaecol 1990;97:178–180
53. Loy RA, Gallup DG, Hill JA, Holzman GM, Geist D. Pelvic abscess: examination and transvaginal drainage guided by real time ultrasonography. South Med J 1989;82:788–790
54. Nosher JL, Winchman HK, Needell GS. Transvaginal pelvic abscess drainage with US guidance. Radiology 1987;165:872–873
55. Bennett JD, Kozak RI, Taylor BM, Jory TA. Deep pelvic abscesses: transrectal drainage with radiologic guidance. Radiology 1992;185:825–828
56. Nelson AL, Sinow RM, Oliak D. Transrectal ultrasonographically guided drainage of gynecologic pelvic abscesses. Am J Obstet Gynecol 2000;182:1382–1388

18 Clinical Perspective: Pelvic Pain (Gynecology)

C. Paul Perry

Chronic pelvic pain in women is a common and disabling condition. It is defined as pelvic pain, which has been present for 6 months or longer. Two to ten percent of all gynecologic office consultations are for chronic pelvic pain and 20% of all laparoscopic evaluations are performed for chronic pelvic pain. It is estimated that 10 million women suffer from this condition and that 7 million do not seek help. The economic impact of this condition is astonishing. The annual medical cost for diagnosis and treatment of chronic pelvic pain is estimated to be approximately $1.2 billion. The cost of lost productivity in these patients is estimated to be $15 billion annually. In contrast to episodic and acute pain, chronic pain is almost always continuous and unresponsive to conventional diagnosis and treatment. If unrelieved, it can potentially result in long-term disability, depression, and neurologic changes.

Chronic pelvic pain (CPP) can be caused by numerous organic pathologies usually accompanied with variable psychologic dysfunctions. The most commonly made diagnosis in chronic pelvic pain is endometriosis (31%). After evaluation, up to 61% of patients are found to have no explanation for their pain. The majority remains undiagnosed or improperly diagnosed.[1] Many improperly diagnosed patients will undergo misdirected therapy. These and other patients often abandon their pursuit of medical help due to the fact that they never receive an explanation or any treatment for their pain.

The majority of women with no obvious pathologic cause for their pain may be suffering from pelvic congestion syndrome (PCS). Pelvic congestion is defined as the presence of enlarged venous complexes of the reproductive tissues with impaired circulation and drainage. This can produce pain alone or an association with other more common pathologies (e.g., endometriosis, adhesions, etc.). PCS is a diagnosis that was proposed over 100 years ago, but is only recently regaining some legitimacy. Richet is credited with first describing this condition as a case of "tubo-ovarian varicocele."[2] Before the days of laparoscopy and venography, Howard Taylor described this syndrome and gained some credibility in the medical community of the 1950s. However, due to assumptions regarding the psychosexual component of this illness and the fact that stress always aggravates the pain, many physicians saw this as a purely psychosomatic illness.[3,4] The resurgence of pelvic congestion as a legitimate cause of chronic pelvic pain is due to the elegant and systematic work of Beard's group at St. Mary's Hospital in London.[3]

Starting in the 1970s and proceeding through the present, the clinical characteristics, methods and criteria for diagnosis, and psychological components have been addressed in the United Kingdom without totally being accepted by the American academic and medical practicing community. Until recently, gynecologists in the United States have viewed PCS as rare, psychosomatic, or imaginary. Our view is certainly evolving. Better clinical data with a clear association between symptoms, diagnostic criteria, and treatment outcomes has won the respect of many including the American College of Obstetrics and Gynecology.[5] To this we and our patients owe a great debt to Dr. Richard Beard's group in the United Kingdom.[6]

■ Pathogenesis

A recent prevalence study suggests that 9.9% of women will have radiologic evidence of pelvic varicosities and 59% of these patients will be symptomatic. The importance of this finding is supported by the fact that up to 77% of these symptomatic patients might benefit from therapy.[7] Several possible etiologies for the venous congestion and pelvic pain associated with PCS have been classified by El-Minawi into categories including anatomic dysfunction, orgasmic dysfunction, hormonal dysfunction, psychosomatic dysfunction, and iatrogenic dysfunction.[8] Unfortunately, these are not complete and do not singularly explain all the clinical findings of pelvic congestion, each failing in some respect.

Anatomic Dysfunction

The rich anastomotic venous plexuses of the pelvic viscera include ovarian, paraovarian, uterine, bladder, rectal, and vulvar veins. The vulvar and uterine veins normally drain into the internal iliac veins. Anatomically, the left ovarian vein drains into the left renal vein and then into the inferior vena cava while the right ovarian vein drains directly into the inferior vena cava. Vascular connections exist between the bladder and rectal venous complexes as well with the veins of the upper thigh. These channels are relatively valveless and are gravity and vascular-tone dependent for their circulation.

Anatomic studies have shown that 13 to 15% of women lack valves in the left ovarian vein; the corresponding figure for the right ovarian vein is 6%. When present, 43% of the valves on the left and 35 to 41% on the right are incompetent. Mean values of ovarian venous diameter are 3.8 mm in the presence of competent valves and 7.5 mm when the valves are incompetent due to resulting reflux and congestion within the vein. The upper limit of the normal diameter for ovarian veins is considered to be 5 mm.[9]

The structure of the human ovarian vein has been studied with transmission electron microscopy. This has revealed that the vein has typical venous endothelium that is immediately adjacent to the first of three smooth layers; no elastic lamina separates the endothelium from the inner layer of smooth muscle. Thinning of the inner circular layer of smooth muscle can be seen with advancing age.[10] The middle smooth muscle layer consists of a circular arrangement of fibers. The outer layer of smooth muscle is arranged longitudinally with collagen and with autonomic nerves penetrating throughout the muscle.

Anatomic dysfunction is thought by most to play a role in the development of PCS. Pelvic varicosities are thought to be due primarily to the effect of gravity on an incompetent venous valvular system. The resultant stasis produces the congestion and pain that is associated with this condition. Parity is a known risk factor in the development of PCS.[11] It is known that pregnancy increases the capacity of the pelvic veins by 60%. When this is combined with the venous kinking of a malpositioned gravid uterus, venous stagnation, flow reversal, and pelvic varicosities are likely to occur.

Allen and Master's controversial theory regarding a "fascial defect" producing uterine malposition and congestion has been discounted.[12] However, an additional anatomic relationship between retroversion of the uterus with pelvic pain and dilated pelvic veins has been established.[13] Extensive cadaver dissections of pelvic venous vasculature have confirmed the scarcity of valves in these veins. These studies have led to the conclusion that genetic structural venous wall anomalies are a major contributing factor in the development of pelvic varicosities.[14] The nutcracker syndrome, which is compression of the left renal vein by the superior mesenteric artery, can lead to high pressure within the left ovarian vein and pelvic varicosities.[15–17]

Orgasmic Dysfunction

When a female patient is sexually stimulated up to, but not reaching, orgasm (the plateau phase of a woman's sexual response), some pain caused by vasocongestion may be felt in the pelvic viscera. Whether or not this can produce permanent vascular changes remains unknown.

Psychosomatic Dysfunction

In 1949, Taylor wrote that "psychiatric disturbances, usually of an emotional character, are a common accompaniment of pelvic congestion."[4] It was his opinion that an important factor in the etiology of pelvic congestion was "the effect of a primary state of emotional tension" on the smooth muscle and secretory cells of the pelvis in producing psychosomatic disturbances.[4] Later studies seem to confirm psychosomatic contribution to pelvic pain in that women who suffered from chronic pelvic pain were psychologically different from women without pain. They tended to be more neurotic and to have abnormal attitudes toward their own and their partner's sexuality.[3] This caused pelvic congestion to be considered by some as a purely psychiatric condition (pelipathia vegetativa). Beard and colleagues partially confirmed this by finding that women with pelvic congestion tended to be more neurotic and were in less satisfying relationships.[18] As El-Minawi points out, this proposition brings up the old adage regarding the "chicken and the egg." It is true that these women will have some psychologic overlay, but we have learned that the stress of chronic pain itself induces many of these social and psychologic consequences.

Hormonal Dysfunction

Women with pelvic congestion have a higher incidence of multicystic ovaries, enlarged uteri, and thickened endometrium, which are all findings that may be hormonally induced. On ultrasound, up to 56% of women with pelvic varicosities and pain were found to have polycystic or multicystic ovaries.[19] Taylor and Beard mentioned the possibility that this condition might be related to hormonal sensitivity because it is virtually unknown in postmenopausal women. Reginald et al found that by inhibiting the effect of estrogen with medroxyprogesterone acetate (MPA), a decrease in the degree of pelvic congestion can be demonstrated on venography. In addition, the majority of these women experienced symptomatic relief when compared with controls.[20]

Iatrogenically Induced Dysfunction

Tubal ligation procedures and the use of intrauterine devices for contraception have both been theorized to be associated with PCS. In one series, 60% of patients with pelvic congestion were found to have had undergone a tubal ligation procedure.[21] These patients were also found to have a greater volume of peritoneal transudate with fluid containing higher levels of 6 keto-prostaglandin α than controls. These patients were symptomatic 16 to 39% of the time. An additional study demonstrated venographically (95%) and laparoscopically (52%) that there is an association between PCS and the Lippes loop.[8] Larger studies have yet to verify any of these causes.

Neuropathic Dysfunction

Janicki has postulated that the pain and vasodilatation of pelvic congestion is actually a manifestation of a visceral complex regional pain syndrome.[22] As nociceptive signals from any pelvic pain pathology are transmitted to the dorsal horn receptor cells of the spinal cord, antidromic transmission to pelvic vasculature produces venous changes. Endothelial release of neurotransmitters then produces the pain and tenderness associated with PCS.

Stones et al have identified several neurotransmitters produced by the abnormal vessels seen in PCS, which may play a role in the pathogenesis of this syndrome. These include adenosine 5' triphosphate, substance P, endothelin, vasopressin, calcitonin gene-related peptide and nitric oxide.[23–26] As a result, it has been theorized that PCS may actually be an epiphenomenon, and that venous congestion may be a consequence of pain experienced elsewhere in the body. It is possible that a vascular disturbance at the ovarian or uterine arteriolar level results in the release of these endothelial factors, which excite sensory nerves in the outer layer of smooth muscle in the ovarian veins and cause vasodilatation through release of nitric oxide. The presence of a relevant mediator, such as substance P, in the endothelium of the human ovarian vein has been described and can evoke endothelium-mediated vasorelaxation in organ bath preparations. The release of substance P and ATP under conditions of shear stress has also been demonstrated from the perfused human ovarian vascular bed. The release of nitric oxide has been shown to evoke pain in an in vivo study of human dorsal hand veins.[24]

Conversely, the reduction of pain through venoconstriction has been documented as well. Reginald et al[27] found that the changes of PCS can be temporarily reversed with dihydroergotamine administered intravenously. This was demonstrated by observing symptoms and findings during transuterine venography. Pelvic pain was significantly improved after dihydroergotamine infusion when compared with the administration of a placebo. In addition, there was a mean reduction of 35% in the diameter of the pelvic veins measured and the observation that contrast medium cleared rapidly. These results confirm an association between demonstrable pelvic congestion and pain.[27]

■ Symptoms

Pain is the definitive symptom of PCS. It is usually described as a dull ache with intermittent acute exacerbations. Usually one side will predominate, but on careful questioning, symptoms are also felt on the other side as well. The acute exacerbation of pain will often have a sharp quality. Because irritable bowel syndrome and endometriosis can also be present, these pain generators may confuse the patient and clinician alike. A low backache is often present. The aches and pains of PCS are exacerbated by anything that increases venous pressure, including standing, walking, prolonged sitting, sexual intercourse, and vigorous sports activities. These patients ultimately learn to avoid the activities associated with pain and become deconditioned.[28]

Both deep thrust dyspareunia (71 to 78%) and postcoital aching (65%) are common complaints associated with PCS as well. This invariably produces sexual dysfunction with associated social and interpersonal ramifications. Patients may also develop penetration dyspareunia from vulvovestibulitis as a result of their chronic visceral pain.[29] Menstrual disorders such as menorrhagia and menometrorrhagia occur in up to 54% of patients. Intermenstrual bleeding may be present in up to 25% of patients. Dysmenorrhea of the congestive type will usually begin up to 1 week before menses (89%) and is described as cramping in a low lateral location. This is very similar to the predysmenorrhea of patients with endometriosis.

Gastrointestinal and urinary tract symptoms are common as well. Bloating, nausea, and diffuse abdominal cramping are common. Urinary frequency and urgency may be noted as well. These symptoms are probably a function of the venous engorgement within the perivesicle and perirectal spaces. Interstitial cystitis, being among the common pain generators in CPP, must not be overlooked in these patients.[30] Headache, fatigue, and insomnia may be due to a general autonomic dysfunction. Fibromyalgia can be present in many of these patients.[8,22]

■ Physical Examination

An abdominal examination will produce tenderness over the ovarian points. These lie at the junction of the upper and middle third of a line drawn from the anterior superior iliac spine and the umbilicus (**Fig. 18.1**). This point is at the level of the ovarian vein crossing into the bony pelvis. The compression induced by an examination increases the venous pressure, which exacerbates the ovarian tenderness.[9]

On inspection of the external genitalia, superficial varicosities may be noted. Vulvovestibulitis may be present by Q-tip test.[29] Visualization of the cervix may reveal cyanosis and an increase in cervical mucous production. The uterus and/or ovaries are tender on examination. The uterus may be retroverted. The combination of tenderness on abdominal palpation over the ovarian point and a history of postcoital ache was 94% sensitive and 77% specific for discriminating pelvic congestion from other causes of pelvic pain in the study by Beard et al.[31] In contrast, Taylor

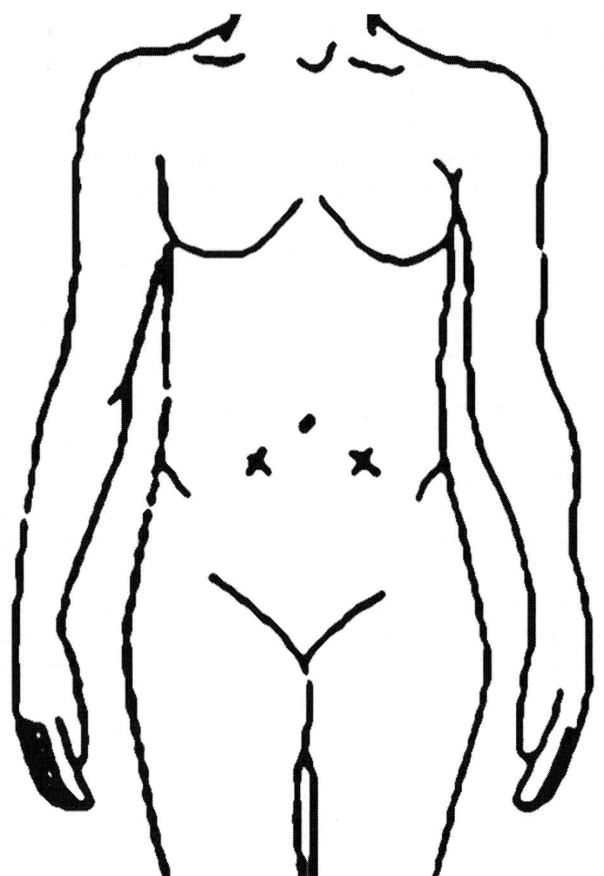

Fig. 18.1 In patients with pelvic congestion, abdominal examination will often produce tenderness over the ovarian points. This lies at the junction of the upper and middle third of a line drawn from the anterior superior iliac spine and the umbilicus.

reported the most reliable sign to be tenderness of the posterior parametrium and the uterosacral ligaments (80%).

■ Diagnostic Studies

The twofold criteria of enlarged veins together with reduced circulation require a dynamic diagnostic study that can measure both. Laparoscopy is typically performed as part of the evaluation of a patient with chronic pelvic pain. This procedure is usually done in the Trendelenburg position with increased intraabdominal pressure. This can result in venous collapse and a false-negative impression during laparoscopy. Women with chronic pain found to have normal pelvic anatomy at laparoscopy may have undiagnosed venous congestion, which will remain undiagnosed without proper imaging techniques. If an experienced observer reverses the head down position and decreases the insufflation pressure, a more accurate picture can be achieved. By lifting the fallopian tubes to visualize the paraovarian varicosities between the tubes and the ovaries, suspicion of pelvic congestion may be affirmed.

Imaging studies, including percutaneous venography, ultrasonography, computerized tomography (CT), magnetic resonance imaging (MRI), and radionuclear studies have all been described as potentially helpful in patients with PCS.[32–35] To date, these all lack the clinically verified criteria, precision, and dynamic quality of transcervical myometrial venography.[36]

Venography should be considered the diagnostic study of choice. Pelvic venography can be performed percutaneously or transcervically (transuterine) by myometrial extravasation. Ducuing was reportedly the first to attempt pelvic venography and in 1954, Guilhem and Baux used the technique of directly injecting the myometrium.[37] This technique was further refined to include a special transcervical needle.[38] Beard and colleagues described a transuterine venogram scoring system, which permitted an objective standard for pelvic venography (**Table 18.1**).[6] By measuring the maximum diameter and the time necessary for the contrast to clear, the score can range from 3 to 9, with a score of 3 to 4 being normal and a score of 5 to 9 suggesting increasingly severe pelvic congestion.

A transcervical, transuterine approach is much less expensive and less invasive than a percutaneous transvenous approach. The patient is placed in the dorsal lithotomy position and a vaginal speculum exposes the cervical os. This is cleansed with povidone antiseptic solution and a special double-lumen needle (Cook Urological Inc., Bloomington, IN) is employed (**Fig. 18.2**). The needle is passed through the cervix via a concentric metal sheath that covers all but the final 0.5 cm tip. Twenty to 30 mL of water-soluble dye is injected into the fundal myometrium under fluoroscopic guidance. The use of two 10 mL syringes is recommended to decrease the manual force required for myometrial injection. Most patients will require conscious sedation for this procedure. It may also be performed under general anesthesia with a C-arm in the operative suite before diagnostic/operative laparoscopies.

The first image is taken immediately and then at 20-second intervals for up to 60 seconds. We usually administer an oral antibiotic prophylactically. Beard's criteria for pelvic congestion are then used to score the degree of congestion (normal, moderate, or extensive). We prefer transuterine injection because it demonstrates the uterine vein component of PCS, which might continue even after ovarian vein ligation or embolization. In fact, the continuing effect of a uterine vein component of PCS may explain why the therapies that address only the ovarian component of congestion might produce inadequate pain relief.

With the percutaneous venous approach, sterile technique must be strictly maintained. After the venous system is accessed via the common femoral or internal jugular veins, the ovarian veins are then selectively catheterized and imaged. Unless the patient is tilted head up, incomplete visualization of the uterine and paraovarian veins may result. Kennedy and Hemingway described the radiologic criteria for congestion including maximal diameter of the ovarian veins of 10 mm, congestion of the ovarian venous plexus, filling of the veins across the midline, or filling of vulvar and thigh varicosities.[39] Unlike the transcervical procedure, however, no clinical validation studies have been reported to date with percutaneous venography.

■ Treatment

Reginald et al found that dihydroergotamine decreased the congestion and pain associated with PCS. Because this effect is only transient, no therapeutic modality has been able to take advantage of this phenomenon. Reginald and colleagues treated 22 PCS patients with 30 mg of medroxyprogesterone acetate (MPA) daily; 17 patients achieved a reduction in the pelvic venography score.[20] Of these patients, 75% had a corresponding reduction in the degree of pain they were experiencing. It is not known whether this is due to the estrogen-blocking effect of MPA or whether inhibition of the neurotransmitters occurred in these abnormal veins. This form of therapy is even more successful when combined with psychotherapy. Farquhar et al, in the only randomized control trial for medical treatment of PCS, confirmed the effectiveness of this treatment regimen.[40] Weight gain and depression have been reported by those patients not tolerating MPA. Gonadotropic-releasing hormone agonist (GnRHa) in a randomized control study has shown a statistically significant advantage and longer lasting pain reduction after 6 months of therapy without estrogen add-back therapy.[41] In an earlier study, Gangar et al utilized a GnRHa along with estrogen (1 mg) and MPA (5 mg) add-back, but failed to show added benefit with this approach.[42]

Patients who do not respond to conservative medical therapy can be considered for more invasive treatment from a percutaneous, laparoscopic, or open surgical approach. Embolization, which was first described in 1993 by Edwards et al[43] has been reviewed in Chapter 16. Pain response to embolotherapy has been reported to be up to 83%, with minimal complications reported in association with this procedure.[44–46] Although Taylor[4] decried surgical treatment for PCS, ligation of the ovarian veins can be successfully done through a McBurney incision or may be performed laparoscopically. In the small number of patients reported to have undergone this procedure, good pain relief was achieved.[9]

Laparoscopic venous ligation techniques may also prove effective after larger clinical trials have been completed.[47] Uterine suspension should be performed laparoscopically in patients with a retroverted uterus and deep thrust dyspareunia.[48] Hysterectomy with bilateral salpingo-oophorectomy has been used successfully in some patients. Beard reported 36 women who had failed medical management and went on to hysterectomy with bilateral salpingo-oophorectomy. All patients except one experienced good pain relief one year after surgery.[49] However, because these patients are often young, more conservative initial therapy is more appropriate than hysterectomy. Recently, laparoscopically directed sclerotherapy into the perivascular space has been reported to relieve the symptoms associated with venous congestion.[50]

■ Conclusions

The widely variable symptoms and the strong association with psychologic disturbances have caused many gynecologists to question the legitimacy of the pelvic congestion syndrome.[8,9] However, a preponderance of clinical evidence has validated the history, physical examination findings, and radiologic findings associated with PCS and the diagnosis and treatment options that can address the associated symptoms.[5]

PCS is more common than previously assumed. In patients with chronic pelvic pain and no visible pathology at laparoscopy, transcervical pelvic venography should be performed. Also, those patients with other pain generators not responding to conventional therapy should be studied when indicated by history or physical examination. Medical therapy with MPA or GnRHa should be given for at least 3 to 6 months before the use of more invasive therapy is considered. Laparoscopic venous ligation or embolotherapy should be selected for those patients not responding to medical management. Women's health care providers should become more educated about this condition and approach its diagnosis and management with an open mind. Only then will we see a reduction in the suffering of these patients.

Table 18.1 Beard's Criteria for Pelvic Congestion: (A) Scoring System for Assessing Pelvic Venography and (B) Atlanta I Criteria for Pelvic Varicosity Pain Syndrome

	Score		
A	1	2	3
Maximal diameter of ovarian veins (mm)	1–4	5–8*	>8*
Time to disappearance of contrast medium after injection (seconds)	0	20	40
Ovarian plexus congestion	Normal	Moderate	Extensive
Total score	1–4	5–8	>8

B

Terminology: Pelvic congestion syndrome (PCS) should be changed to pelvic varicosity pain syndrome (PVPS) in light of misunderstanding of PCS by many clinicians.

Consensus statement: Pelvic varicosity pain syndrome (PVPS) is a valid diagnosis for the production of chronic pelvic pain in women. It is important that all four of these criteria are present before making the diagnosis. Currently, the only diagnostic study that confirms varicosities with delayed emptying is transcervical venography.

Definition: Pelvic varicosity syndrome (PVPS) is defined by four major criteria:

1. Chronic pelvic pain
2. Ovarian or uterine varicosities
3. Delayed emptying of veins
4. Tenderness of uterus or adnexa

Clinical Presentation

- History
- Chronic pelvic pain
- May or may not include
  - Premenstrual exacerbations
  - Aggravated by prolonged physical activity
  - Decreased pain when lying down
  - Postcoital pain
  - Intermittent episodes of acute severe pain
  - Deep dyspareunia
  - Pain that may move from side to side
- Physical examination
- Tenderness of uterus or adnexa
- May or may not include
  - Tenderness to deep palpation at Beard's Point: a point 2/3 of the way from the anterior superior iliac spine to umbilicus
  - Cervical motion tenderness
- Diagnostic studies
- Studies that demonstrate varicosities and delayed emptying
  - Transcervical venography
- Studies that demonstrate venous dilation, but not delayed emptying
  - Transvenous retrograde venography
  - Pelvic ultrasound with or without Doppler
  - MRI with or without contrast
  - CT with or without contrast
- Treatment
- Level I evidence (U.S. Preventative Task Force)
  - Oral medroxyprogesterone acetate
  - GnRHa

Table 18.1 (*Continued*)

B
Level III Evidence (US Preventative Task Force)
Embolotherapy
Ovarian vein ligation
Hysterectomy with bilateral salpingo-oophorectomy

*A value of 5 or more gave a diagnostic sensitivity of 91% and specificity of 89% for the pelvic pain syndrome.
Abbreviations: CT, computed tomography; MRI, magnetic resonance imaging; GnRHa, gonadotropic-releasing hormone agonist.
Source: (A) Adapted from Beard RW, Highman JH. Diagnosis of pelvic varicosities in women with chronic pelvic pain. Lancet 1984, ii: 946–9. (B) International Pelvic Pain Society. Symposium and Consensus Statement on Pelvic Congestion Syndrome. Atlanta, GA. January 27, 2007. Participants: Fred Howard, MD, Rochester, NY; Richard Marvel, MD, Baltimore, MD; Alfredo Nieves, MD; Chattanooga, TN; C. Paul Perry, MD, Birmingham, AL; Howard Sharp, MD, Salt Lake City, UH.

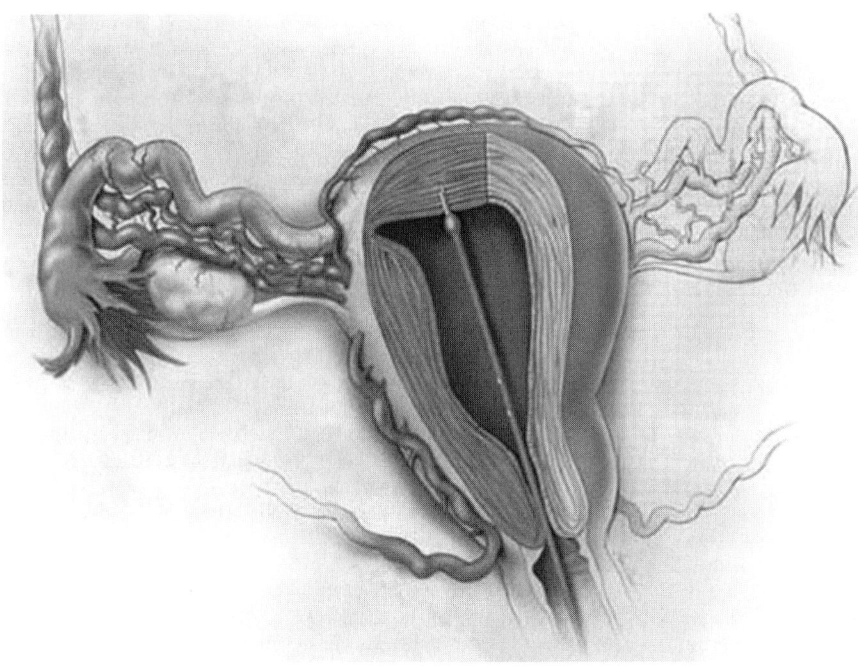

Fig. 18.2 Transcervical venography needle. The needle is passed through the cervix via a concentric metal sheath that covers all but the final 0.5 cm tip. Twenty to 30 mL of water-soluble dye is injected into the fundal myometrium under fluoroscopic guidance.

References

1. Scialli AR. Chronic Pelvic Pain. An Integrated Approach. Philadelphia, PA: WB Saunders; 1998
2. Richet MA. Traite Pratique d'Anatomie Medico-Chirugicale. Paris: E. Chamerot Libraire Editeur, 1875
3. Beard RW, Belsey EM, Lieberman BA, Wilkinson JC. Pelvic pain in women. Am J Obstet Gynecol 1977;128:566–570
4. Taylor HC. Vascular congestion and hyperemia, their effect on structure and function in the female reproductive organs: Part II. Am J Obstet Gynecol 1949;57:637–653
5. ACOG Committee on Practice Bulletins--Gynecology. Chronic pelvic pain. ACOG Practice Bulletin: Clinical Management Guidelines for Obstetrician-Gynecologists, Number 51. Obstet Gynecol 2004;103:589–605
6. Beard RW, Highman JH, Pearce S, Reginald PW. Diagnosis of pelvic varicosities in women with chronic pelvic pain. Lancet 1984;2:946–949
7. Belenky A, Bartal G, Atar E, Cohen M, Bachar GN. Ovarian varices in healthy female kidney donors: incidence, morbidity, and clinical outcome. AJR Am J Roentgenol 2002;179:625–627
8. El-Minawi AM. Pelvic varicosities and pelvic conngestion syndrome. In: Howard FM, Perry CP, El-Minawi AM, Carter JE, eds. Pelvic Pain: Diagnosis and Management. Philadelphia: Lippincott Williams & Wilkins; 2000:171–183
9. Metzger DA. Pelvic congestion. In: Steege J, Metzger DA, Levy B, eds. Chronic Pelvic Pain: An Integrated Approach. Philadelphia: WB Saunders;1999:191–196
10. Stones RW, Turmaine M, Beard RW, Burnstock G. The fine structure of human ovarian vein. J Anat 1994;185:285–294
11. Capasso P, Simons C, Dondelinger RF, Henroteaux D, Gaspard U. Treatment of symptomatic pelvic varices by ovarian vein embolization. Cardiovasc Intervent Radiol 1997;20:107–111
12. Allen WM. Chronic pelvic congestoin and pelvic pain. Am J Obstet Gynecol 1971;109:198–202
13. Truc JB, Musset R. Pathologie de tissue cellulaire pelvien et grosssesse. In: De Brux J, ed. Le Tissue Cellulaire Pelvien. Paris: Masion; 1973
14. LePage PA, Villaiconcio JL, Gomez ER, Sheridan MN, Rich NM. The valvular anatomy of the iliac venous system and its clinical implications. J Vasc Surg 1991;14:678–683
15. Ahmed K, Sampath R, Khan MS. Current trends in the diagnosis and management of renal nutcracker syndrome: a review. Eur J Vasc Endovasc Surg 2006;31:410–416
16. Rudloff U, Holmes RJ, Prem JT, Faust GR, Moldwin R, Siegel D. Mesoaortic compression of the left renal vein (nutcracker syndrome): case reports and review of the literature. Ann Vasc Surg 2006;20:120–129

17. Koc Z, Ulusan S, Tokmak N, Oguzkurt L, Yildirim T. Double retroaortic left renal veins as a possible cause of pelvic congestion syndrome: imaging findings in two patients. Br J Radiol 2006;79:e152–e155
18. Beard R, Reginald PW, Pearce S. Psychological and somatic factors in women with pain due to pelvic congestion. Adv Exp Med Biol 1988;245:413–421
19. Adams J, Reginald PW, Franks S, Wadsworth J, Beard RW. Uterine size and endometiral thickness and the significance of cystic ovaries in women with pelvic pain due to congestion. Br J Obstet Gynaecol 1990;97:583–587
20. Reginald PW, Adams J, Franks S, Wadsworth J, Beard RW. Medroxyprogesterone acetate in the treatment of pelvic pain due to venous congestion. Br J Obstet Gynaecol 1989;96:1148–1152
21. El-Minawi MF, Mashhor N, Reda MS. Pelvic venous changes after tubal sterilization. J Reprod Med 1983;28:641–648
22. Janicki TI. Re: Current concepts of pelvic congestion and chronic pelvic pain. JSLS 2002;6:90–91
23. Stones RW, Vials A, Milner P, Beard RW, Burnstock G. Release of vasoactive agents from the isolated perfused human ovary. Eur J Obstet Gynecol Reprod Biol 1996;67:191–196
24. Kindgen-Milles D, Arndt JO. Nitric oxide as a chemical link in the generation of pain from veins in humans. Pain 1996;64:139–142
25. Stones RW, Thomas DC, Beard RW. Suprasensitivity to calcitonin gene-related peptide but not vasoactive intestinal peptide in women with chronic pelvic pain. Clin Auton Res 1992;2:343–348
26. Stones RW, Loesch A, Beard RW, Burnstock G. Substance P: endothelial localization and pharmacology in the human ovarian vein. Obstet Gynecol 1995;85:273–278
27. Reginald PW, Beard RW, Kooner JS, et al. Intravenous dihydroergotamine to relieve pelvic congestion with pain in young women. Lancet 1987;2:351–353
28. Stones RW. Pelvic vascular congestion-half a century later. Clin Obstet Gynecol 2003;46:831–836
29. Perry CP. Vulvodynia. In: Howard FM, Perry CP, El-Minawi AM, Carter JE, eds. Pelvic Pain: Diagnosis and Treatment. Philadelphia: Lippincott Williams & Wilkins; 2000: 201–210
30. Chung MK, Chung RP, Gordon D. Interstitial cystitis and endometriosis in patients with chronic pelvic pain: the "evil twins" syndrome. JSLS 2005;9:25–29
31. Beard RW, Reginald PW, Wadsworth J. Clinical features of women with chronic lower abdominal pain and pelvic congestion. Br J Obstet Gynaecol 1988;95:153–161
32. Liu SZ, Chou CP, Lion WS, Huang JS, Pan HB. Pelvic congestion syndrome–findings on multi-detector row computerized tomography: a case report. Kaohsiung J Med Sci 2003;19:569–573
33. Siddall KA, Rubens DJ. Multidetector CT of the female pelvis. Radiol Clin North Am 2005;43:1097–1118
34. Park SJ, Lim JW, Ko YT, et al. Diagnosis of pelvic congestion syndrome using transabdominal and transvaginal sonography. AJR Am J Roentgenol 2004;182:683–688
35. Nascimento AB, Mitchell DG, Holland G. Ovarian veins: magnetic resonance imaging findings in an asymptomatic population. J Magn Reson Imaging 2002;15:551–556
36. Perry CP. Current concepts of pelvic congestion and chronic pelvic pain. JSLS 2001;5:105–110
37. Wegryn SP, Harron RA. Pelvic phlebography. Obstet Gynecol 1960;15: 73–76
38. Bellina JH, Dougherty CM, Mickal A. Transmyometrial pelvic venography. Obstet Gynecol 1969;34:194–199
39. Kennedy A, Hemingway A. Radiology of ovarian varices. Br J Hosp Med 1990;44:38–43
40. Farquhar CM, Rogers V, Franks S, Pearce S, Wadsworth J, Beard RW. A randomized controlled trial of medroxyprogesterone acetate and psychotherapy for the treatment of pelvic congestion. Br J Obstet Gynaecol 1989;96:1153–1162
41. Soysal ME, Soysal S, Vicdan K, Ozer S. A randomized controlled trial of goserelin and medroxyprogesterone acetate in the treatment of pelvic congestion. Hum Reprod 2001;16:931–939
42. Gangar KF, Stones RW, Saunders D, et al. An alternative to hysterectomy? GnRH analogue combined with hormone replacement therapy. Br J Obstet Gynaecol 1993;100:360–364
43. Edwards RD, Robertson IR, MacLean AB, Hemingway AP. Case report: pelvic pain syndrome–successful treatment of a case by ovarian vein embolization. Clin Radiol 1993;47:429–431
44. Takahashi H, Mitsushima M, Okada N, et al. Role of interaction with vinculin in recruitment of vinexins to focal adhesions. Biochem Biophys Res Commun 2005;336:239–246
45. American College of Obstetricians and Gynecologists. Uterine leiomyomata. In: 1999 Compendium of Selected Publications. ACOG Technical Bulletin Number 192. Washington, DC: The American College of Obstetricians and Gynecologists;1994:863–870
46. Kim HS, Malhotra AD, Rowe PC, Lee JM, Venbrux AC. Embolotherapy for pelvic congestion syndrome: long-term results. J Vasc Interv Radiol 2006;17:289–297
47. Gettman MT, Lotman Y, Cadeddu J. Laparoscopic treatment of ovarian vein syndrome. JSLS 2003;7:257–260
48. Perry CP, Presthus J, Nieves A. Laparoscopic uterine suspension for pain relief: a multicenter study. J Reprod Med 2005;50:567–570
49. Beard RW, Kennedy RG, Gangar KF, et al. Bilateral oophorectomy and hysterectomy in the treatment of intractable pelvic pain associated with pelvic congestion. Br J Obstet Gynaecol 1991;98:988–992
50. Ghosh A, Shafie-Pour H, Ayers KJ. Laparoscopic sclerotherapy in a case of pelvic congestion syndrome. BJOG 2006;113:610–611

V Spine Interventions

19 Clinical Review: Osteoporosis

Michael F. Holick

Osteoporosis is the most common metabolic bone disease worldwide.[1–4] It is estimated that 25 million Americans are at risk for osteoporosis. Osteoporosis is more common in women than adult onset diabetes, heart disease, and stroke combined. Osteoporosis by definition means that both the matrix and mineral content of the skeleton has declined to the degree where there is loss of architectural integrity increasing risk of fracture.

The prevalence of osteoporosis increases progressively with age, and by the age of 80, 25% of women and 15% of men will have had a hip fracture.[1–5] Approximately 33% of women 60 to 70 years of age and 66% of those 80 years of age or older have osteoporosis.[1–4] Forty-seven percent of women and 22% of men 50 years of age or older will sustain an osteoporotic fracture.[2,4] Although loss of bone mineral density (BMD) per se is considered by many to be a benign disease of little consequence, an osteoporotic fracture can cause chronic debilitating pain, diminished quality of life, and even death. Approximately 1.5 million skeletal fractures occur in women annually in the United States, many of which can be attributed to osteoporosis. Two hundred fifty-thousand hip fractures occur annually, and ~20% of these patients will die within the first year from complications of the fracture and 50% never regain their previous quality of life.[2,4,5] Approximately 8 to 10 billion dollars are spent annually for the acute care of patients with hip fracture. As the U.S. population ages by 2020, it is estimated that $120 billion dollars a year will be spent for acute and chronic care of these patients.[2,3]

■ Risk Factors

Classically, osteoporosis is associated with a thin white female who has been postmenopausal for 10 to 15 years (**Fig. 19.1**). However, all men and women are at risk for developing osteoporosis. Some of the more common causes associated with osteopenia and osteoporosis include early age of onset for menopause, history of amenorrhea or oligomenorrhea during the second and third decades, hypogonadism, family history, poor lifetime intake of calcium, and chronic vitamin D deficiency (**Table 19.1**).[2,4,6] In addition, heavy cigarette smoking, premature graying of the hair (50% of the hair turns gray by the age of 40 years), several endocrinopathies including hyperthyroidism and primary hyperparathyroidism, genetic diseases of collagen synthesis, i.e., Ehlers–Danlos syndrome and osteogenesis imperfecta as well as chronic glucocorticoid and antiseizure therapy are major risk factors for this debilitating disease (**Tables 19.1** and **19.2**).[2,4,6,7]

■ Pathophysiology

The major precipitating cause of osteoporosis in women is loss of ovarian function.[2–4] Calcium and vitamin D deficiency in addition to aging will also cause a significant reduction in BMD.[2,4,7–9] For men and women, estrogen plays an essential role in bone remodeling.[2,4] Osteoblasts that make the collagen matrix for bone mineralization have receptors for estrogen. Estrogen regulates bone mineralization and demineralization by coupling osteoblastic and

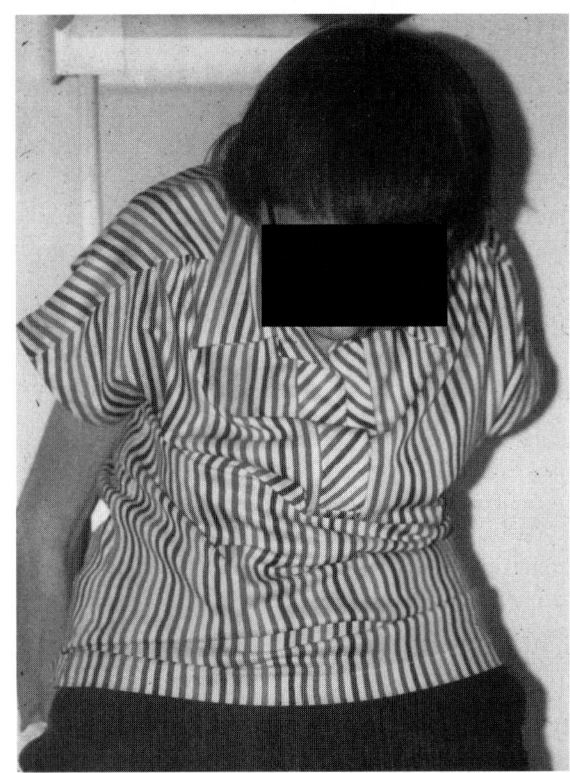

Fig. 19.1 Elderly woman presenting with severe kyphosis consistent with wedge fractures of her cervical and thoracic spine. Her only complaint was that she could not look up any longer. (Copyright Michael F. Holick, PhD, MD, 2007. Reprinted with permission.)

Table 19.1 Risk Factors for Development of Osteoporosis

Risk factor
Early menopause (natural or surgical)
Amenorrhea or oligomenorrhea in second and third decades
Thin body habitus
Family history
Inadequate lifelong calcium intake (<800 mg/day)
Chronic vitamin D deficiency
Hypogonadism
Cigarette smoking
Premature graying (50% of hair turns gray before age 40)
Steroid and antiseizure therapy
Excessive thyroid hormone replacement
Immobilization

osteoclastic activity. Estrogen deficiency causes an uncoupling of this process leading to an imbalance resulting in an increase in osteoclastic activity (bone resorption). This ultimately causes the dissolution of the matrix and mineral.

As women enter menopause, they begin to lose on average 2 to 4% of their bone mass each year. This is unrelenting and continues for at least a decade, causing a 30 to 40% reduction in BMD. Aging also plays a role by decreasing bone mineral density on average of 0.5 to 1% per year after the age of 50 years. Chronic calcium deficiency results in transient decreases in blood ionized calcium levels, which are immediately corrected by increased production of parathyroid hormone (PTH). PTH stimulates the production of osteoclasts that dissolve bone, causing both osteopenia and osteoporosis. Similarly, vitamin D deficiency results in a decrease in intestinal calcium absorption, which leads to a compensatory increase in PTH levels resulting in the same destruction of the skeleton (**Fig. 19.2**).[2,4,7]

Calcium, Vitamin D, and Bone Physiology

The body obtains all of its calcium from the diet. The hormone responsible for providing the body with its calcium requirement is vitamin D. Vitamin D coming from either exposure to sunlight or from diet requires two successive hydroxylations. The first occurs in the liver to form 25-hydroxyvitamin D [25(OH)D], the major circulating form of vitamin D. This is the form of vitamin D that is used to measure a person's vitamin D status. 25(OH)D, however, is biologically inactive and requires activation (hydroxylation) in the kidneys to form 1,25-dihydroxyvitamin D [$1,25(OH)_2D$], the biologically active form of vitamin D (**Fig. 19.2**).[7]

$1,25(OH)_2D$ production is controlled by serum PTH, calcium, phosphorus, and fibroblast growth factor 23 (FGF-23). Hypocalcemia and hypophosphatemia will stimulate

Table 19.2 Causes of Osteoporosis and Osteopenia

Cause
Common
Vitamin D deficiency
Calcium deficiency
Estrogen deficiency
Testosterone deficiency
Thyrotoxicosis (natural or TSH-suppressive doses of thyroxine)
Hyperadrenocorticism (Cushing syndrome)
Hyperparathyroidism
Chronic glucocorticoid and antiseizure medication use
Immobilization
Less common
Malabsorption
Vitamin C deficiency (scurvy)
Chronic heparin administration
Systemic mastocytosis
Adult hypophosphatasia
Chronic renal failure
Primary biliary cirrhosis
Cancer
Chronic obstructive lung disease
Rheumatoid arthritis
Inherited
Osteogenesis imperfecta
Ehlers–Danlos syndrome
Marfan syndrome
Homocystinuria

the kidney's production of $1,25(OH)_2D$ and FGF-23 will reduce it. $1,25(OH)_2D$ interacts with its vitamin D receptor (VDR) in the small intestine to enhance the absorption of dietary calcium and phosphorus (**Fig. 19.2**).[7] Only 10 to 15% of dietary calcium and 60% of dietary phosphorus is absorbed in the absence of vitamin D. $1,25(OH)_2D$ enhances intestinal calcium absorption to 30 to 40% and phosphorus absorption to ~ 80%.[7]

Vitamin D deficiency results in secondary hyperparathyroidism. PTH increases tubular reabsorption of the calcium in the kidneys, stimulates the kidneys to produce $1,25(OH)_2D$ and stimulates osteoblasts through its receptor to increase the expression of receptor activator of NFκB (RANK) ligand (RANKL). The preosteoclast that has the RANK interacts with RANKL on the osteoblast which, in turn, induces it to become a mature osteoclast (**Fig. 19.3**). Once mature, it secretes hydrochloric acid and variety of enzymes including collagenases to dissolve the bone matrix and mineral to release calcium into the circulation.[2,4,7]

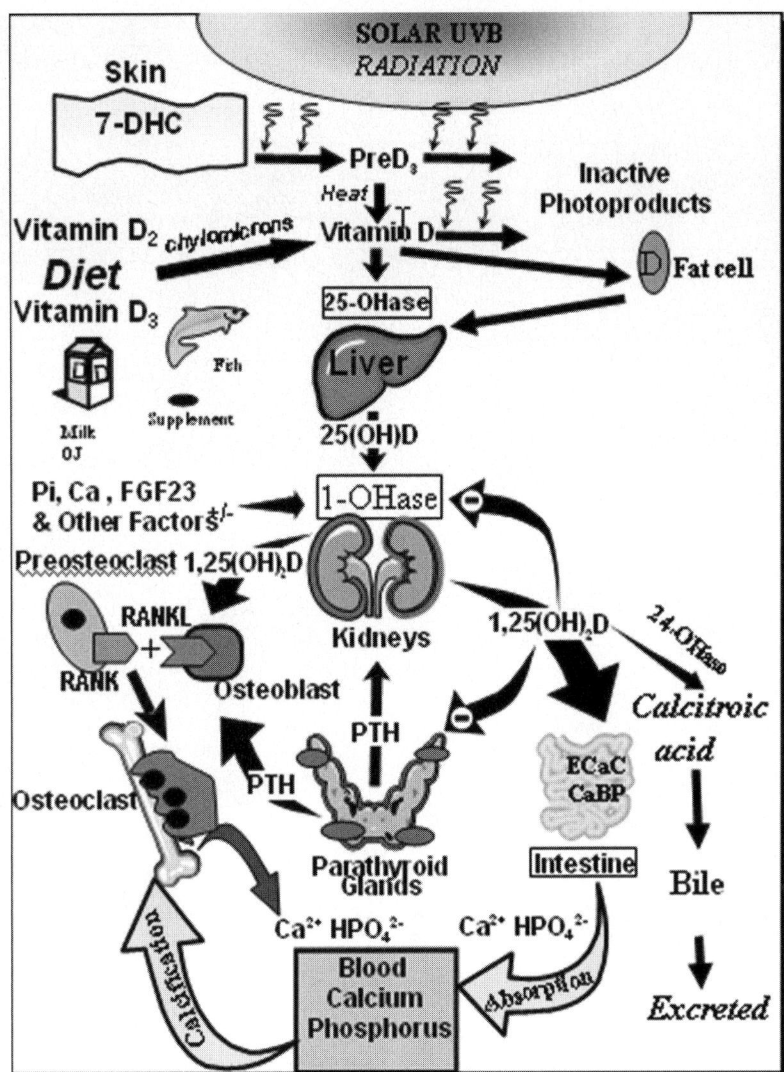

Fig. 19.2 Schematic representation of the synthesis and metabolism of vitamin D for regulating calcium, phosphorus, and bone metabolism. During exposure to sunlight, 7-dehydrocholesterol (7-DHC) in the skin is converted to previtamin D_3 (preD_3). PreD_3 immediately converts by a heat-dependent process to vitamin D_3. Excessive exposure to sunlight degrades previtamin D_3 and vitamin D_3 into inactive photoproducts. Vitamin D_2 and vitamin D_3 from dietary sources are incorporated into chylomicrons, transported by the lymphatic system into the venous circulation. Vitamin D (D represents D_2 or D_3) made in the skin or ingested in the diet can be stored in and then released from fat cells. Vitamin D in the circulation is bound to the vitamin D binding protein, which transports it to the liver where vitamin D is converted by the vitamin D-25-hydroxylase (25-OHase) to 25-hydroxyvitamin D [25(OH)D]. This is the major circulating form of vitamin D that is used by clinicians to measure vitamin D status (although most reference laboratories report the normal range to be 20 to 100 ng/mL, the preferred healthful range is 30 to 60 ng/mL). 25(OH)D is biologically inactive and must be converted in the kidneys by the 25-hydroxyvitamin D-1α-hydroxylase (1-OHase) to its biologically active form 1,25-dihydroxyvitamin D [1,25$(OH)_2$D]. Serum phosphorus, calcium, fibroblast growth factor (FGF-23) and other factors can either increase (+) or decrease (−) the renal production of 1,25$(OH)_2$D. 1,25$(OH)_2$D feedback regulates its own synthesis and decreases the synthesis and secretion of parathyroid hormone (PTH) in the parathyroid glands. 1,25$(OH)_2$D increases the expression of the 25-hydroxyvitamin D-24-hydroxylase (24-OHase) to catabolize 1,25$(OH)_2$D and 25(OH)D to the water-soluble biologically inactive calcitropic acid, which is excreted in the bile. 1,25$(OH)_2$D enhances intestinal calcium absorption in the small intestine by stimulating the expression of the epithelial calcium channel (ECaC; also known as transient receptor potential cation channel subfamily V member 6 [TRPV6]) and the calbindin 9K (calcium-binding protein; CaBP). 1,25$(OH)_2$D is recognized by its receptor in osteoblasts causing an increase in the expression of receptor activator of NFκB ligand (RANKL). Its receptor RANK on the preosteoclast binds RANKL, which induces the preosteoclast to become a mature osteoclast. The mature osteoclast removes calcium and phosphorus from the bone to maintain blood calcium and phosphorus levels. Adequate calcium and phosphorus levels promote the mineralization of the skeleton and maintain neuromuscular function. (Copyright Michael F. Holick, PhD, MD, 2007. Reprinted with permission.)

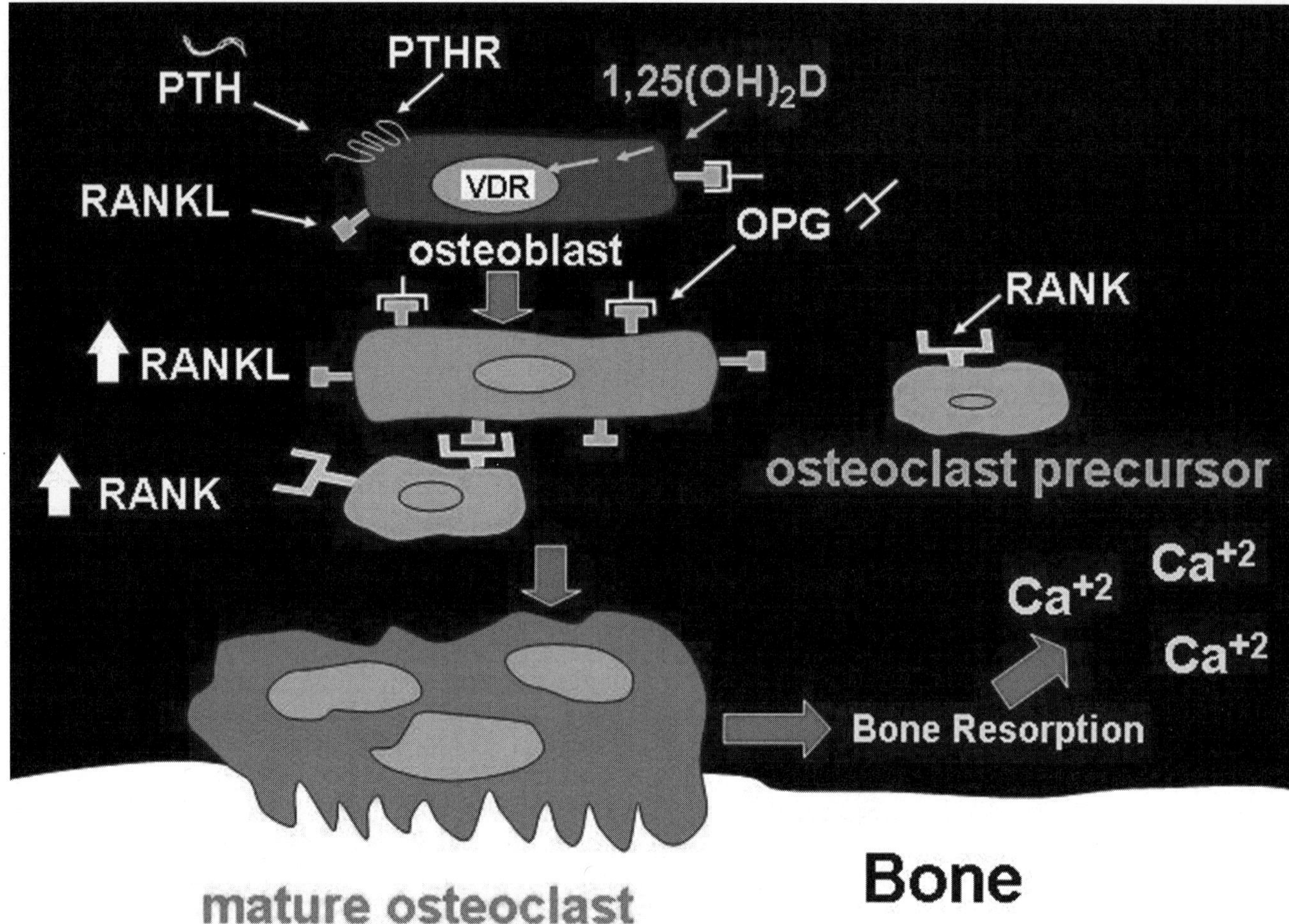

Fig. 19.3 1,25$(OH)_2D$ and parathyroid hormone (PTH) stimulation of the mobilization of calcium from the skeleton through interactions with their respective receptors on osteoblasts, which induce expression of the receptor activator of nuclear factor $-\kappa B$ (RANK) ligand (RANKL). The receptor activator of nuclear factor $-\kappa B$ on immature osteoblasts binds to the receptor activator of nuclear factor $-\kappa B$ ligand, which causes the cells to mature and coalesce with other osteoclast precursors to become mature multinuclear osteoclasts. (Copyright Michael F. Holick, PhD, MD, 2007. Reprinted with permission.)

■ Using Dual Energy X-Ray Absorptiometry

Before the advent of bone densitometry, the radiologist made the diagnosis of osteoporosis either based on the presence of a nontraumatic fracture in the spine or by observing a decrease in the density of the skeleton relative to soft tissue density in an x-ray. However, a patient needs to lose 30 to 50% of the skeletal mass before this can be detected by a radiograph (**Fig. 19.4**). Dual energy x-ray absorptiometry (DEXA), which was introduced more than 20 years ago, uses two x-ray beams with different energy levels. When soft tissue absorption is subtracted out, the BMD can be determined from the absorption of each beam by bone. The most common sites for measuring BMD are the lumbar spine and the hip (**Fig. 19.5**).[2,4,6] However, the proximal and mid-radius and ulna BMD can be determined as well as whole body calcium and fat content. The World Health Organization has defined osteoporosis as a T-score (standard deviation from the maximum BMD in healthy young, 20 to 30 year olds matched for sex and race) <2.5 or less. Osteopenia was defined as a T-score of −1 to −2.5. The amount of radiation dose from a DXA is −1/10th of a standard chest x-ray, and, therefore, is of little concern.[2,4,6]

Although BMD is the single most accurate predictor of fracture risk, it should be noted that BMD per se does not necessarily mean that the patient suffers from osteoporo-

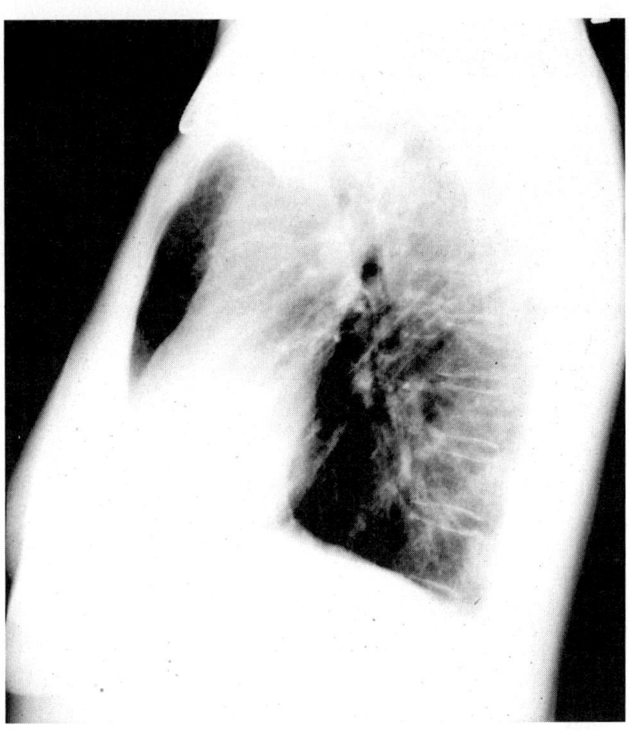

Fig. 19.4 Lateral radiograph of an osteoporotic woman with lower back pain radiating down her left leg to the knee. Note severe osteopenia of the thoracic and lumbar vertebral bodies with wedge-shaped compression fractures. Marked osteopenia of the tubercular bone with preservation of the rim of cortical bone gives rise to classic fish-mouth appearance between two vertebral bodies, evidence of vertebral collapse and compression fractures. (Copyright Michael F. Holick, PhD, MD, 2007. Reprinted with permission.)

sis, i.e., loss of bone mineral and bone matrix. Osteomalacia, which is commonly due to vitamin D deficiency, is caused by a mineralization defect of the skeleton (i.e., that the osteoblasts laid down the bone matrix, but it was not mineralized). As far as an x-ray is concerned, there is no bone mineral present in matrix of the osteomalacic bone, and thus appears as low BMD. It is not possible to distinguish osteoporosis and osteomalacia based on an x-ray or by BMD. The only proven method is to do a bone biopsy and stain the sample for mineral and matrix.[7]

Bone Mineral Density and Fracture Risk

Because BMD only provides an estimate of the bone mineral content and no information about the architecture or the stability of the combined matrix and mineral, it is, therefore, not at all surprising that the proportion of fractures attributable to DEXA defined osteoporosis (T-score < 2.5) is modest. A recent study suggested that 10 to 44% of fractures occurred in patients who had a T-score of <2.5.[2] However, it is recognized that the lower the T-score the higher the risk of fracture. Furthermore, aging also plays a significant role in fracture risk and a person 60 years of age compared with an 80 year old with the same T-score has a 30% less likelihood of experiencing a fracturing.[2–4] Thus, other aspects including bone strength, bone architecture as well as soft tissue surrounding the bone all influence the risk of fracture. Muscle weakness, increased body sway, and poor eyesight are among the many causes of falls which is the largest cause of injury in older people and a major cause of low trauma fracture. It has been estimated that 5 to 6% of falls result in fracture in older persons and that 1 to 2% of these are hip fracture.[2–4]

■ Prevention

Calcium, Vitamin D, and Estrogen Supplementation

Adequate calcium and vitamin D intake throughout life is one of the most important contributions for maintaining bone health. Vitamin D and calcium deficiency during infancy and childhood will prevent maximum growth and bone mineral density that is determined by the person's genetics. Typically, peak bone mass is attained after puberty and begins to diminish after 30 years of age. A low calcium intake and vitamin D deficiency will result on average in a 0.25 to 0.5% decrease in BMD/year. Although this appears to be inconsequential when it is multiplied by 20 or 30 years, upwards of 10 to 15% of skeletal mass can potentially be lost during the third and fourth decades due to inattention to dietary calcium and vitamin D intake.

In 1997, the Institute of Medicine released recommendations for adequate intake for calcium and vitamin D.[10] All men and women 50 years of age and older should ingest 1200 mg of calcium each day. Most experts still agree that the calcium recommendations are reasonable and should be followed. However, most experts also agree that the recommended intakes for vitamin D (i.e., 200 IU/d for all children and adults up to the age of 50 years, 400 IU and 600 IU/d for adults 51 to 70 years and 71+ years respectively) are woefully inadequate. It's been recommended that without adequate sun exposure, which is the major source of vitamin D for most humans, at least 1000 IU of vitamin D/day is required for both children and adults to sustain a 25(OH)D level > 30 ng/mL.[7,9] The National Osteoporosis Foundation recently came out with the recommendation that all postmenopausal women should receive 800 IU of vitamin D/day.

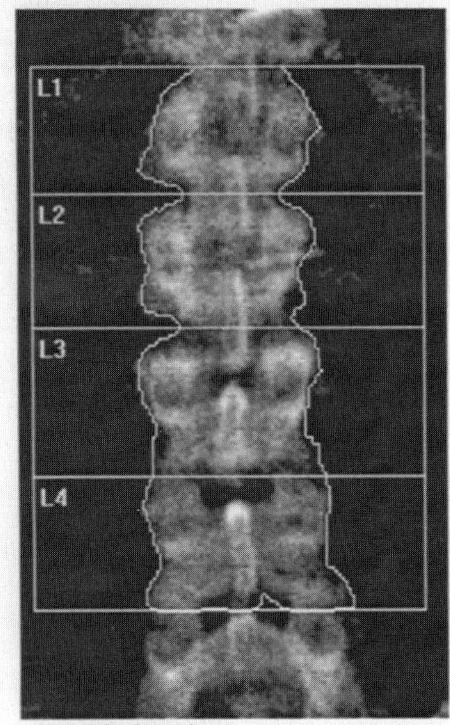

DXA Results Summary:

Region	Area (cm²)	BMC (g)	BMD (g/cm²)	T - score	Z - score
L1	15.34	13.36	0.870	-2.2	-1.9
L2	17.09	17.50	1.024	-1.6	-1.3
L3	20.36	20.00	0.983	-2.1	-1.8
L4	20.75	19.73	0.951	-2.8	-2.5
Total	**73.54**	**70.58**	**0.960**	**-2.2**	**-1.9**

Total BMD CV 1.0%, ACF = 1.029, BCF = 1.018, TH = 7.381
WHO Classification: Osteopenia
Fracture Risk: Increased

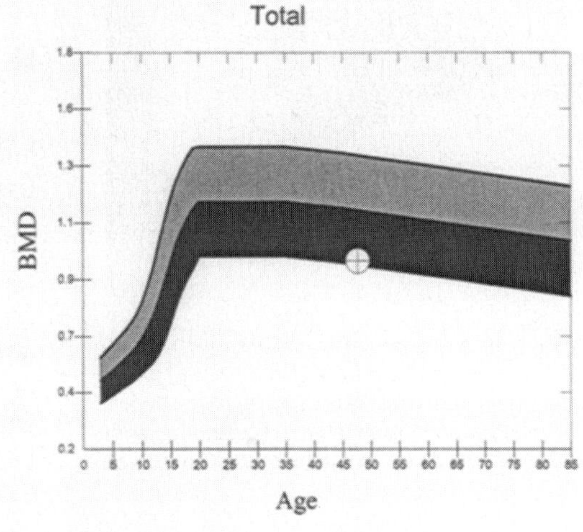

A

Fig. 19.5 (A) Bone mineral density report in a postmenopausal woman with osteopenia of L2–L4 spine.

Adolescent girls who suffer from amenorrhea or oligomenorrhea should consider some type of estrogen replacement therapy to help maximize their bone growth and maintain bone formation activity. Reducing other risk factors as noted in **Tables 19.1** and **19.2** are also important for prevention of osteopenia and osteoporosis. Most important is to discourage cigarette smoking and to increase calcium and vitamin D intake for all patients, especially those who are on antiseizure medications or glucocorticoids.

Weight-Bearing Exercise

It is well documented that weight lifters who put an enormous amount of stress on their skeletons increase the BMD in the bones that are stressed as a result of the weight lifting.[2–4,11] Unloading of the skeleton results in significant mobilization of calcium from the skeleton. Astronauts, on average, lose ~0.1% of their skeletal mass per month in a weightless environment. This is the reason why swimming does not improve bone density whereas it improves muscle tone and muscle strength. It is, however, weight-bearing exercise that is important for the maintenance of skeletal health. The "jarring" activity on the skeleton that occurs during weight-bearing exercise is translated to bone cells to increase bone formation. This is why the radius and ulna BMD are higher in the dominant forearm of professional tennis players compared with their nondominant forearm. Volleyball players who put an enormous amount of stress on their skeleton by their jumping activity also have excellent BMD in the hip and spine. However, any gain in BMD due to weight bearing is lost once the weight-bearing activity is stopped. Patients at strict bed rest lose ~0.1 to 1.0% BMD each month.[4]

I recommend to my patients, especially those with osteoporosis of their spine, not to lift with their back but

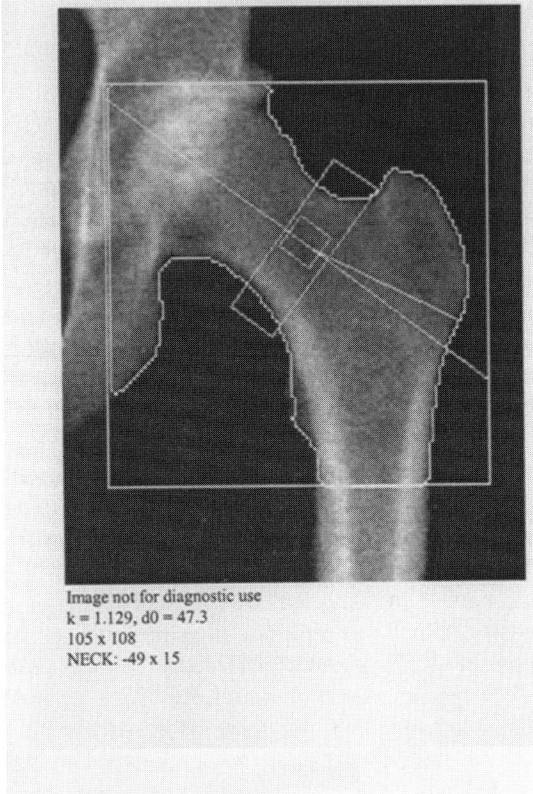

DXA Results Summary:

Region	Area (cm²)	BMC (g)	BMD (g/cm²)	T-score	Z-score
Neck	5.32	4.26	0.801	-1.7	-0.7
Troch	10.11	6.55	0.648	-1.7	-0.9
Inter	20.04	24.27	1.211	-0.7	-0.2
Total	**35.47**	**35.08**	**0.989**	**-1.1**	**-0.4**
Ward's	1.16	0.66	0.571	-2.1	-0.7

Total BMD CV 1.0%, ACF = 1.029, BCF = 1.018, TH = 6.457
WHO Classification: Osteopenia
Fracture Risk: Increased

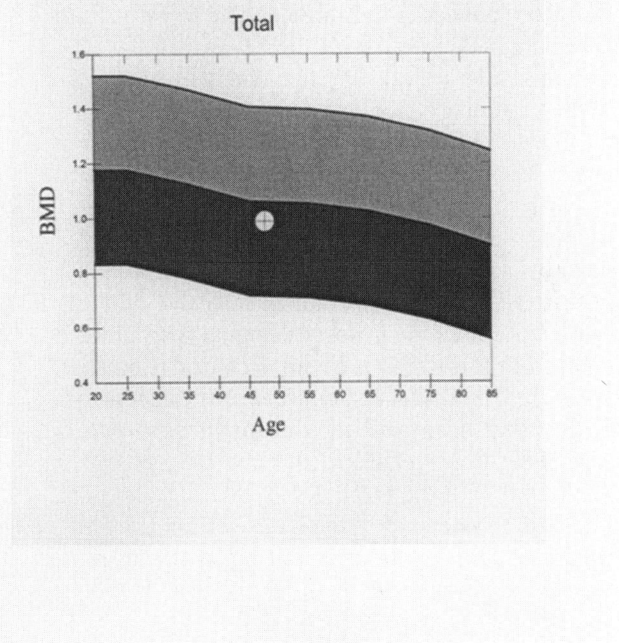

B

Fig. 19.5 *(Continued)* **(B)** Femoral neck bone density. (Copyright Michael F. Holick, PhD, MD, 2007. Reprinted with permission.)

rather with their legs. And not to lift more than 10 to 15 pounds if they had a previous fragility fracture. I also recommend that if they are using a training facility, not to lift weights with their shoulders or to push up weights with their legs; which potentially could cause a compression fracture in the spine. Because it is the direct stress of muscle action and gravity for enhancing BMD, it is not possible for the skeleton to be globally affected by exercise. Only the parts of the skeleton that are being stimulated by the exercise will increase BMD in response to it. Thus, weight-bearing exercise in moderation should be encouraged to increase muscle tone and improve cardiovascular function. Walking 3 to 5 miles a week, preferably on pavement, will improve muscle tone and muscle strength in the hip girdle muscles, and thus decrease risk of sway and falling; which is the major precipitating cause of fracture. It will also maintain BMD in the lumbar spine and hips.

■ Treatment

Calcium and Vitamin D

Vitamin D deficiency is one of the most common associated causes for osteopenia and osteoporosis. The easiest way to treat vitamin D deficiency is to quickly fill up the vitamin D tank by giving the patient 50,000 IU of vitamin D_2 once a week for eight weeks.[7] Since the patient presented with vitamin D deficiency, it is likely that the patient will become vitamin D deficient once the treatment is concluded because the cause(s) have not been rectified. Therefore, after being treated for their vitamin D deficiency and raising their blood levels of 25(OH)D > 30 ng/mL, patients should be given 50,000 IU of vitamin D_2 once every 2 weeks or 1,000 IU vitamin D_3/day as maintenance therapy.

The patient should also be encouraged to increase their dietary intake of calcium.[2,4,12] Milk, which is an excellent source of calcium, contains 250 mg in 8 oz of whole milk and 300 mg and 100 IU respectively in 8 oz of skim milk. Orange juice fortified with calcium and vitamin D is also an excellent source of calcium (300 mg in 8 oz). Kale and broccoli do contain calcium, but 10 cups of these vegetables a day are required to provide a 1000 mg of calcium. Spinach contains calcium as well, but is not a good dietary source because the high oxalate content in the spinach irreversibly binds the calcium, and thus it is not bioavailable. Yogurt, cheeses, and bones in sardines are also additional sources of dietary calcium. Because all adults over the age of 50 should ingest 1200 mg of calcium/day, supplementation is recommended if they are not able to get it from dietary sources.

There are a variety of calcium supplements available today. Calcium carbonate, calcium citrate, calcium gluconate, and calcium phosphate are some of the forms of calcium available in supplements. If the calcium product is chewed such as Tums (calcium carbonate; GlaxoSmithKline, Brentford, London, UK) or dissolved in the mouth as some of the candied forms, for example, Viactive (McNeill Nutritionals, Ft. Washington, PA), the calcium is bioavailable whether taken with or without food. Most calcium pills swallowed are dissolved in the stomach by stomach acid. However, patients with achlorhydria cannot dissolve calcium carbonate pills; this means that the calcium in these pills is not bioavailable. However, if an achlorhydric patient takes the calcium pill with the meal, then as the meal is being "ground up" in the stomach so too is the calcium pill. Thus, achlorhydric patients can be given calcium carbonate pills, but they should always take them with a meal. It should also be noted that taking all of the calcium at one time is less efficiently absorbed than if it is taken 2 or 3 times/day in smaller amounts. Thus, I typically recommend that patients take their calcium supplement with their meal both to insure its absorption and also as a means of having the patients keep it as part of their routine. This will make them less likely to forget taking their calcium supplement.

There has been concern that increasing calcium intake will increase the risk of kidney stones. However, increasing calcium intake decreases the risk of kidney stones unless you have had one. This is based on the realization that it is hyperabsorption of oxalate that is often responsible for increased risk of kidney stones, and that by increasing calcium intake, the calcium in the intestine binds oxalate irreversibly, thus preventing its absorption. For patients with a history of calcium containing kidney stones, they still need to have adequate calcium intake. I typically recommend that they take calcium citrate. The citrate will chelate the calcium in the ultrafiltrate and urine and help prevent it from binding oxalate, which can precipitate stone development.

Bisphosphonate Therapy

Patients with osteoporosis who have had adequate calcium and vitamin D intake may need pharmacologic intervention to increase BMD and decrease the risk of fracture. In the early 1990s, a new class of drugs known as bisphosphonates was introduced as a novel approach for treating osteopenia and osteoporosis.[13–15] A bisphosphonate, by definition, consists of two phosphate groups that are connected with a carbon. On the carbon atom is a variety of different substituents that make bisphosphonates different from each other. The first oral bisphosphonate introduced in the United States for the treatment of osteoporosis was alendronate. It was observed that 10 mg of alendronate once a day for 3 years increased BMD in the lumbar spine by ~6 to 8% on average and decreased the risk of vertebral fractures by more than 50%. Hip bone density increased an average of 4 to 6% in 3 years, and there was approximately a 50% reduction in risk of hip fracture.[2,13,15]

Risedronate (5 mg/day) was also found to be effective in increasing spinal and hip bone densities and decreasing the risk of vertebral and nonvertebral fractures (**Table 19.3**).[2,14,15] Because bisphosphonates are deposited in the bone and have a long half-life, it was observed that giving a total weekly dose was as effective as taking a daily dose. Thus, alendronate (70 mg/week) and risedronate (35 mg/week) were approved for the prevention and treatment of osteoporosis. Recently, ibandronate (150 mg/monthly) was approved for the prevention of vertebral fractures.[16]

The exact mechanism by which bisphosphonates work is not fully understood. However, what is known is that bisphosphonates inhibit osteoclastic bone resorption by either causing them to be released from the bone or causing them to die. Thus, osteoblasts lay down matrix which is mineralized unimpeded by osteoclasts. This is the reason why on average there is a 2 to 3% per year increase in BMD in the lumbar spine and 1 to 2% increase in BMD in the hips when patients are given a bisphosphonate with adequate calcium and vitamin D.

Bisphosphonates are very safe to use. One study reported that patients on alendronate for 10 years continued to benefit by either increasing or maintaining their BMD in the hip and spine and maintaining a suppression of bone resorption.[2,17] The major side-effects of bisphosphonates that should prompt cessation are severe myalgias and arthralgias. Another side effect that is potentially life threatening is erosion of the lower esophagus. This usually presents itself as symptoms of gastritis, but can be silent. It occurs in no more than 2 to 3% of patients and can be product specific (i.e., some patients on alendronate have GI symptoms whereas on risedronate they do not and vice versa).[2] Osteoporosis of the jaw is seen in cancer patients

Table 19.3 Medications Approved by the Food and Drug Administration (FDA) for the Treatment or Prevention of Postmenopausal Osteoporosis

Drug	Method of Administration and Dose	Reduction in Risk of Fracture	Side Effect	FDA Approval
Bisphosphonates	Oral			
Alendronate	70 mg weekly, 10 mg daily	Vertebral, nonvertebral, fracture, hip	Esophagitis, myalgias arthralgias	For treatment and prevention
Risedronate	35 mg weekly, 5 mg daily	Vertebral, nonvertebral, fracture	Esophagitis, myalgias arthralgias	For treatment and prevention
Ibandronate	150 mg monthly, 2.5 mg daily	Vertebral fracture	Esophagitis, myalgias arthralgias	For treatment and prevention
Bisphosphonates	IV			
Zoledronic acid	5 mg IV once a year	Vertebral, hip	Arthralgias	For treatment
Estrogens	Oral or transdermal			
17β-estradiol	Oral, 0.5–2 mg/d, or transdermal twice weekly	No data from randomized, controlled trials	Risk of DVT; risk of cardiovascular disease; cancer of breast, uterus, and ovaries	Approved for prevention only
Conjugated equine estrogens	Oral, 0.3–1.25 mg daily	Vertebral, nonvertebral, and hip fracture (at dose of 0.625 mg daily)	Risk of DVT; risk of cardiovascular disease; cancer of breast, uterus, and ovaries	Approved for prevention only
SERM	Oral			
Raloxifene	60 mg daily	Vertebral fracture only	Hot flashes, nausea, DVT, leg cramps	For treatment and prevention
Calcitonin				
Miacalcitonin	Subcutaneous or intranasal, 100–200 IU	Vertebral fracture only	Nasal stuffiness, rhinitis, nausea	Approved for treatment only
Anabolic agent	Subcutaneous			
PTH (1–34) (teriparatide)	20 µg sq daily	Vertebral and nonvertebral fracture	Hypercalcemia, hypercalciuria, nausea, leg cramps	Approved for treatment only; generally used for severe osteoporosis

Abbreviations: DVT, deep vein thrombosis; PTH, parathyroid hormone; SERM, selective estrogen-receptor modulators; SQ, subcutaneous.

who receive intravenous bisphosphate treatment for hypercalcemia, but not in postmenopausal patients on an oral bisphosphonate.[2]

Patients who take an oral bisphosphonate must take it on empty stomach and with a full glass of water and remain sitting or standing for at least 30 minutes before reclining to minimize esophageal reflux and the potential for the drug to cause esophageal irritation and erosion. Under the ideal circumstances ~ 0.7% of the bisphosphonate is absorbed into the circulation.

In the United States, intravenous zoledronic acid (5 mg) once a year was approved for the treatment of osteoporosis.[18] Patients unable to tolerate any oral bisphosphonate because of gastrointestinal symptoms have also received intravenous pamidronate (30 mg/3 months), but this is not an approved use for this medication in the United States.[2,4]

Both intravenous bisphosphonates have been shown to maintain or increase BMD in the lumbar spine and hip and reduce risk of fractures (**Table 19.3**).

Hormone Replacement and SERM Therapy

Menopause is one of the precipitating causes for increased bone loss due to the lack of estrogen and increased bone resorption activity of osteoclasts. Estrogen replacement slows bone resorption and reduces the incidence of new vertebral fractures by ~50%.[2,4,19,20] Women in the Women's Health Initiative who took 0.625 mg of conjugated estrogen and 5 mg of a progestin daily had a 33% reduction in hip fracture. Because of concern that women in this study on hormone replacement therapy had a 25% increase risk of developing breast cancer, many physicians stopped using hormone replacement therapy as a means of helping maintain BMD in postmenopausal women. Because of this study, lower doses of hormone replacement therapy (HRT) have been used and found to be effective in maintaining or marginally increasing BMD, but there is no data available on fracture prevention using this regimen. However, many physicians now use conjugated estrogen/progestin of (0.3 mg/1.5 mg). This strategy is also helpful in minimizing menopausal symptoms (**Table 19.3**).[2]

To combat the issue of HRT and breast cancer, a drug was developed that had selective estrogen-like effects on bone with no activity either in the breasts or on the uterus. These drugs are known as selective estrogen-receptor modulators (SERM) and the one approved in the United States is raloxifene. Like estrogen, raloxifene inhibits bone resorption and either maintains or marginally increases BMD in the lumbar spine. It also decreases the risk of vertebral fractures by 40% in osteoporotic women.[2,21] There is no evidence that this drug decreases the risk of nonvertebral fractures. There is, however, the additional benefit of a reduced risk of breast cancer with long-term use of this SERM, but the downside is that it can precipitate or worsen menopausal hot flashes.[22]

Calcitonin

Calcitonin is a 32 amino acid residue peptide secreted by the C-cells in the thyroid gland. Calcitonin receptors are present on the surface of osteoclasts and calcitonin decreases osteoclastic activity and bone resorption. Calcitonin is effectively used for the acute treatment of hypercalcemia because of its inhibitory activity on osteoclasts. However, when osteoclasts are continually exposed to calcitonin, they respond by internalizing their receptor and become resistant to it. There is only one study that has reported that intranasal calcitonin at 200 IU/day decreased the risk of vertebral fractures. It did not have any effect on reducing risk of nonvertebral fractures, and no other studies have substantiated this potential benefit.[23] As a result, it has lost favor and has been replaced with bisphosphonate therapy or other therapies in this population.[2]

■ Anabolic Agents

Fluoride is known to stimulate osteoblastic activity, and thus it was thought that sodium fluoride would be an ideal drug to treat osteoporosis. However, in a randomized trial, patients on sodium fluoride not only had dramatic increases in bone mineral density, but also increased number of nonvertebral fractures. The likely cause was that fluoride was incorporated into the bone and the fluorohydroxyapatite did not provide as much structural support as calcium hydroxyapatite. Thus, fluoride is no longer used.

Parathyroid hormone (1–34) [PTH (1–34)] was approved for the treatment and prevention of osteoporosis. Unlike bisphosphonates, which inhibit bone resorption and do not stimulate osteoblastic activity, PTH (1–34) (teriparatide) interacts with its receptor on osteoblasts to stimulate osteoblastic activity. In a randomized clinical trial over ~18 months, there was a dramatic 10 to 14% increase in vertebral bone density and a 3 to 5% increase in total hip bone density. Twenty micrograms of PTH (1–34)/day administered subcutaneously was also shown in the same study to reduce risk of vertebral and nonvertebral fractures by more than 50%.[24]

It is recommended that PTH (1–34) be used for 18 to 24 months. The reason is that when rats received 30 to 60 times the amount of PTH (1–34) daily they had a marked increase in developing osteosarcomas. As a result, there is a black box warning on the PTH (1–34) drug label. However, this drug was approved because it was known that rats are prone to developing osteosarcomas spontaneously and patients with chronic secondary and primary hyperparathyroidism who often sustain elevated levels of PTH for decades do not have an increased risk of developing osteosarcomas.

The major side effects of PTH (1–34) are muscle cramping especially in the lower legs, which often resolves within a few days, transient hypercalcemia typically seen within 4 hours after the injection that resolves by 24 hours, and hypercalciuria.[2,24] Once the treatment is completed, the patient should be placed on a bisphosphonate to preserve the gains made in bone density.[25]

■ Conclusions

Osteoporosis and osteopenia is a significant health problem worldwide that continues to increase in incidence as the world's population ages.[2–4,26,27] A major effort should be made in developing prevention strategies because most humans, if they have an adequate calcium and vitamin D intake and exercise, will attain a bone mass that if sustained throughout life will either prevent or markedly decrease risk of fracture. Patients with osteopenia and osteoporosis should be evaluated for primary and secondary risk factors and causes. A thyroid-stimulating hormone level should always be obtained in these patients to rule out silent hyperthyroidism. There is no need to obtain a PTH level if a serum calcium is normal. However, if the calcium is elevated, a PTH level is indicated to rule out primary hyperparathyroidism. A 25(OH)D level should be obtained as well to determine the patient's vitamin D status. This will allow for correction of a vitamin D deficiency before instituting osteoporosis therapy. Physical activity (typically walking 3 to 5 miles/week) is recommended to help maintain muscle mass in the lower back and hip region, to decrease the risk of falling, and to help maintain BMD at both skeletal sites.

Pharmacologic intervention is warranted in patients who have osteoporosis and have additional risk factors that put them at risk for fracture. Patients with osteoporosis and nontraumatic fractures should be aggressively treated. Adequate calcium and vitamin D intake along with a bisphosphonate is often the first line of therapy.[2–4,12–18,28,29] Alternatively, in perimenopausal and early postmenopausal women, adequate calcium, vitamin D, and either HRT or SERM is a good alternative to help maintain BMD.[2–4,19–21] Patients who fail bisphosphonate therapy,who are unable to tolerate the bisphosphonate therapy, or who are having vertebral fractures on bisphosphonate therapy should be considered for PTH (1–34).[2,24] This anabolic drug is very effective in enhancing osteoblastic activity, thereby markedly decreasing the risk of both vertebral and nonvertebral fractures within a relatively short period.

Acknowledgments

This work was supported in part by NIH grant M01RR00533.

References

1. Office of the Surgeon General. Bone health and osteoporosis: a report of the Surgeon General. Rockville, MD: Department of Health and Human Services, 2004; 436
2. Rosen CJ. Postmenopausal osteoporosis. N Engl J Med 2005;353:595–603
3. NIH Consensus Development Panel on Osteoporosis Prevention, Diagnosis, and Therapy. Osteoporosis prevention, diagnosis, and therapy. JAMA 2001;285:785–795
4. Holick MF. Evaluation and treatment of disorders in calcium, phosphorus, and magnesium metabolism. In: Noble J, ed. Textbook of Primary Care Medicine. 3rd ed. St. Louis, MO: Mosby, Inc.; 2001:886–898
5. Cummings SR, Nevitt MC, Browner WS, et al. Risk factors for hip fracture in white women. N Engl J Med 1995;332(12):767–773
6. Raisz LG. Screening for osteoporosis. N Engl J Med 2005;353:164–171
7. Holick MF, Vitamin D. Deficiency. N Engl J Med 2007;357:266–281
8. LeBoff MS, Kohlmeier L, Hurwitz S, Franklin J, Wright J, Glowacki J. Occult vitamin D deficiency in postmenopausal US women with acute hip fracture. JAMA 1999;281:1505–1511
9. Boonen S, Bischoff-Ferrari HA, Cooper C, et al. Addressing the musculoskeletal components of fracture risk of calcium and vitamin D: a review of the evidence. Calcif Tissue Int 2006;78(5):257–270
10. Standing Committee on the Scientific Evaluation of Dietary Reference Intakes, Food and Nutrition Board Institute of Medicine 1997. Vitamin D. In: Dietary Reference Intakes for Calcium, Phosphorus, Magnesium, Vitamin D, and Fluoride. Washington, DC: National Academy Press; 1999:250–287
11. Kelley GA, Kelley KS. Efficacy of resistance exercise on lumbar spine and femoral neck bone mineral density in premenopausal women: a meta-analysis of individual patient data. J Womens Health (Larchmt) 2004;13:293–300
12. Shea B, Wells G, Cranney A, et al. Meta-analyses of therapies for postmenopausal osteoporosis. VII. Meta-analysis of calcium supplementation for the prevention of postmenopausal osteoporosis. Endocr Rev 2002;23(4):552–559
13. Black DM, Cummings SR, Karpf DB, et al. Randomized trail of effect of alendronate on risk of fracture in women with existing vertebral fractures. Lancet 1996;348(9041):1535–1541
14. Harris ST, Watts NB, Genant HK, et al. Effects of risedronate treatment on vertebral and nonvertebral fractures in women with postmenopausal osteoporosis: a randomized controlled trial. JAMA 1999;282(14):1344–1352
15. Cummings SR, Karpf DB, Harris F, et al. Improvement in spine bone density and reduction in risk of vertebral fractures during treatment with antiresorptive drugs. Am J Med 2002;112(4):281–289
16. Chesnut CH III, Skag A, Christiansen C, et al. Effects of oral ibandronate administered daily or intermittently on fracture risk in postmenopausal osteoporosis. J Bone Miner Res 2004;19(8):1241–1249
17. Harris WH, Heaney RP. Skeletal renewal and metabolic bone disease. N Engl J Med 1969;280(4):193–202
18. McClung M, Recker R, Miller P, et al. Intravenous zoledronic acid 5 mg in the treatment of postmenopausal women with low bone density previously treated with alendronate. Bone 2007;41(1):122–128
19. Lindsay R, Gallagher JC, Kleerekoper M, Pickar JH. Effect of lower doses of conjugated equine estrogens with and without medroxyprogesterone acetate on bone in early postmenopausal women. JAMA 2002;287:2668–2676
20. Guyatt GH, Cranney A, Griffith L, et al. Summary of meta-analyses of therapies for postmenopausal osteoporosis and the relationship between bone density and fractures. Endocrinol Metab Clin North Am 2002;31(3):659–679 xii
21. Ettinger B, Black DM, Mitlak BH, et al. Reduction of vertebral fracture risk in post-menopausal women with osteoporosis treatment with raloxifene: results from a 3-year randomized clinical trial. JAMA 1999;282(7):637–645 [Erratum, JAMA 1999; 282(22):2124]
22. Cummings SR, Eckert S, Krueger KA, et al. The effect of raloxifene on risk of breast cancer in postmenopausal women: results from the MORE randomized trial. JAMA 1999;281(23):2189–2197 [Erratum, JAMA 1999; 282(22):2124]
23. Chesnut CH III, Silverman S, Andriano K, et al. A randomized trial of nasal spray salmon calcitonin in postmenopausal women with established osteoporosis: the Prevent Recurrence of Osteoporotic Fractures Study. Am J Med 2000;109(4):267–276
24. Neer RM, Arnaud CD, Zanchetta JR, et al. Effect of parathyroid hormone (1–34) on fractures and bone mineral density in post-menopausal women with osteoporosis. N Engl J Med 2001;344(19):1434–1441
25. Rittmaster RS, Bolognese M, Ettinger MP, et al. Enhancement of bone mass in osteoporotic women with parathyroid hormone followed by alendronate. J Clin Endocrinol Metab 2000;85(6):2129–2134
26. Chesnut C, Jajumdar S, Gardner J, et al. Assessment of bone quality, quantity, and turnover with multiple methodologies at multiple skeletal sites. Adv Exp Med Biol 2001;496:95–97
27. Gabriel SE, Tosteson AN, Leibson CL, et al. Direct medical costs attributable to osteoporotic fractures. Osteoporos Int 2002;13(4):323–330
28. Ensrud KE, Barrett-Connor EL, Schwartz A, et al. Randomized trial of effect of alendronate continuation versus discontinuation in women with low BMD: results from the Fracture Intervention Trial long-term extension. J Bone Miner Res 2004;19(8):1259–1269
29. McClung MR, Geusens P, Miller PD, et al. Effect of risedronate on the risk of hip fracture in elderly women. N Engl J Med 2001;344(5):333–340

20 Compression Fractures: Vertebroplasty

David F. Kallmes

The care of patients suffering from painful, osteoporotic vertebral fractures has been revolutionized by the development of percutaneous vertebroplasty. Prior to the era of vertebroplasty, these patients usually were managed using a combination of analgesics, bedrest, and bracing. The attendant morbidity of these measures was essentially unavoidable because surgical intervention was rarely, if ever, undertaken. Watchful waiting and suffering was the typical scenario for patients with painful, osteoporotic vertebral fractures.

Percutaneous vertebroplasty comprises the injection of medical polymers or cements, usually polymethylmethacrylate (PMMA), into a fractured vertebra. Initially used in spinal tumors in France in the 1980s,[1] the technique was applied to osteoporotic fractures by Dion and Jensen at the University of Virginia in 1993. In a small series of patients published in 1997, these latter authors noted improvement in pain in 90% of patients, with little procedure-related morbidity.[2] The procedure has disseminated rapidly throughout the United States in the past decade for several reasons. First, at the time this procedure became commonly offered, there were no satisfactory alternative therapies. Second, the procedure is fairly easy to perform. Third, the apparent efficacy as reported in numerous reports is outstanding. Last, Medicare currently reimburses for the procedure in most areas of the country. Upwards of 80,000 vertebroplasty procedures are performed annually, and most likely the numbers of procedures will only increase in the future.

■ Patient Selection

Vertebroplasty is typically offered to patients suffering from painful, spontaneous, vertebral compression fractures, usually resulting from systemic osteoporosis. In the majority of such patients, pain will relent within 6 to 8 weeks, so many vertebroplasty practitioners will recommend delaying the procedure until pain persists for at least 6 weeks. It remains unclear why a subset of patients fails to achieve spontaneous regression of pain from osteoporotic fractures, but this subset is the most appropriate group of patients to offer vertebroplasty and the one most likely to benefit from this procedure.

History and Physical Examination

Patients with compression fractures due to osteoporosis typically complain of midline back pain that is severe and worsens with activity. In the mid- and upper thoracic region, patients also complain of radicular-type pain with radiation around the rib cage. In the lumbar region, especially with severe fractures, there may be some component of radicular pain. However, signs or symptoms that suggest spinal cord compression are considered contraindications to vertebroplasty.[3] Most patients are maintained with oral analgesics, often narcotics, for control of the associated pain. Thus, it may be useful to instruct referring physicians to have the patients hold their analgesics on the day that they present for a vertebroplasty evaluation so that pain patterns are not masked by their pain medication.

In this group of patients, physical examination often elicits pain on palpation over the spinous process of the affected vertebra or vertebrae.[2] However, such a physical finding is not required for offering the procedure; patients without pain on palpation over the fracture may still gain relief from vertebroplasty.[4]

Imaging

In patients with a clear-cut history and with a plain radiograph showing a new vertebral compression fracture, it is reasonable to proceed directly to vertebroplasty without other imaging modalities. In practice, however, the majority of patients being considered for vertebroplasty will have other spinal imaging performed. Commonly, a magnetic resonance imaging (MRI) scan will be performed as it has been found to be useful in several scenarios. Patients with multiple fractures of varying age can pose a problem for an interventionalist who may find it difficult to identify the fracture or fractures responsible for the patient's pain. Most practitioners consider the finding of marrow edema

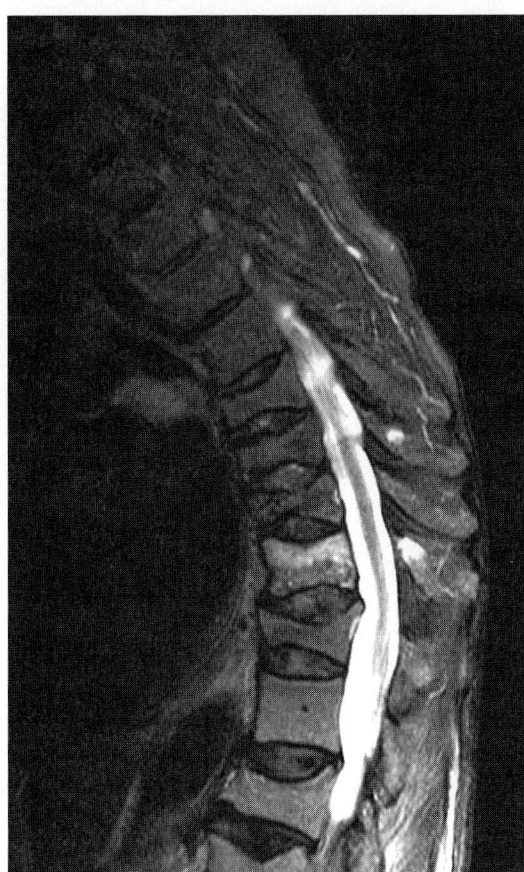

Fig. 20.1 A 79-year-old woman with severe midthoracic back pain and multiple thoracic compression fractures. Sagittal T2-weighted magnetic resonance image shows high-signal edema within the compression fracture at T10, while multiple other fractures show no edema. Patient underwent T10 vertebroplasty with good result.

on MRI as a marker for a painful vertebra, so all edematous fractures will likely be treated and nonedematous fractures would not be treated (**Fig. 20.1**). However, there remains no good study to prove the hypothesis that marrow edema indicates a pain-generating fracture; and vertebrae with normal marrow signal, without edema, have also shown good response to vertebroplasty.[5] Intraosseous cavities or clefts, historically considered as Kümmell osteonecrosis, are readily identified on MRI and can be a target for cement infusion (**Fig. 20.2**).[6] Another potential strength of MRI is that it can allay fears of an underlying neoplasm and can assess for compression of the spinal canal or nerve roots. MRI can also assess for related pain-generating lesions such as spinal stenosis and disk pathology.

Patients who cannot undergo MRI are often referred for bone scanning. At least one series of patients treated based on elevated activity on bone scan showed good relief following vertebroplasty.[7] A bone scan may be more physiologically relevant than an MRI because uptake on bone scan indicates ongoing bone turnover in a healing fracture, whereas MRI simply shows edema (**Fig. 20.3**). However, the anatomic detail offered by a bone scan is substantially inferior to MRI, and often exact identification of abnormal levels may be difficult on bone scan imaging, especially in the upper thoracic region. Other imaging modalities such as computed tomography are rarely performed as part of a workup prior to vertebroplasty, but may be useful to assess the integrity of the posterior cortex of the involved vertebral body.

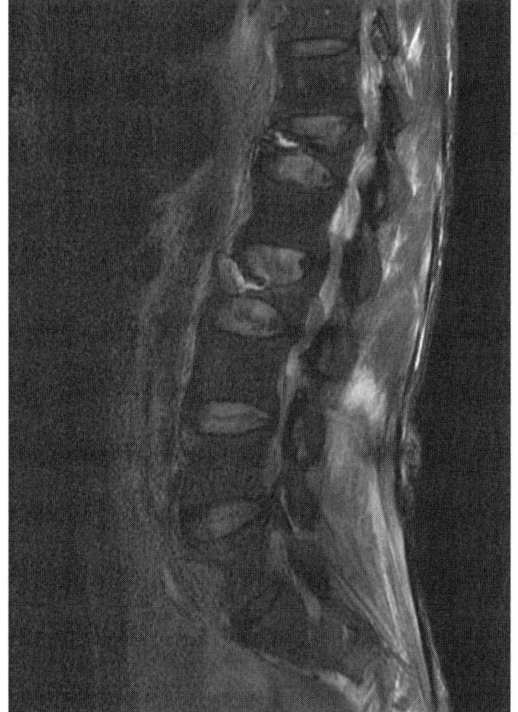

A

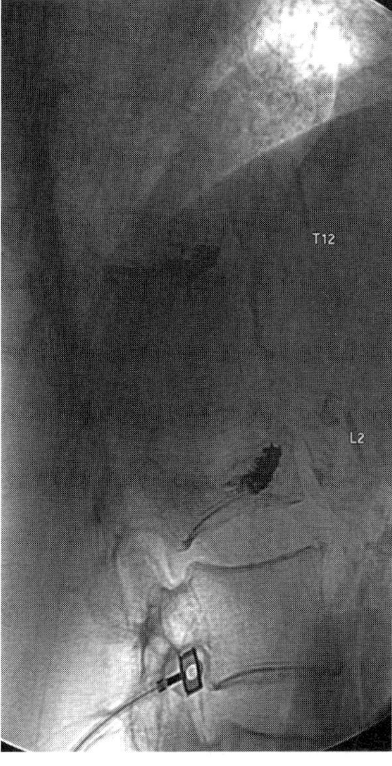

B

Fig. 20.2 A 56-year-old man with severe back pain. **(A)** Sagittal T2-weighted magnetic resonance image shows severe compression fractures at T12 and L2. At both levels there are fluid-filled cavities within the verebral bodies, indicating osteonecrosis. **(B)** Postvertebroplasty radiograph shows barium-opacified polymethylmethacrylate (PMMA) at both levels.

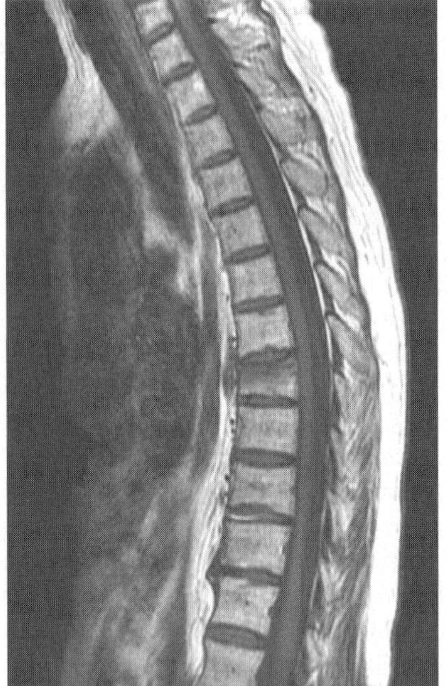

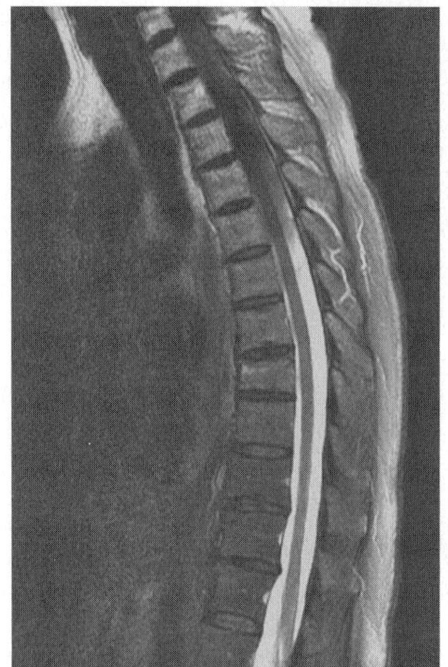

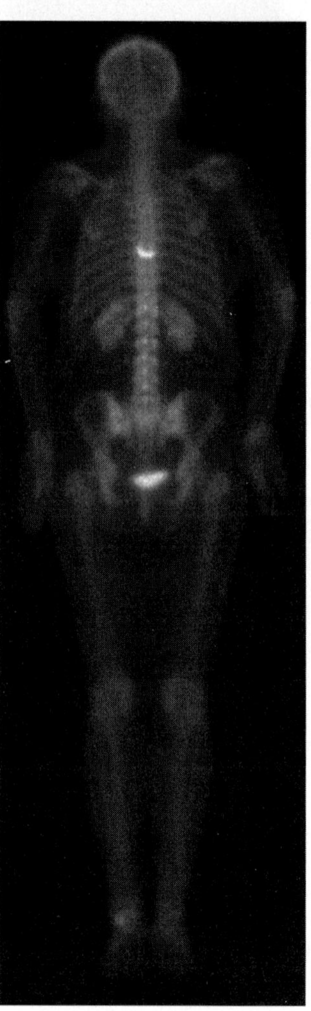

Fig. 20.3 A 70-year-old woman with severe back pain. **(A)** Sagittal T1-weighted and **(B)** T2-weighted magnetic resonance images show mild edema under the superior endplate at T9. **(C)** Anteroposterior image from radionuclide bone scan shows intense uptake at T9. Patient improved following T9 vertebroplasty.

Laboratory Evaluation

All patients presenting with spontaneous vertebral fractures and osteopenia should be evaluated for osteoporosis. Indeed, medical treatment of osteoporosis should be initiated because it can reduce the risk of a new fracture by 50% or more. Therefore, all patients should be counseled that, while vertebroplasty can potentially alleviate current pain, optimal care must include treatment of their underlying osteoporosis.

Any patient with a suspected systemic infection should be fully evaluated prior to vertebroplasty because instillation of PMMA in the setting of bacteremia could lead to seeding of the cement. Infection of PMMA in vertebroplasty, though rare, may lead to the need for vertebrectomy.[8] It is also prudent to assess for a potential coagulopathy and to hold anticoagulants and antiplatelets, except aspirin, during the periprocedural period.[9]

■ Technique

Vertebroplasty is usually performed under fluoroscopic guidance and many busy centers perform the procedure in a dedicated, biplane angiography suite with high-quality fluoroscopic imaging. Patients are placed in the prone position and are administered intravenous sedation and analgesics. Rarely, for underlying comorbidities such as pulmonary compromise, is vertebroplasty done under general anesthesia.

After sterile preparation, a biopsy needle, either 11 or 13 g, is placed into the anterior portion of the center of the target vertebral body using a transpedicular approach. The transpedicular approach allows for reliable avoidance of structures such as the thecal sac or nerve roots during transit to the vertebral body. In the thoracic region, a parapediculate approach can be used, as long as care is taken to avoid the pleura. In early series, an intraosseous venogram was performed to identify sites of potential cement leakage, but this practice has largely been abandoned.

Vertebroplasty Materials

Polymers

The vast majority of vertebroplasty procedures are currently performed with PMMA.[2] PMMA is an acrylic polymer that is supplied as a liquid monomer and powdered polymer. After mixing the liquid and solid components, a highly exothermic reaction follows that gradually results in hardening of the material. The material is usually injectable for 10 to 15 minutes and is fully hardened within one hour. The mechanism of action of PMMA in treating painful fractures remains unclear, and may be related either to stabilization of microfractures or microinstability, or related to thermal or chemical injury to pain receptors. Most practitioners favor the former theory over the latter.

Opacifiers

Safe vertebroplasty can only be performed with highly radiopaque materials because the practitioner aims to maximize intraosseous delivery while minimizing extraosseous extravasation to veins, neural foramina, the epidural space, or the disk space. Powdered barium is the most commonly used opacifying agent, typically mixed as a 30% by volume component. Other agents such as tantalum are also available. Irrespective of type, the opacifying agent must allow ready identification of extraosseous leakage, even in the lower lumbar region, which is often hampered by substantial overlying soft tissues.

Antibiotics

As noted above, intraosseous infection is a devastating, although rare, complication of vertebroplasty. Based on the orthopedics literature, early practitioners of vertebroplasty routinely added gentamicin or tobramycin to the cement mixture as a prophylactic measure against infection. Our own experience has shown that tobramycin may markedly alter the viscosity of the PMMA mixture, with diminished working time. Some practitioners use intravenous antibiotics aimed at skin contaminants in lieu of antibiotics within the cement.

Alternative Materials

The only U.S. Food and Drug Administration (FDA-) approved material for vertebroplasty remains PMMA at the time this chapter is being prepared. However, at least one investigational device exemption (IDE) trial for a non-PMMA material is currently under way and may result in more approvals in the near future.[10] The relative merits of the new materials as compared with PMMA remain unknown at this time.

Material Injection

Once the needle is in place, ideally in the central aspect of the ventral vertebral body, the barium-opacified material is slowly infused under constant lateral fluoroscopy. Infusion rates are approximately 1 cc/min or slower (**Fig. 20.4**). Extraosseous extravasation should result in immediate cessation of injection. The most common routes of leakage are into epidural or paravertebral veins, which can connect directly to the inferior vena cava.[11] Leakage into the venous system may result in cement pulmonary embolism.[12] Intermittent anteroposterior fluoroscopy may be useful to identify leakage into the veins lateral to the spinal column. Leakage of cement into the disk space is common, and small amounts of such leakage not only may be benign, but may also allow treatment of fracture lines that extend to the endplate. However, larger amounts of extravasation into the disk space may predispose to new-onset fractures.

The infusion is stopped when the cement reaches the posterior one-quarter of the vertebral body, or when extraosseous extravasation continues even after waiting several minutes for interval hardening of the cement (**Fig. 20.5**).[13] The needle can be withdrawn during infusion to help avoid ongoing extraosseous extravasation. After termination of the infusion, the needle should be slowly withdrawn under constant lateral fluoroscopy to avoid leaving a tract of hardened cement in the subcutaneous tissues.

In most cases a single injection per level is satisfactory.[14] If cross-midline flow of cement is not achieved, some practitioners will place a second needle through the contralateral pedicle to fill the remainder of the vertebral body. Imaging of the second infusion is usually compromised by the indwelling cement from the first injection, so oblique views may be needed to track cement distribution.

There is no absolute upper limit to the number of levels that can be treated in a single session. Most practitioners will routinely treat three or four levels, usually by placing all needles and then injecting each level with a single batch of PMMA. There is some concern about systemic effect of PMMA infusion because hemodynamic parameters such as oxygen tension and blood pressure have been compromised by PMMA instillation in orthopedic procedures.[15] Leakage of the liquid monomer has been implicated as a mediator of these systemic effects, but such effects are rare in vertebroplasty.

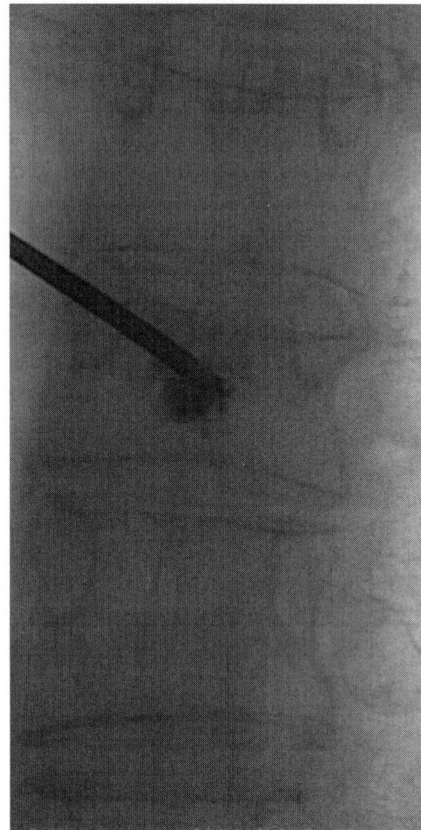

A

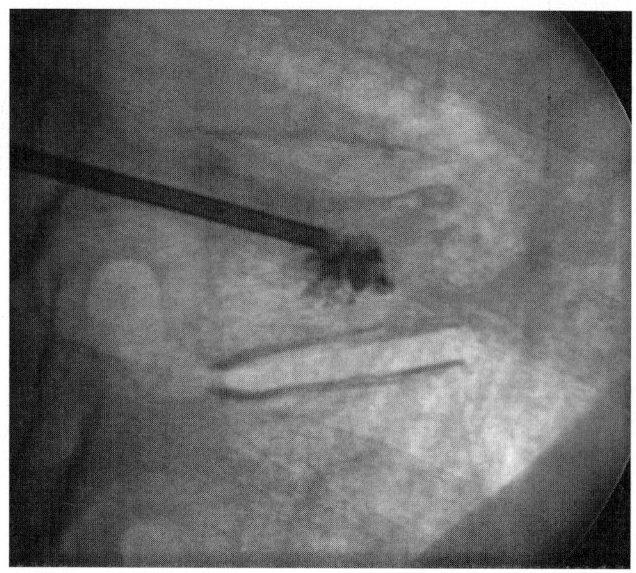

B

Fig. 20.4 A 70-year-old woman with severe back pain. **(A)** Anteroposterior and **(B)** lateral radiographs with the needle in place within the T9 pedicle, with the tip of the needle centered in the ventral aspect of the vertebral body as polymethylmethacrylate is infused.

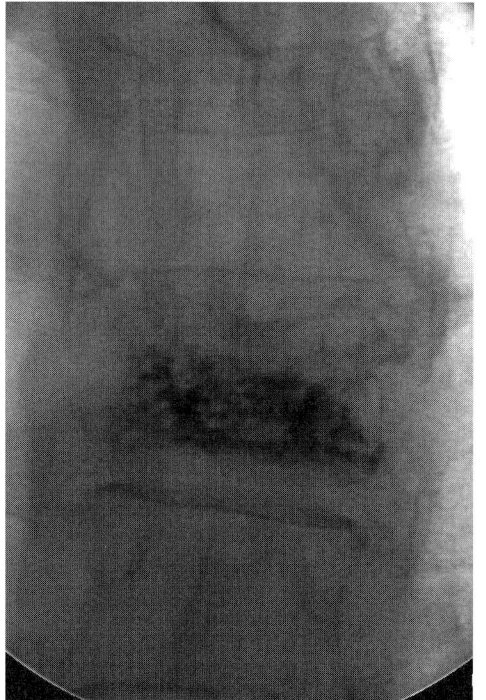

A

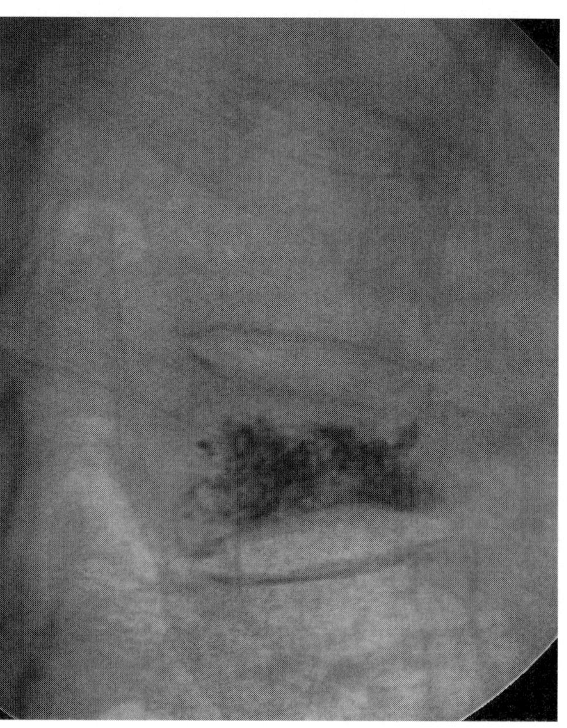

B

Fig. 20.5 A 68-year-old woman with severe back pain. **(A)** Anteroposterior and **(B)** lateral radiographs following T7 vertebroplasty shows barium-opacified polymethylmethacrylate completely within the vertebral body, without extravasation.

■ Postprocedural Care

Patients typically are left at bedrest for 1 to 2 hours, after which time they can be mobilized and discharged. Periprocedural pain is usually managed with acetaminophen or, in severe cases, with Toradol (Roche Pharmaceuticals, Nutley, NJ). No specific imaging follow-up is required.

■ Results

There are numerous case series showing excellent pain relief from vertebroplasty.[16–18] In general, pain is markedly diminished immediately after the procedure and quality of life improves.[19,20] However, even though most practitioners are convinced of the procedure's efficacy and safety, there are few controlled trials available, and none has been compared with placebo. Diamond et al[21] compared a cohort of patients undergoing early vertebroplasty for new compression fractures and compared them to a group that was offered the procedure but deferred. Although pain was better in the treatment group several days after the procedure, by 6 weeks the groups were similar in regards to pain. Do et al[22] randomized patients to either receive vertebroplasty or to undergo 6 weeks of continued medical therapy, followed by vertebroplasty if needed. This study showed marked improvement in the treatment group, but no improvement in the medical therapy arm, which then, in most cases, was offered vertebroplasty that relieved the pain.

To improve the understanding of the true efficacy of vertebroplasty, at least two randomized, controlled trials are currently underway comparing vertebroplasty to "simulated" vertebroplasty, in which no cement is actually infused. These trials will further delineate the treatment effect of PMMA in treating fractures.

■ Complications

Vertebroplasty remains safe in experienced hands. Large series have reported complication rates on the order of 3%, with serious complications on the order of 1% or less.[23] The most frequent adverse event is that of rib fractures, which occur secondary to placing severely osteopenic patients on the fluoroscopy table prior to and during the procedure.[2] Epidural or neural foraminal cement infusion may cause extremely painful radiculopathies that require surgical removal of the hardened cement.

New-Onset Fractures

One area of ongoing research in vertebroplasty is in answering the question, "Does vertebroplasty increase the risk for new fractures, as compared to patients not undergoing vertebroplasty?"[24] The stiffness profile of PMMA is different from that of normal bone, and computer modeling using finite element analysis has suggested that elevated stresses may be placed on adjacent vertebra following vertebroplasty by the indwelling cement.[25] Numerous series have been published documenting the incidence of new-onset fractures following vertebroplasty, with most series showing ~20% incidences of new fractures within 1 year of the procedure.[24,26] Of note, the majority of these new fractures involve the vertebral bodies immediately adjacent to treated levels, suggesting causation between the cement and the new fracture. However, it is also known that osteoporotic fractures even in the absence of vertebroplasty tend to cluster in the midthoracic region and in the thoracolumbar region, so the preponderance of adjacent level fractures perhaps is expected. In any event, it likely is prudent to educate vertebroplasty candidates to the potential for new-onset fractures and to stress the need, as described above, for systemic osteoporotic therapies.

■ Alternative Procedures

Balloon-assisted vertebroplasty, or kyphoplasty, is a closely related procedure initially developed in hopes of allowing reduction of kyphosis angle in vertebral fractures. Kyphoplasty comprises inflation of noncompliant balloons within the vertebral body, followed by cement infusion and is discussed in more detail within a separate chapter in this text. The procedure was originally espoused as a method to restore vertebral body height and correct kyphotic angulation, to restore vertebral biomechanics and potentially alleviate extra-spinal dysfunction such as restrictive lung and abdominal pathologies. Most case series of kyphoplasty report pain relief that is similar in degree to that seen with vertebroplasty.[27,28] The height restoration achieved with kyphoplasty is modest, on the order of 3 to 4 mm, and correction of kyphotic angulation is rare.[29] The cost of kyphoplasty is substantially higher than that of vertebroplasty. Enrollment in a large, European trial comparing kyphoplasty to medical management has recently been completed, but no data are yet available. There are at least two trials currently underway in the United States comparing kyphoplasty to vertebroplasty, but these trials are at an early stage.

■ Conclusions

Percutaneous vertebroplasty represents an important advance in the treatment of painful, osteoporotic fractures. Efficacy is reportedly high, and the procedure can be carried out safely by a wide range of practitioners. Ongoing questions remain, however, including which material is ideal, whether vertebroplasty or kyphoplasty is superior, and what role nonspecific factors such as patient expectation play in observed outcomes.

References

1. Galibert P, Deramond H, Rosat P, Le Gars D. Preliminary note on the treatment of vertebral angioma by percutaneous acrylic vertebroplasty. Neurochirurgie 1987;33(2):166–168
2. Jensen ME, Evans AJ, Mathis JM, Kallmes DF, Cloft HJ, Dion JE. Percutaneous polymethylmethacrylate vertebroplasty in the treatment of osteoporotic vertebral body compression fractures: technical aspects. AJNR Am J Neuroradiol 1997;18(10):1897–1904
3. Mathis JM, Barr JD, Belkoff SM, Barr MS, Jensen ME, Deramond H. Percutaneous vertebroplasty: a developing standard of care for vertebral compression fractures. AJNR Am J Neuroradiol 2001;22(2):373–381
4. Gaughen JR Jr, Jensen ME, Schweickert PA, Kaufmann TJ, Marx WF, Kallmes DF. Lack of preoperative spinous process tenderness does not affect clinical success of percutaneous vertebroplasty. J Vasc Interv Radiol 2002;13(11):1135–1138
5. Voormolen MH, van Rooij WJ, Sluzewski M, et al. Pain response in the first trimester after percutaneous vertebroplasty in patients with osteoporotic vertebral compression fractures with or without bone marrow edema. AJNR Am J Neuroradiol 2006;27(7):1579–1585
6. Do HM, Jensen ME, Marx WF, Kallmes DF. Percutaneous vertebroplasty in vertebral osteonecrosis (Kummell's spondylitis). Neurosurg Focus 1999;7(1):e2
7. Maynard AS, Jensen ME, Schweickert PA, Marx WF, Short JG, Kallmes DF. Value of bone scan imaging in predicting pain relief from percutaneous vertebroplasty in osteoporotic vertebral fractures. AJNR Am J Neuroradiol 2000;21(10):1807–1812
8. Vats HS, McKiernan FE. Infected vertebroplasty: case report and review of literature. Spine 2006;31(22):E859–E862
9. Layton KF, Kallmes DF, Horlocker TT. Recommendations for anticoagulated patients undergoing image-guided spinal procedures. AJNR Am J Neuroradiol 2006;27(3):468–470
10. Gheduzzi S, Webb JJ, Miles AW. Mechanical characterisation of three percutaneous vertebroplasty biomaterials. J Mater Sci Mater Med 2006;17(5):421–426
11. Hiwatashi A, Ohgiya Y, Kakimoto N, Westesson PL. Cement leakage during vertebroplasty can be predicted on preoperative MRI. AJR Am J Roentgenol 2007;188(4):1089–1093
12. Righini M, Sekoranja L, Le Gal G, Favre I, Bounameaux H, Janssens JP. Pulmonary cement embolism after vertebroplasty. Thromb Haemost 2006;95(2):388–389
13. Kallmes DF, Schweickert PA, Marx WF, Jensen ME. Vertebroplasty in the mid- and upper thoracic spine. AJNR Am J Neuroradiol 2002;23(7):1117–1120
14. Kim AK, Jensen ME, Dion JE, Schweickert PA, Kaufmann TJ, Kallmes DF. Unilateral transpedicular percutaneous vertebroplasty: initial experience. Radiology 2002;222(3):737–741
15. Kaufmann TJ, Jensen ME, Ford G, Gill LL, Marx WF, Kallmes DF. Cardiovascular effects of polymethylmethacrylate use in percutaneous vertebroplasty. AJNR Am J Neuroradiol 2002;23(4):601–604
16. Evans AJ, Jensen ME, Kip KE, et al. Vertebral compression fractures: pain reduction and improvement in functional mobility after percutaneous polymethylmethacrylate vertebroplasty retrospective report of 245 cases. Radiology 2003;226(2):366–372
17. McGraw JK, Lippert JA, Minkus KD, Rami PM, Davis TM, Budzik RF. Prospective evaluation of pain relief in 100 patients undergoing percutaneous vertebroplasty: results and follow-up. J Vasc Interv Radiol 2002;13(9 Pt 1):883–886
18. Zoarski GH, Snow P, Olan WJ, et al. Percutaneous vertebroplasty for osteoporotic compression fractures: quantitative prospective evaluation of long-term outcomes. J Vasc Interv Radiol 2002;13(2 Pt 1): 139–148
19. McKiernan F, Faciszewski T, Jensen R. Quality of life following vertebroplasty. J Bone Joint Surg Am 2004;86-A(12):2600–2606
20. Trout AT, Kallmes DF, Gray LA, et al. Evaluation of vertebroplasty with a validated outcome measure: the Roland-Morris Disability Questionnaire. AJNR Am J Neuroradiol 2005;26(10):2652–2657
21. Diamond TH, Champion B, Clark WA. Management of acute osteoporotic vertebral fractures: a nonrandomized trial comparing percutaneous vertebroplasty with conservative therapy. Am J Med 2003;114(4): 257–265
22. Do HM, Kim BS, Marcellus ML, Curtis L, Marks MP. Prospective analysis of clinical outcomes after percutaneous vertebroplasty for painful osteoporotic vertebral body fractures. AJNR Am J Neuroradiol 2005;26(7):1623–1628
23. Nussbaum DA, Gailloud P, Murphy K. A review of complications associated with vertebroplasty and kyphoplasty as reported to the Food and Drug Administration medical device related web site. J Vasc Interv Radiol 2004;15(11):1185–1192
24. Trout AT, Kallmes DF. Does vertebroplasty cause incident vertebral fractures? A review of available data. AJNR Am J Neuroradiol 2006;27(7):1397–1403
25. Baroud G, Nemes J, Heini P, Steffen T. Load shift of the intervertebral disc after a vertebroplasty: a finite-element study. Eur Spine J 2003;12(4):421–426 Epub 2003 Apr 1
26. Syed MI, Patel NA, Jan S, Harron MS, Morar K, Shaikh A. New symptomatic vertebral compression fractures within a year following vertebroplasty in osteoporotic women. AJNR Am J Neuroradiol 2005;26(6):1601–1604
27. Gill JB, Kuper M, Chin PC, Zhang Y, Schutt R Jr. Comparing pain reduction following kyphoplasty and vertebroplasty for osteoporotic vertebral compression fractures. Pain Physician 2007;10(4):583–590
28. Taylor RS, Taylor RJ, Fritzell P. Balloon kyphoplasty and vertebroplasty for vertebral compression fractures: a comparative systematic review of efficacy and safety. Spine 2006;31(23):2747–2755
29. Lieberman IH, Dudeney S, Reinhardt MK, Bell G. Initial outcome and efficacy of "kyphoplasty" in the treatment of painful osteoporotic vertebral compression fractures. Spine 2001;26(14):1631–1638

21 Vertebral Compression Fractures: Kyphoplasty

Wayne J. Olan and Joey Marie Robinson

Kyphoplasty is an established treatment for painful osteoporotic and pathologic compression fractures of the spine. First developed in the mid-1990s shortly after the development of vertebroplasty, and initially adopted by spine surgeons, kyphoplasty is now practiced increasingly by interventional radiologists. This procedure, like vertebroplasty, involves the percutaneous injection of bone cement into a fractured vertebral body. However, kyphoplasty also aims to reduce the fracture and restore endplate alignment and vertebral body height through the use of an inflatable bone tamp (balloon). The tamp is used to compress the cancellous bone to create a cavity and possibly realign the endplate of the vertebral body once the cavity is created. Polymethylmethacrylate (PMMA) is then injected into the cavity to stabilize the fracture. Safety, efficacy and positive results for pain relief have been reported widely in the literature throughout this decade.[1–8]

■ Background

Vertebral compression fractures (VCF) caused by osteoporosis, tumors, malignancies, and other pathologies have a devastating impact on quality of life for patients. There is general consensus among physicians treating VCF patients that a significant reduction in quality of life and "downward spiral" of general health is associated with vertebral compression fractures. The pain associated with these fractures leads to loss of mobility and independence. For patients with osteoporosis, restricted movement further exacerbates the underlying disease, as less demand is placed on the skeletal structure and bone regeneration further decreases. Subsequent fractures of the spine as well as hip and other fractures are common among patients with untreated vertebral compression fractures.[9]

Most patients with a symptomatic VCF are treated with medical therapy, which includes bed rest, analgesics, and rehabilitation. Medical therapy is only partially effective at addressing symptoms with many patients having persistent pain and some degree of functional limitation.[10] One of the potential results of a fracture in the thoracic and lumbar spine is kyphosis, which changes the patient's center of gravity and puts the patient at greater risk of a fall. Kyphosis also limits the function of vital organs; restricted pulmonary function[11–14] and compromised digestion due to kyphosis have long been documented anecdotally and are currently being studied. Clinically significant correction of the local deformity has been demonstrated throughout the literature in retrospective studies; however, at present, the clinical benefit of vertebral body fracture reduction on overall sagittal alignment is speculative.[15] Clearly, further clinical studies regarding these issues would be of value to referring and treating physicians, as well as patients.

■ Patient Selection

Patient selection begins with a thorough history and physical examination; patients presenting with palpable, focal back pain should be referred for imaging. Plain film x-rays are often adequate to identify vertebral compression fractures. Further imaging studies, particularly magnetic resonance imaging (MRI), computed tomography (CT), and bone scan may be required to help the treating physician determine whether fracture reduction will be possible, which depends largely on the acuity of the fracture and density of the bone. Fractures treated within 4 to 6 weeks of the event have been shown to have greater restoration of vertebral body height and fracture reduction.[16]

The majority of acute osteoporotic and pathologic fractures from T7 to L5 can be treated safely. However, relative contraindications for kyphoplasty include vertebra plana or compression severe enough to prohibit insertion of the instruments. Exclusion criteria include asymptomatic VCFs; presence of osteomyelitis or systemic infection; retropulsed bone fragments; or epidural extension of tumor at the fractured level. Treatment of VCFs with retropulsed fragments or tumors intruding into the epidural space may result in cord compression during inflation of the balloon bone tamp. However, kyphoplasty is often considered a safer option than vertebroplasty for patients with degenerative VCFs of pathologic origin such as multiple myeloma. The cavity created by the balloon bone tamp may provide a more secure reservoir for the bone cement and may reduce risk of cement leakage in these specific cases (**Fig. 21.1**).

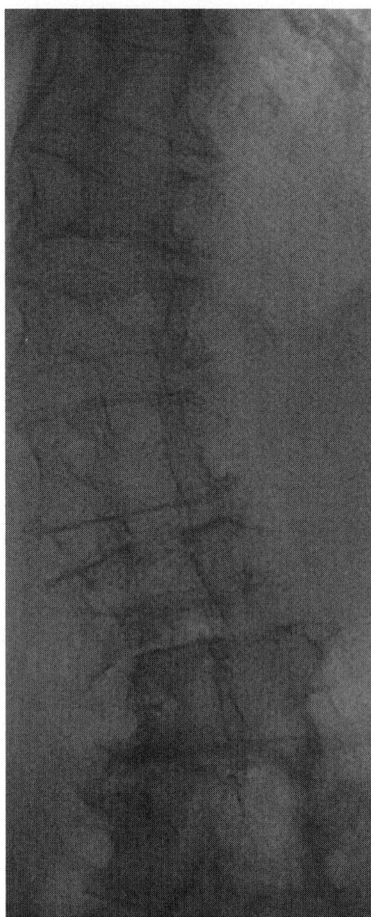

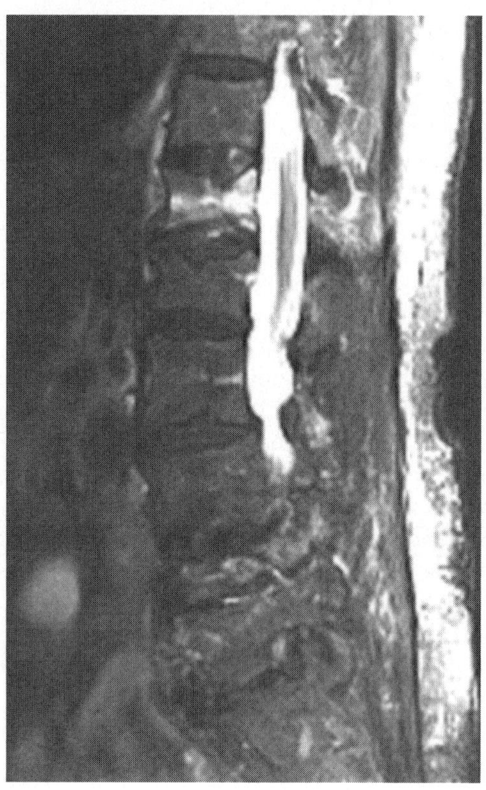

A B

Fig. 21.1 Imaging of T12 vertebral compression fracture (VCF) in a 90-year-old female patient. VCFs can often be identified in plain film x-rays or under fluoroscopy **(A)**; magnetic resonance imaging **(B)** can better determine the acuity of the fracture and potential for fracture reduction and kyphosis correction through kyphoplasty. (Images courtesy of Orlando Ortiz, MD, MBA, FACR.)

■ Technique

High-resolution biplane or C-arm fluoroscopy is essential to safe performance of percutaneous vertebral augmentation. Placement of instruments and injection of cement must be visualized in multiple planes throughout the procedure. Percutaneous vertebral augmentation requires informed consent of the patient prior to the procedure. Kyphoplasty is increasingly performed with the patient under conscious sedation, typically with an intravenous combination of Fentanyl (Janssen Pharmaceutica, Beerse, Belgium) and Versed (Hoffman LaRoche, Nutley, NJ), rather than general anesthesia. This, however, is at the discretion of the operator and is typically addressed with the patient in advance of the procedure. Use of general anesthesia may include several factors, including the patient's general health, comorbidities, and the ability of the patient to tolerate the prone position and remain still throughout the procedure. Many operators order the administration of conscious sedation prior to the patient being situated prone on the table. Kyphoplasty is performed under strict aseptic conditions; the operator and assisting staff follow sterile operating procedure. Because of the use of imaging equipment, care is also taken to protect the physician, staff, and patient through radiologic barriers including lead aprons, thyroid shields, and mobile barriers. Increasing use of lead barriers to absorb scatter radiation as well as pulsed fluoroscopy have demonstrated significant decrease in radiation exposure to the operator, staff, and patients.[17]

With the patient positioned prone on the table with the spine at the isocenter of the C-arm, the fracture is identified fluoroscopically. Local anesthesia is then administered thoroughly to the points of entry in the skin, subcutaneous tissues, and periosteum of the area being treated. A small incision is made in the skin where 11 g or 9 g diamond tip needles are inserted and guided fluoroscopically to the vertebra. Access to the vertebral body is typically transpedicular, although parapedicular and posterolateral approaches are also possible and may be preferable in patients with narrow or absent pedicles. Initially, kyphoplasty was a bilateral procedure; however, operators increasingly evaluate each fracture to determine the optimal fracture reduction and cement distribution. In some cases, unilateral needle placement and balloon tamp inflation provides optimal endplate alignment and equivalent pain relief.[18]

Minor variants of the kyphoplasty procedure may be employed; Kyphon (Sunnyvale, CA) offers a variety of components in kyphoplasty kits, as well as custom kits, to accommodate operator preference and the specific requirements of each case. In general, after the needles are placed, the stylus from one is removed, an inflatable bone tamp is introduced through the cannula and inflated in the vertebral body, and then the opposite side is treated in the identical fashion. The first balloon tamp is then removed, and a mixture of viscous, barium-enhanced PMMA cement is delivered into the resulting cavity in small increments under frequent fluoroscopic observation. The second tamp is removed and cement is delivered into the second cavity. Some operators may elect to alter the order of cavity filling, or may use only one bone tamp if the topography of the fracture and endplate realignment can best be achieved with a single-cavity fill. After the initial fill of the cavity, most operators partially withdraw the cannula and deliver additional cement; this practice ensures a more complete fill of the cavity, reducing the risk of refracture of the vertebral body (**Fig. 21.2** and **Fig. 21.3**). The cannulas are removed, gentle pressure is applied to the skin for 2 to 5 minutes, and the area is simply bandaged. PMMA sets quickly at human body temperature; the exact rate depends on the manufacturer (**Fig. 21.4**). The patient is kept still in prone position until

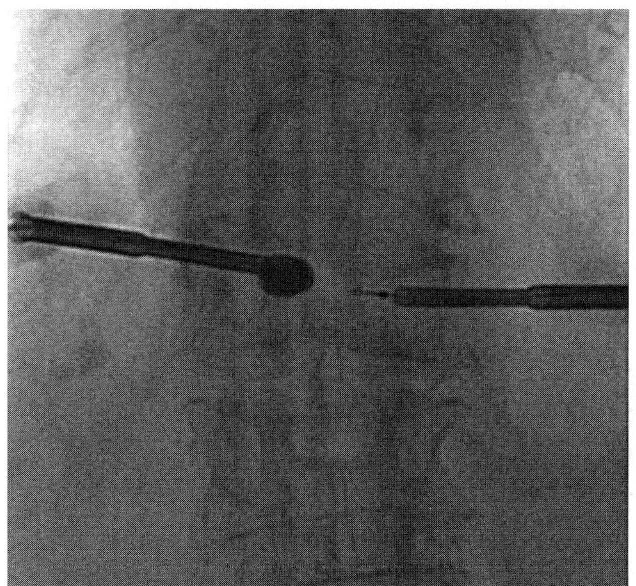
A

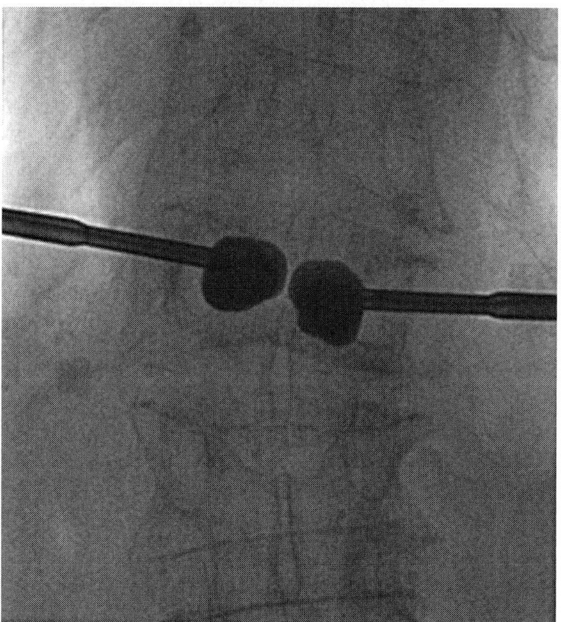
B

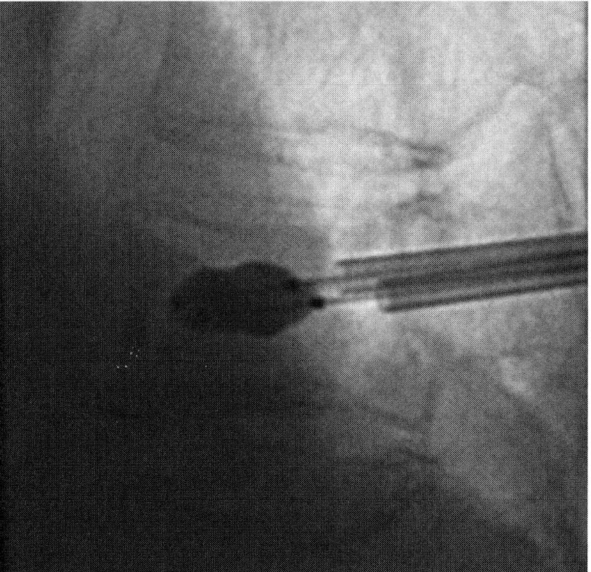
C

Fig. 21.2 **(A)** Bilateral placement and **(B,C)** inflation of balloon bone tamps prior to inflation. Note deformity of the vertebral body prior to fracture reduction **(Fig. 21.1)**. **(B)** Inflated bone tamps may elevate the endplates and provide partial correction for the deformity. (Images courtesy of Orlando Ortiz, MD, MBA, FACR.)

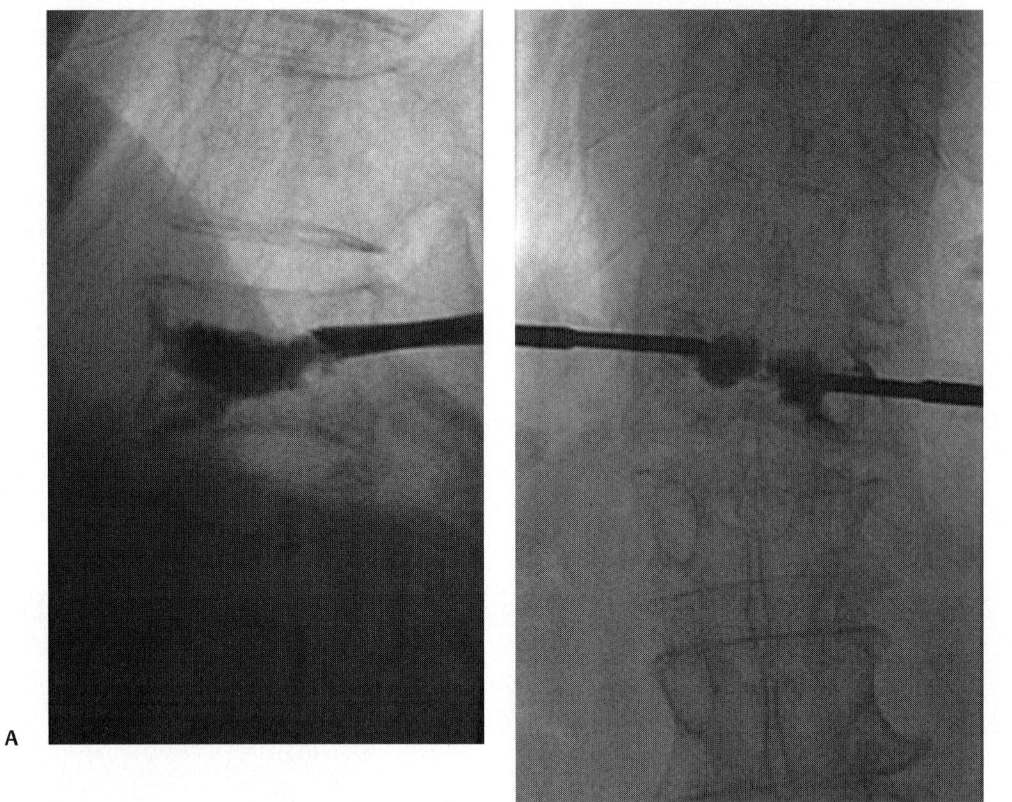

Fig. 21.3 (A) Lateral and **(B)** anteroposterior views: cement delivery into the cavities created by the bone tamps stabilizes the fracture. (Images courtesy of Orlando Ortiz, MD, MBA, FACR.)

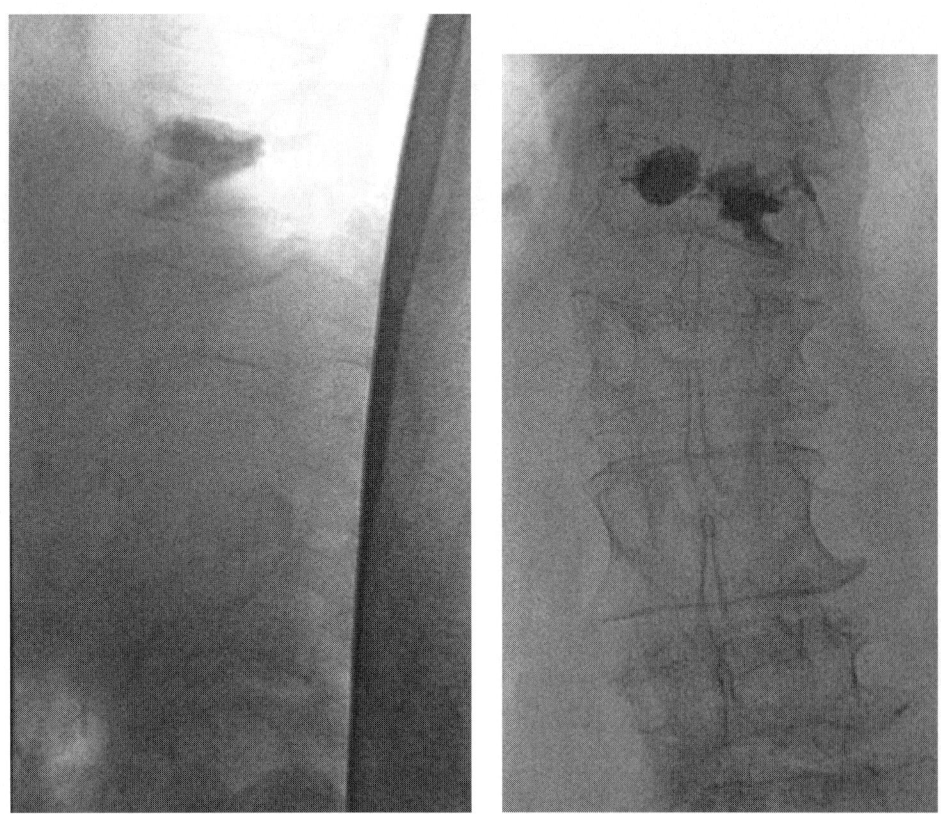

Fig. 21.4 Plain films of the spine demonstrating how cement fills both cavities after the procedure. The stabilized vertebral body has retained the minor fracture reduction achieved by the balloon bone tamps. (Images courtesy of Orlando Ortiz, MD, MBA, FACR.)

the remaining cement on the prep table is fully set. The entire procedure typically lasts ~30 minutes for each level being treated, although operators with extensive experience have been able to reduce the procedure time substantially. The patient is kept in a recovery room under observation for 1 to 4 hours before being released to continue recovery at home, where general activity should be limited for a few days, and resumed gradually thereafter.

Kyphoplasty is a technically challenging procedure, with potentially catastrophic outcomes if it is not performed correctly. Therefore, it should be practiced only after thorough training, which preferably includes the successful completion of a hands-on, cadaver-based kyphoplasty course taught by highly experienced instructors. Practice and operator training standards established for vertebroplasty should be considered of equal importance for the practice of kyphoplasty given that the key points of safety and efficacy are equivalent between the two procedures.[19]

■ Results

The effectiveness of kyphoplasty for treating pain is well-documented in the literature.[2,3,5,7,20,21] Reports of excellent or complete pain relief in 70 to 94% of patients, with significant complication rates below 3% have been described in multiple studies. In one recent meta-analysis involving 168 studies of vertebroplasty and kyphoplasty, the mean improvement in Visual Analog Scale (VAS) scores following kyphoplasty was 4.6, with a 7.0% rate of cement leakage.[20] Another recent meta-analysis involving 21 studies of vertebroplasty and kyphoplasty noted an improvement of more than 5 points (~50%) on the VAS scale following kyphoplasty in 263 patients.[6] Compared with medical therapy, kyphoplasty significantly improves pain, functionality, and health-related quality of life.[22] In addition, kyphoplasty improves vertebral height and the kyphotic angle of the spine.

There is a significantly higher incidence of cement leakage seen in association with vertebroplasty than kyphoplasty.[22] This may be due to the creation of the cavity and the use of more viscous cement in kyphoplasty.[23] It is worth noting that the cement leakages associated with kyphoplasty are rarely clinically significant, not problematic to the patient, and evident only under radiographic examination. This differs from the leaks seen after vertebroplasty, in which 3% are symptomatic, the results of which can include pulmonary embolism, nerve root pain, or radiculopathy.[22] In addition, the incidence of new vertebral fractures, both total and adjacent, is slightly higher after kyphoplasty than vertebroplasty.

Clinical studies regarding the long-term clinical impact of fracture reduction and endplate realignment are still required to provide definitive data regarding this critical aspect of kyphoplasty. Complication rates associated with vertebral augmentation remain low, although case studies of catastrophic or serious complications such as permanent neurologic deficit continue to be reported in the literature.[24] Patient selection, physician training, and quality of equipment continue to be the critical factors of the safety of vertebral augmentation.

■ Postprocedure Care and Management

Following kyphoplasty for osteoporotic fracture(s), the patient should be referred for treatment of the underlying disease. The natural course of untreated osteoporosis, as outlined in a previous chapter, will inevitably lead to subsequent fractures. The literature reviewing clinical evidence debates the use of oral medications to control osteoporosis, which include bisphosphonates [under brand names Fosamax (Merck & Company Inc., Whitehouse Station, NJ), Boniva (Roche Laboratories Inc., Nutley, NJ), Actonel (Proctor & Gamble Pharmaceuticals, Cincinnati, OH), Miacalcin (Novartis Pharmaceuticals, East Hanover, NJ)], hormone replacement therapies [estrogens with or without progestins, and parathyroid hormone under brand name Forteo (Eli Lilly & Co., Indianapolis, IN)], and selective estrogen receptor modulators [SERMs; raloxifene under brand name Evista (Eli Lilly & Co., Indianapolis, IN)].[25–28] In many cases, occupational therapy is appropriate to help patients learn how to perform tasks of everyday living more safely and reduce the risk of further fractures.[29,30]

■ Conclusions

Kyphoplasty is a safe and effective treatment for painful osteoporotic and pathologic vertebral compression fractures, and provides potential restoration of vertebral endplate alignment that may restore sagittal alignment and biomechanical integrity of the spine. The ability to provide permanent pain relief and restore the patient's independence and quality of life depends on well-trained physicians skilled in imaging-guided interventions using high-quality equipment. Further studies, particularly randomized clinical trials, are required to establish the long-term clinical benefits of fracture reduction and kyphosis correction.

Acknowledgments

The authors of this chapter wish to thank Orlando Ortiz, MD, MBA, FACR, for his generous contribution of images.

References

1. Theodorou DJ, Wong WH, Duncan TD, Garfin SR, Theodorou SJ, Stoll T. Percutaneous balloon kyphoplasty: a novel technique for reducing pain and spinal deformity associated with osteoporotic vertebral compression fractures (abstr). Radiology 2000;217:511
2. Lieberman IH, Dudeney S, Reinhardt M-K, et al. Initial outcome and efficacy of kyphoplasty in the treatment of painful osteoporotic vertebral compression fractures. Spine 2001;26(14):1631–1638
3. Lieberman IH, Dudeney S, Reinhardt MK, Bell G. New technologies in spine: kyphoplasty and vertebroplasty for the treatment of painful osteoporotic compression fractures. Spine 2001;26(14):1631–1638
4. Phillips FM, Ho E, Campbell-Hupp M, McNally T, Todd Wetzel F, Gupta P. Early radiographic and clinical results of balloon kyphoplasty for the treatment of osteoporotic vertebral compression fractures. Spine 2003;28(19):2260–2265 discussion 2265–7
5. De Negri P, Tirri T, Paternoster G, Modano P. Treatment of painful osteoporotic or traumatic vertebral compression fractures by percutaneous vertebral augmentation procedures: a nonrandomized comparison between vertebroplasty and kyphoplasty. Clin J Pain 2007;23(5):425–430
6. Gill JB, Kuper M, Chin PC, Zhang Y, Schutt R Jr. Comparing pain reduction following kyphoplasty and vertebroplasty for osteoporotic vertebral compression fractures. Pain Physician 2007;10(4):583–590
7. Pateder DB, Khanna AJ, Lieberman IH. Vertebroplasty and kyphoplasty for the management of osteoporotic vertebral compression fractures. Orthop Clin North Am 2007;38(3):409–418
8. Taylor RS, Fritzell P, Taylor RJ. Balloon kyphoplasty in the management of vertebral compression fractures: an updated systematic review and meta-analysis. Eur Spine J 2007;16(8):1085–1100
9. U.S. Department of Health and Human Services, Office of the Surgeon General. Bone Health and Osteoporosis, A Report of the Surgeon General. Rockville, MD: U.S. Department of Health and Human Services, Office of the Surgeon General; 2004
10. Philips FM. Minimally invasive treatment of osteoporotic vertebral compression fractures. Spine 2003; 28(15, Suppl)S45–S52
11. Leech JA, Dulberg C, Kellie S, et al. Relationship of lung function to severity of osteoporosis in women. Am Rev Respir Dis 1990;141(1):68–71
12. Lyles KW, Gold DT, Shipp KM, et al. Association of osteoporotic vertebral compression fractures with impaired functional status. Am J Med 1993;94(6):595–601
13. Schlaich C, Minne HW, Bruckner T, et al. Reduced pulmonary function in patients with spinal osteoporotic fractures. Osteoporos Int 1998;8(3):261–267
14. Kado DM, Prenovost K, Crandall C. Narrative review: hyperkyphosis in older persons. Ann Intern Med 2007;147(5):330–338
15. Pradhan BB, Bae HW, Kropf MA, Patel VV, Delamarter RB. Kyphoplasty reduction of osteoporotic vertebral compression fractures: correction of local kyphosis versus overall sagittal alignment. Spine 2006;31(4):435–441
16. Crandall D, Slaughter D, Hankins PJ, Moore C, Jerman J. Acute versus chronic vertebral compression fractures treated with kyphoplasty: early results. Spine J 2004;4(4):418–424
17. Ortiz AO, Natarajan V, Gregorius DR, Pollack S. Significantly reduced radiation exposure to operators during kyphoplasty and vertebroplasty procedures: methods and techniques. AJNR Am J Neuroradiol 2006;27(5):989–994
18. Ortiz AO, Zoarski GH, Beckerman M. Kyphoplasty. In: Semba CP, Katzen BT, eds. Techniques in Vascular and Interventional Radiology. Philadelphia, PA: WB Saunders; 2002:239–249
19. Barr J, Mathis J, Barr M, et al. Percutaneous Vertebroplasty Standards of Practice. In: ACR Standards. Reston, VA: American College of Radiology; 2000
20. Eck JC, Nachtigall D, Humphreys SC, Hodges SD. Comparison of vertebroplasty and balloon kyphoplasty for treatment of vertebral compression fractures: a meta-analysis of the literature. Spine J 2007; 8(3):488–497 Epub 2007 May 29
21. Lewis G. Percutaneous vertebroplasty and kyphoplasty for the standalone augmentation of osteoporosis-induced vertebral compression fractures: present status and future directions. J Biomed Mater Res B Appl Biomater 2007;81(2):371–386
22. Taylor RS, Taylor RJ, Fritzell P. Balloon kyphoplasty and vertebroplasty for vertebral compression fractures: a comparative systematic review of efficacy and safety. Spine 2006;31:2747–2755
23. Heini PF, Orler R. Kyphoplasty for treatment of osteoporotic vertebral fractures. Eur Spine J 2004;13:184–192
24. Patel AA, Vaccaro AR, Martyak GG, et al. Neurologic deficit following percutaneous vertebral stabilization. Spine 2007;32(16):1728–1734
25. Tang BM, Eslick GD, Nowson C, Smith C, Bensoussan A. Use of calcium or calcium in combination with vitamin D supplementation to prevent fractures and bone loss in people aged 50 years and older: a meta-analysis. Lancet 2007;370(9588):657–666
26. Strampel W, Emkey R, Civitelli R. Safety considerations with bisphosphonates for the treatment of osteoporosis. Drug Saf 2007;30(9): 755–763
27. Moro Alvarez MJ, Diaz-Curiel M. Pharmacological treatment of osteoporosis for people over 70. Aging Clin Exp Res 2007;19(3):246–254
28. Malden NJ, Pai AY. Oral bisphosphonate associated osteonecrosis of the jaws: three case reports. Br Dent J 2007;203(2):93–97
29. Daley T, Cristian A, Fitzpatrick M. The role of occupational therapy in the care of the older adult. Clin Geriatr Med 2006;22(2):281–290 viii
30. Woodland JE, Hobson SJ. An occupational therapy perspective on falls prevention among community-dwelling older adults. Can J Occup Ther 2003;70(3):174–182

22 Clinical Perspective: Spine Interventions (Orthopedic Surgery)

Burt Yaszay and Jeffrey M. Spivak

Every year in the United States, more than 700,000 vertebral compression fractures occur secondary to osteoporosis.[1] This is in addition to those that are attributed to metastatic vertebral lesions. Significant morbidity can result from both the related pain and deformity associated with these compression fractures. Studies have shown that vertebral compression fractures can lead to decreased physical function, quality of life, and even survival.[2,3]

The majority of patients that suffer a compression fracture experience acute pain at the time of initial injury. This pain may be initially severe; however, it typically resolves in most patients over the course of weeks to months. Many patients respond to mild analgesics and remain quite functional during this acute episode. However, for some patients the pain can be incapacitating in nature and can ultimately become a chronic problem. Although not completely understood, the development of chronic pain in association with a vertebral compression fracture can be multifactorial.[4] There may be progression of the fracture with further bony collapse. Incomplete healing of the fracture can lead to a pseudoarthrosis and a sense of instability or motion through the vertebrae. Finally, the kyphotic deformity that often results from a compression fracture can alter the biomechanics of the spine leading to fatigue of spinal extensor muscles and strain on other dynamic stabilizers of the axial skeleton. Severe kyphosis can also result in discomfort from impingement of the rib cage on the pelvis.

In addition to pain, the kyphotic deformity resulting from a compression fracture can have other negative clinical consequences for the patient. Kyphosis shifts the sagittal vertical axis (patient's center of gravity) anteriorly. This loss of sagittal balance and a decrease in vertebral height can cause a loss of physical height, diminished pulmonary function, compression of abdominal organs, and poor appetite.[2] This is supported by the increased mortality rate from pulmonary complications that is seen in elderly women with five or more thoracic compression fractures.[5] In addition, kyphosis displaces compressive forces anteriorly on other vertebral bodies, which can lead to additional fractures. The risk of developing a new fracture is increased following a vertebral compression fracture, especially at adjacent levels. Psychosocial effects include limitations in functional abilities and a poor perception of general health.[2]

Because the symptoms resolve in the majority of patients with a compression fracture, the mainstay of treatment is nonoperative and includes analgesics, bracing, and progressive mobilization.[6] Medical evaluation and management of the patient's osteoporosis must be undertaken if not done previously, to help minimize the risk of additional fractures. For those patients that have failed nonoperative management due to severe incapacitating pain, progressive collapse and/or wedging, or chronic pain with nonunion, more invasive procedures of vertebral cement augmentation can be very helpful to provide the desired outcome of pain relief. Some physicians caring for patients with osteoporotic vertebral compression fractures prefer to be even more aggressive, recommending cement augmentation early in the course of all fractures, to not miss those fractures which will go on to progressive collapse and wedging and become too severe for such treatment.

Since the 1990s, percutaneous vertebral augmentation has become increasingly popular for the treatment of these refractory cases.[7] Originally described for the treatment of malignant vertebral lesions, vertebroplasty refers to the percutaneous injection of a hardening substance (a "cement"), which is injected into the structurally compromised vertebral body and then hardens, providing immediate stability and augmenting the strength of the vertebral body.[8] As far back as the 1980s, it was noted that patients that had acrylic cement injected to strengthen vertebral bodies with angiomas also had an analgesic effect with improvement in their pain. As a result, the indications for vertebroplasty were expanded to include painful osteoporotic vertebral compression fractures.

Introduced clinically in 1998, kyphoplasty is similar to vertebroplasty in that it involves the percutaneous injection of acrylic cement into a mechanically compromised or fractured vertebral body.[9] However, prior to the injection, a percutaneous inflatable balloon tamp is placed within the vertebral body and inflated, achieving additional restoration of vertebral collapse and wedging and creating a central cavity with impacted bone margins. The subsequent void can then be filled with partially cured (thicker or more viscous) cement through a low pressure injection. This may diminish the risk of unwanted extravasation of cement that is seen more commonly with vertebroplasty.

The most commonly used material in vertebroplasty or kyphoplasty is polymethylmethacrylate (PMMA). Typically referred to as acrylic bone cement, it is initially a liquid when first mixed that then polymerizes and hardens through an exothermic reaction. It is felt to be bioinert and does not reabsorb over time. It is also much more rigid (lower modulus of elasticity) than the native vertebral body bone.

■ Patient Selection

Indications and Contraindications

The indications for vertebroplasty and kyphoplasty continue to evolve. In our practice, the most common clinical use for percutaneous vertebral augmentation is the treatment of painful or kyphotic vertebral compression fractures from osteoporosis or osteolytic lesions. Vertebroplasty is used primarily to relieve pain despite the fact that the mechanism for the pain relief associated with this procedure is not completely understood. One possible explanation is that the bone cement provides immediate immobilization of the fracture and augments the mechanical strength of the affected vertebrae. Another theory is that the heat from the PMMA's exothermic reaction may desensitize the fractured bone. Although the mechanism may be multifactorial, partial to complete pain relief commonly occurs within 24 to 72 hours.[10]

Vertebroplasty does not have any significant ability to improve vertebral height that is intrinsic to the procedure. It relies more on the dynamic mobility that is seen with many of these fractures.[11] Proper positioning of a patient for the procedure in an antikyphotic position may partially restore vertebral height and improve wedging, especially in relatively acute or unstable fractures. This increase can then be maintained by the solidified bone cement.

In addition to providing significant pain relief equal to that of vertebroplasty, kyphoplasty has the added capability of decreasing kyphosis and restoring vertebral body height through the use of a single or paired inflatable balloon tamp.[9] Inflation of the properly positioned balloons elevates the endplate and creates a walled-off cavity, which is then supported by the injected cement. If performed within 3 months of the fracture occurrence, kyphoplasty has been shown to diminish kyphosis by up to 50%.[12] Therefore, in light of these benefits, we consider kyphoplasty to be the preferred technique for the kyphotic compression fracture.

The original indication for percutaneous vertebral augmentation is in the management of painful metastatic vertebral lesions.[6] Again, it is unclear how augmentation procedures result in pain control for these patients. Neoplasms are not usually innervated and therefore are not directly painful. Instead, the pressure from the expanding mass or the impending fracture of the weakened bone may be the source of pain. In addition, the tumor cells may secrete local mediators that induce pain. Similar to what is observed in compression fractures, stabilization and desensitization of the bone may be responsible for the diminished pain. An additional source of relief may be from an antitumoral effect of the injected cement. Whether from heat production, toxicity of the PMMA polymers, or local ischemia, a direct cytotoxic effect has been suggested by the decreased local recurrence rate following percutaneous vertebral augmentation.[13] Interestingly, the relief of pain following vertebroplasty has not been correlated with the type of lesion or the amount of PMMA injected into the vertebral body.[14] Excluding those patients that suffer an associated compression fracture, deformity correction is not typically needed in patients with a metastatic vertebral lesion. Therefore, vertebroplasty has been the treatment of choice in the published literature. Some studies demonstrate sustained pain relief in greater than 70% of the treated cancer patients.[15,16]

Other indications for percutaneous vertebral augmentation are rare. These include Kümmell disease (avascular necrosis of the vertebral body) and painful nonmalignant lesions such as vertebral body hemangiomas. The scope of pathologies that percutaneous vertebral augmentation can treat continues to expand.

The contraindications for vertebroplasty and kyphoplasty include both local vertebral anatomy as well as systemic considerations. Ideally, there should not be local disruption of the posterior vertebral body cortex because this can lead to a leak of PMMA into the spinal canal, which can result in neurologic injury. Cortical disruption can be determined by radiographic imaging such as computed tomography (CT) or suggested by preexisting neurologic injury from either the fracture or the tumor mass. The finding of cortical disruption, however, is a relative contraindication because practitioners with significant experience may perform cement injections in these patients with caution using real-time fluoroscopy during injection. Kyphoplasty may be the safer of the two procedures for these patients due to the walled-off nature of the cavity created and the more viscous cement injected, which has less of a tendency to spread after placement. Other local contraindications include instances where the trocar cannot be safely placed into the vertebral body. These include vertebral height loss to less than one-third of normal or vertebra plana.[6] Finally, fractures that have completely healed as demonstrated by radiographic studies do not benefit from a percutaneous vertebral augmentation. No studies have demonstrated improvement in pain or local deformity in a healed fracture.

Systemic contraindications for percutaneous vertebral augmentation involve the general health of the patient. They include coagulopathy, sepsis, spinal infections, and cardiopulmonary compromise. One study suggested no deleterious cardiovascular effects of PMMA when used for vertebroplasty; however, others have found intraoperative alterations in cardiovascular function following other uses of PMMA.[17,18] This has led to the recommendation to avoid these procedures in patients with low cardiopulmonary reserve. Others recommend limiting the number of fractures treated at one setting to diminish the load of PMMA to the cardiopulmonary system.

■ Patient Evaluation

The initial assessment of the patient with a vertebral compression fracture includes a thorough history and physical examination. Information regarding the onset of symptoms and the nature of the inciting trauma should be evaluated. If the patient has a history of osteoporosis or malignancy then this will aid in the diagnosis and selection of additional forms of treatment before or after percutaneous vertebral augmentation. Otherwise, risk factors for osteoporosis or malignancy should be assessed because a compression fracture is commonly the first presentation of the underlying disease. The physical examination should evaluate the patient for changes in height as well as alterations in normal spinal curvatures. Palpation of the back may illicit tenderness over the involved spinous processes. Finally, a thorough neurologic examination should be documented.

Once a vertebral compression fracture is suspected, appropriate radiographic studies should then be performed. Plain films, including anteroposterior and lateral views centered on the painful area, will typically demonstrate a collapsed vertebral body. A standing lateral radiograph of the entire spine will allow for the assessment of any changes in sagittal alignment of the spine, and may also diagnose older compression deformities that may never have been symptomatic. Flexion and extension views of the spine may demonstrate any associated instability and can sometimes show gapping of the fracture on extension indicative of nonunion.

After the diagnosis of a compression fracture is made by plain radiographs, magnetic resonance imaging (MRI) is often ordered as the next diagnostic test. This will confirm the presence of the fracture and potentially give insight into its etiology. Bone marrow changes in the fractured vertebrae or in the remaining portions of the spine can suggest a metastatic or infiltrative process, as does the presence of a significant perivertebral soft tissue component. A fluid-filled vertebral cleft is indicative of a simple compression fracture. If a neurologic deficit is found on physical exam, the MRI is used to assess for any neurologic compression within the spinal canal and foramina. An MRI will also help determine if a fracture has healed or is still metabolically active. Indications of an active fracture on MRI include increased signal intensity on the T2-weighted images and decreased signal intensity on T1-weighted images. This is particularly important in determining if a fracture is the source of the patient's pain, especially in the setting of multiple fractures seen on plain films. For those patients where a better assessment of the vertebral cortex is needed, a CT scan is very helpful. Sclerosis along the fracture site can help determine the chronicity of the injury. Sagittal reconstructions can better define the fracture and assess the involvement of the posterior vertebral cortex.

Imaging studies can also be used to classify a thoracic or lumbar fracture according to the injury pattern of a vertebra's three columns.[19] The anterior column refers to the anterior portion of the vertebral body, disk, and anterior longitudinal ligament. The middle column includes the posterior portion of the vertebral body and disk and the posterior longitudinal ligament. The posterior column includes the pedicles and remaining posterior bony and ligamentous elements. A standard osteoporotic compression fracture is usually a failure of the anterior column alone. Any indication of middle column or posterior column injury suggests a more severe and potentially unstable fracture pattern. These higher energy injuries may require more invasive operative treatment than what is used for a "simple" compression fracture.

In those patients that are unable to have an MRI, a technetium-99 labeled bone scan is commonly obtained. Increased signal at multiple noncontiguous sites suggests a systemic process such as malignancy. Similar to an MRI, increased metabolic activity at a particular vertebra can confirm an active fracture and the possible source of the patient's symptoms.

■ Treatment

The initial acute treatment of a newly diagnosed compression fracture is generally nonoperative, except in those rare cases of incapacitating pain or severe wedging. Symptom relief while the fracture heals is achieved with progressive mobilization, analgesic medication, and bracing. For this frail patient population commonly affected by vertebral compression fractures, even these seemingly benign treatments can have significant complications. Bed rest has its associated morbidity including pressure sores, pneumonia, thromboembolic disease, and further bone loss. In the elderly, narcotic medication can cause confusion and increase the risk of falling. Bracing can be poorly tolerated and may lead to skin ulcerations. In addition, patients are often noncompliant with brace use.

During the initial treatment of the symptoms associated with a vertebral compression fracture, it is important to initiate an evaluation and treatment of the underlying disease. In cases of fracture due to osteoporosis, patients should have a dual energy x-ray absorptiometry (DXA) scan and be started on appropriate medications (if not done previously). This has been shown to help minimize the risk of additional fractures over time. If malignancy is suspected, the appropriate referrals should be made to medical oncology for further systemic evaluation. A bone marrow or vertebral biopsy may be needed for tissue diagnosis of a particular neoplasm. Ultimately, a patient's clinical outcome after nonoperative management may be more related to the underlying fracture etiology than to the fracture itself.

The patients that should be considered for percutaneous vertebral augmentation are those patients that are refractory to nonoperative management and have continued symptoms after 3 months of treatment. Depending on the previously discussed indications and morphology of the injury, either a vertebroplasty or kyphoplasty will be performed. Further imaging may be necessary to ensure selection of the appropriate treatment. A hyperextension lateral film over a bolster may demonstrate the anticipated reduction that would occur with positioning. If additional deformity correction is required, then a kyphoplasty would be the recommended procedure. A CT scan should be performed if there is any concern for a posterior vertebral body defect that would allow cement extravasation. Finally, an MRI or bone scan can identify the symptomatic fractures when a patient has multiple compression injuries. Increased signal on a bone scan has been shown to be predictive of a good clinical response to vertebroplasty.[20]

In those rare cases of neurologic compression by fracture fragments or significant spinal instability, a larger reconstructive procedure is likely going to be needed. A spinal instrumentation and fusion with or without decompression may be the only option to allow these patients to mobilize safely. Unfortunately, spine surgery in this patient population has many risks secondary to advanced age and the patient's overall health, as well as the poor bone quality in osteoporosis. For these reasons, major reconstructive spine surgery is avoided if at all possible.

■ Postprocedure Care and Management

Following a percutaneous vertebral body augmentation procedure, patients should be allowed to mobilize immediately. No specific restrictions are placed and bracing generally is not used. For many patients, their preprocedure state may be more limiting than following the injection procedure. Physical therapy can be helpful for improved function, with ambulation training, conditioning exercises, and back strengthening programs all playing important roles after treatment. A cane or walker may be needed initially if the patient was inactive prior to the procedure. Pain relief can be expected within the first 24 to 72 hours in ~80 to 90% of patients, with an anticipated reduction in analgesic use.[10]

Continued medical management of the underlying osteoporosis is also critical to the continued care of the patient. An increased rate of adjacent segment fracture is a theoretical concern following both kyphoplasty and vertebroplasty. The stiffness of the bone cement may result in increased stress causing a fracture at an adjacent osteoporotic vertebra. However, it is unclear whether this adjacent fracture is the result of the augmented vertebra or the result of the natural history of osteoporosis and osteoporotic compression fractures.[6] In either situation, strengthening bone density or at least preventing further bone loss will minimize this risk and is therefore an important component of our treatment algorithm.

■ Future Developments in Kyphoplasty and Vertebroplasty

As further experience is gained with kyphoplasty and vertebroplasty, new ideas and directions are beginning to be explored. The indications for the procedures are continuing to evolve. The use of a vertebral injection next to a fractured vertebra has been contemplated.[6] Prophylactic strengthening of an unfractured osteoporotic vertebra is another possibility. Studies will need to be conducted to determine if this will alter the natural history of the osteoporotic spine and affect clinical outcome. Unfortunately, our healthcare system may not tolerate the financial burden of treating millions of potential osteoporotic patients.

The materials used during these procedures are also being evaluated and are starting to evolve. PMMA may not be the optimal material to use with percutaneous vertebral augmentation. In the case of malignancy, a similar substance with greater antineoplastic properties may prove to be more beneficial. Kyphoplasty or vertebroplasty may become an adjuvant to chemotherapy or radiation therapy for vertebral metastasis. Some work has already explored the use of other injectable substances for the treatment of osteoporosis.[21–23] PMMA is not bioresorbable and will remain with the patient for his or her lifetime. In addition, the exothermic curing reaction may have locally deleterious effects and not be beneficial. Ideally, the injected material would provide the same initial structural support, but would then resorb and allow new bone ingrowth and replacement. Better yet, the material could be a carrier for a bioactive molecule that would counteract the causes of osteoporosis. Ultimately, well-done bench research followed by the appropriate clinical trials will guide the future of percutaneous vertebral augmentation.

■ Conclusions

For the physician who has a patient with a suspected vertebral compression fracture, the initial assessment should include a thorough history and physical followed by the appropriate radiographic evaluation. The uncomplicated patient will be managed with analgesics, orthotics, and medicines for their underlying diagnosis. More aggressive surgery is reserved for those rare cases with neurologic injury or gross instability. If the patient remains incapacitated following adequate nonoperative modalities, then a percutaneous vertebral augmentation is considered. In our practice, we seek to match the appropriate procedure with the patient's indication. Both vertebroplasty and kyphoplasty have demonstrated good clinical efficacy with respect to pain relief in patients with vertebral compression fractures. Kyphoplasty may have an improved safety profile and may be preferred in cases with more advanced kyphotic collapse. As for the future, the treating physician can also expect expanded indications and technical improvements in the procedures and the cements used.

References

1. Spivak JM, Connolly PJ. Orthopaedic Knowledge Update: Spine. 3rd ed. Rosemont, IL: American Academy of Orthopaedic Surgeons; 2006
2. Silverman SL. The clinical consequences of vertebral compression fracture. Bone 1992;13(Suppl 2):S27–S31
3. Gold DT. The clinical impact of vertebral fractures: quality of life in women with osteoporosis. Bone 1996;18:185S–189S
4. Herkowitz HN, Garfin SR, Eismont FJ, et al. Rothman-Simeone The Spine. 5th ed. Philadelphia: Saunders Elsevier; 2006
5. Kado DM, Browner WS, Palermo L, et al. Vertebral fractures and mortality in older women: a prospective study. Study of Osteoporotic Fractures Research Group. Arch Intern Med 1999;159:1215–1220
6. Spivak JM, Johnson MG. Percutaneous treatment of vertebral body pathology. J Am Acad Orthop Surg 2005;13:6–17
7. Mathis JM, Petri M, Naff N. Percutaneous vertebroplasty treatment of steroid-induced osteoporotic compression fractures. Arthritis Rheum 1998;41:171–175
8. Galibert P, Deramond H, Rosat P, et al. Preliminary note on the treatment of vertebral angioma by percutaneous acrylic vertebroplasty. Neurochirurgie 1987;33:166–168
9. Lieberman IH, Dudeney S, Reinhardt MK, et al. Initial outcome and efficacy of "kyphoplasty" in the treatment of painful osteoporotic vertebral compression fractures. Spine 2001;26:1631–1638
10. Jensen ME, Evans AJ, Mathis JM, et al. Percutaneous polymethylmethacrylate vertebroplasty in the treatment of osteoporotic vertebral body compression fractures: technical aspects. AJNR Am J Neuroradiol 1997;18:1897–1904
11. McKiernan F, Jensen R, Faciszewski T. The dynamic mobility of vertebral compression fractures. J Bone Miner Res 2003;18:24–29
12. Garfin SR, Yuan HA, Reiley MA. New technologies in spine: kyphoplasty and vertebroplasty for the treatment of painful osteoporotic compression fractures. Spine 2001;26:1511–1515
13. Deramond H, Depriester C, Galibert P, et al. Percutaneous vertebroplasty with polymethylmethacrylate. Technique, indications, and results. Radiol Clin North Am 1998;36:533–546
14. Cotten A, Dewatre F, Cortet B, et al. Percutaneous vertebroplasty for osteolytic metastases and myeloma: effects of the percentage of lesion filling and the leakage of methyl methacrylate at clinical follow-up. Radiology 1996;200:525–530
15. Weill A, Chiras J, Simon JM, et al. Spinal metastases: indications for and results of percutaneous injection of acrylic surgical cement. Radiology 1996;199:241–247
16. Fourney DR, Schomer DF, Nader R, et al. Percutaneous vertebroplasty and kyphoplasty for painful vertebral body fractures in cancer patients. J Neurosurg 2003;98:21–30
17. Kaufmann TJ, Jensen ME, Ford G, et al. Cardiovascular effects of polymethylmethacrylate use in percutaneous vertebroplasty. AJNR Am J Neuroradiol 2002;23:601–604
18. Convery FR, Gunn DR, Hughes JD, et al. The relative safety of polymethylmethacrylate. A controlled clinical study of randomly selected patients treated with Charnley and ring total hip replacements. J Bone Joint Surg Am 1975;57:57–64
19. Denis F. The three column spine and its significance in the classification of acute thoracolumbar spinal injuries. Spine 1983;8:817–831
20. Maynard AS, Jensen ME, Schweickert PA, et al. Value of bone scan imaging in predicting pain relief from percutaneous vertebroplasty in osteoporotic vertebral fractures. AJNR Am J Neuroradiol 2000;21:1807–1812
21. Bai B, Jazrawi LM, Kummer FJ, et al. The use of an injectable, biodegradable calcium phosphate bone substitute for the prophylactic augmentation of osteoporotic vertebrae and the management of vertebral compression fractures. Spine 1999;24:1521–1526
22. Belkoff SM, Mathis JM, Jasper LE, et al. An ex vivo biomechanical evaluation of a hydroxyapatite cement for use with vertebroplasty. Spine 2001;26:1542–1546
23. Belkoff SM, Mathis JM, Erbe EM, et al. Biomechanical evaluation of a new bone cement for use in vertebroplasty. Spine 2000;25:1061–1064

23 Clinical Perspective: Spine Interventions (Interventional Neuroradiology)

Gerald Wyse and Kieran Murphy

Osteoporosis is a disease of increased skeletal fragility, low bone mineral density, and micro architectural deterioration.[1] It is a common condition with a broad clinical spectrum ranging from asymptomatic patients to those presenting with a disabling hip fracture. An osteoporosis fracture can be the initial event leading to a clinical medical decline that may often end in disability or death.[2] The morbidity and mortality from an osteoporotic fracture can be equal to that associated with a spontaneous subarachnoid hemorrhage, yet we seldom regard it as a lethal disease. Although the initial orthopedic management may be excellent, the majority of patients never have their underlying bone disease adequately investigated or treated.

Medical treatment for osteoporosis, in the form of calcium supplementation, vitamin D, bisphosphates, and intravenous zoledronic acid has been shown to be effective.[3,4] Vitamin D is essential for skeletal maintenance and absorption of calcium. Recent concerns of an increased risk of breast cancer and cardiovascular disease have caused some to move away from prescribing long-term estrogen treatment for their patients.[5] Medications are a lifetime commitment and poor adherence is common.[6] Lifestyle changes such as avoidance of smoking, excessive alcohol, and participation in weight-bearing exercise are known to help address the complications associated with osteoporosis, but are difficult to maintain. This is why there is a role for minimally invasive image-guided therapy to be used as both a primary or adjunctive treatment for such a devastating disease. These procedures can improve patient outcome and quality of life with minimal procedural complications.

In the era of image-guided therapy, a complete reevaluation of the historic, outdated, mechanical approach to the biomechanics of spine and bone disease is required. An understanding of bone metabolism and the need for bone-like compliant materials that mimic the beautiful engineering of the native architecture is necessary. Taking the heart as an example, image-guided therapy has helped us move from invasive and often brutal coronary bypass surgery to a 2-day hospital stay and a 5 mm incision associated with angioplasty and stent placement. Presently, we are at the same stage of development for spine image-guided therapy that cardiology was at 20 years ago. Using a multidisciplinary approach, image-guided therapy for osteoporosis has enormous potential. Precise and accurate needle and device placement using image guidance and the importance of understanding the physics involved means that radiologists have a fundamental role to play in the treatment of osteoporosis. In the future, the development and innovation of these techniques will help the many women and men who suffer from osteoporosis.

■ Osteoporosis: A Global Problem

The number of people who suffer from osteoporosis is staggering. Think for a moment of the 400,000 patients with end-stage renal disease on dialysis in the United States[7] who suffer from metabolic bone disease but have contraindications to bisphosphates. Similarly, there are 1.5 million dialysis patients worldwide with renal osteodystrophy due to one or a combination of secondary hyperparathyroidism, adynamic bone disease, and osteomalacia. There are 350,000 people on dialysis in the United States alone with secondary hyperparathyroidism.

Patients with end-stage renal disease are not the only patients to be concerned about. In addition to the above, consider women who have had anorexia during childhood or early adult life that never achieved adequate bone density. Millions of Asian women have had osteomalacia or rickets from childhood depravation during times of civil war in Asia, Vietnam, or the Middle East. All of these people are at increased risk for skeletal fractures, especially of the vertebral bodies, hip, and wrist.[8,9] Osteoporosis is therefore a global problem.

Measurement of bone mineral density at the lumbar spine and proximal femur by dual energy absorptiometry is a reliable way to assess patients for osteoporosis.[9,10] However, a bone density measurement, in and of itself, does not tell the full story for these patients. Other risk factors for an osteoporotic fracture need to be identified such as previous fragile fractures, silent vertebral fractures, and falls secondary to balance disorders.[9,11] If we can predict these events, why do we not treat them before they happen? Why do we wait for fractures of significant morbidity and mortality to occur before we procedurally intervene? There is growing evidence for the use of image-guided therapies for the prophylactic augmentation of the hip, the radius, and vertebral bodies at risk for fracture and it is not unreasonable to expect that many practices will be moving in that direction during the coming years.

Bone is not a solid inert object as envisioned by many. It is a dynamic and flexible substance. In fact, bone is a magnificently designed honeycombed structure with weight-bearing properties that can remodel, as our body needs that to occur. It is virtually impossible to mimic. All we can do is try and reproduce its properties as closely as possible. The development of bioactive materials in combination with systemic drug therapy to stimulate bone is required to ensure a new global approach to metabolic bone disease.

Spinal Intervention

There are other areas of spinal intervention that need revisiting. A medical industry costing billions of dollars annually centers around back pain.[12] Many reviews and treatment guidelines deal with the management of back pain, but few focus on patient outcomes.[13] Disk herniation results in prolapsed disk material in the epidural or foraminal space causing nerve root compression or irritation. Although lumbar disk herniation causing radiculopathy is a common disorder, the optimal treatment is still unknown. Surgical and nonsurgical approaches are commonplace and yet, clear and accepted guidelines do not exist. Bladder and bowel dysfunction are considered classic indications for surgical treatment, but this form of presentation is rare. Ninety percent of acute attacks of sciatica caused by disk herniation settle with medical management.[14] Multiple trials have attempted to show a benefit of surgery over conservative management. Surgical discectomy provides faster relief from the acute attack, but this effect is short lived with no long-term benefit.[14–16]

Indeed, all current treatments leave the patient with an element of disability as compared with the population as a whole, which is a continuing source of frustration for those practitioners treating these patients.[16] Most current interventions for disk herniation result in the inevitable initiation of degenerative disk disease with resultant volume loss and an internal disrupted disk. Currently, most surgical interventions initiate this degenerative process. Percutaneous treatments using thermal ablation cause the same problem. A disk herniation really represents a spectrum of disease where a patient goes from having too much disk to too little. We need to develop minimally invasive techniques that preserve the natural architecture of the disk and surrounding structures rather than accelerating degenerative disk disease, which can lead to chronic lower back pain. One such technique is image-guided ozone treatment, which results in a subtle cicatrisation and shrinkage of the disk without affecting the disk and vertebral body end plate.[17] Later in life, as disks dehydrate and lose volume, we may need to develop methods of disk augmentation using materials that interact and incorporate into the native disk such as hydrogels, bioactive materials, and stem cells. A reevaluation of our approach to this disease is needed and again image-guided therapy is sure to play a fundamental role.

Dilatation of the arachnoid and dura that make up the nerve root sheath results in formation of a Tarlov cyst, which contains nerve fibers from the posterior spinal nerves. These are well-circumscribed, thin-walled cysts that are most commonly found on the S2 and S3 nerve roots. Although the majority of these lesions are asymptomatic, they can cause significant problems in women. There is something unique about the female pelvis that leads to the development of symptomatic Tarlov cysts. These cysts act like one-way valves letting cerebrospinal fluid flow in but not out. As these cysts enlarge they can cause symptoms by stretching or compressing adjacent nerve fibers. Extensive erosion of the sacrum is not uncommon and patients may complain of lower back or perineal pain, radiculopathy, paresthesia, or even bladder and bowel symptoms.[18] They are a debilitating cause of pain that is often overlooked or misdiagnosed as degenerative disk disease. Surgical treatments are complex and invasive requiring sacral laminectomies with cyst fenestration or resection. Using a minimally invasive technique, needles are placed within the cyst using computed tomography (CT) fluoroscopic guidance. The cysts are then drained and partially refilled with fibrin-based tissue adhesive. CT fluoroscopy provides a minimally invasive solution with a successful outcome in the majority of patients.

Conclusions

Spinal pathology results in debilitating symptoms from a wide range of complex disorders. The way we view, investigate, and treat these disorders needs to evolve to improve patient outcomes and alleviate symptoms. We need to rethink what we think we know about the spine. Image-guided therapy offers a huge potential in curing spinal pathology and improving quality of life in a way that is sympathetic to the form and function of the skeleton. We need to move beyond the masonry and scaffolding approach to bone therapy of the current practitioners and apply the creative innovative minds of image-guided therapy to these challenges.

References

1. Consenus Development Conference. Prophylaxis and treatment of osteoporosis. Am J Med 1991;90(90):107–110
2. Solomon DH, Finkelstein JS, Katz JN, Mogun H, Avorn J. Underuse of osteoporosis medications in elderly patients with fractures. Am J Med 2003;115(5):398–400
3. Neer RM, Arnaud CD, Zanchetta JR, et al. Effect of parathyroid hormone (1-34) on fractures and bone mineral density in postmenopausal women with osteoporosis. N Engl J Med 2001;344(19):1434–1441
4. Black DM, Delmas PD, Eastell R, et al. Once-yearly zoledronic acid for treatment of postmenopausal osteoporosis. N Engl J Med 2007;356(18):1809–1822
5. Rosen CJ. Clinical practice. Postmenopausal osteoporosis. N Engl J Med 2005;353(6):595–603
6. Cramer JA, Amonkar MM, Hebborn A, Altman R. Compliance and persistence with bisphosphonate dosing regimens among women with postmenopausal osteoporosis. Curr Med Res Opin 2005;21(9):1453–1460
7. Vonesh EF, Snyder JJ, Foley RN, Collins AJ. Mortality studies comparing peritoneal dialysis and hemodialysis: what do they tell us? Kidney Int Suppl 2006;103:S3–S11
8. Cummings SR, Nevitt MC, Browner WS, et al. Risk factors for hip fracture in white women. Study of Osteoporotic Fractures Research Group. N Engl J Med 1995;332(12):767–773
9. Raisz LG. Clinical practice. Screening for osteoporosis. N Engl J Med 2005;353(2):164–171
10. Genant HK, Cooper C, Poor G, et al. Interim report and recommendations of the World Health Organization Task-Force for Osteoporosis. Osteoporos Int 1999;10(4):259–264
11. Siris ES, Harris ST, Rosen CJ, et al. Adherence to bisphosphonate therapy and fracture rates in osteoporotic women: relationship to vertebral and nonvertebral fractures from 2 US claims databases. Mayo Clin Proc 2006;81(8):1013–1022
12. Katz JN. Lumbar disc disorders and low-back pain: socioeconomic factors and consequences. J Bone Joint Surg Am 2006;88(Suppl 2):21–24
13. Balague F, Mannion AF, Pellisé F, Cedraschi C. Clinical update: low back pain. Lancet 2007;369(9563):726–728
14. Gibson JN, Waddell G. Surgical interventions for lumbar disc prolapse: updated Cochrane Review. Spine 2007;32(16):1735–1747
15. Atlas SJ, Deyo RA, Keller RB, et al. The Maine Lumbar Spine Study, Part II. 1-year outcomes of surgical and nonsurgical management of sciatica. Spine 1996;21(15):1777–1786
16. Thomas KC, Fisher CG, Boyd M, Bishop P, Wing P, Dvorak MF. Outcome evaluation of surgical and nonsurgical management of lumbar disc protrusion causing radiculopathy. Spine 2007;32(13):1414–1422
17. Muto M, Andreula C, Leonardi M. Treatment of herniated lumbar disc by intradiscal and intraforaminal oxygen-ozone (O2-O3) injection. J Neuroradiol 2004;31(3):183–189
18. Acosta FL Jr, Quinones-Hinojosa A, Schmidt MH, Weinstein PR. Diagnosis and management of sacral Tarlov cysts. Case report and review of the literature. Neurosurg Focus 2003;15(2):E15

VI Vein Interventions

24 Clinical Review: Lower Extremity Venous Insufficiency

Chieh-Min Fan

Venous insufficiency is one of the most common medical problems affecting the adult population, and is particularly common in women who have two to three times the risk of developing varicose veins as compared with men. Varicose veins are characterized as either primary (developing de novo) or secondary (the sequelae of traumatic or postthrombotic vein damage). This chapter will review venous anatomy, epidemiology, and pathophysiology of lower extremity venous reflux, as well as the clinical evaluation of patients with varicose veins and venous insufficiency.

■ Epidemiology of Varicose Veins

Lower extremity chronic venous insufficiency (CVI) and varicose veins are among the most common diseases affecting the adult population, estimated to be the seventh most common indication for medical referral in the United States.[1] Despite numerous epidemiological studies, the overall prevalence of CVI is difficult to pinpoint given differences in study design and study populations. In a review of 21 epidemiological studies of varicose veins, Callam et al concluded that the overall prevalence of tortuous visible varicose veins in a Western population greater than 15 years of age was 10 to 15% for men and 20 to 25% for women. **Table 24.1** presents the prevalence of varicose veins by gender as seen in numerous international epidemiological studies.[2]

The development of varicose veins is a multifactorial process, likely reflecting an underlying genetic predisposition for venous insufficiency exacerbated by extrinsic factors. Risk factors that have been implicated in the genesis of primary venous insufficiency and varicose veins include positive family history, increasing parity, increasing age, female gender, obesity, and employment or lifestyle involving prolonged standing or sitting. Of these risk factors, genetic predisposition is clearly one of the most significant. In a study of 67 subject/parent sets compared with 67 control subject/parent sets, Cornu-Thenard et al observed that the presence of varicose veins in one parent was associated with a 25% risk of varicose veins in male offspring and 62% risk in females, and if both parents manifested the disease, the risk in offspring increased to 90%.[3]

Increasing age and lifestyle are both risk factors for varicose vein formation. In the Tampere study[4] in which 3284 men and 3590 women were divided into cohorts of 40, 50, and 60 year olds, the overall prevalence of varicose veins in these age groups were 22, 35, and 41% respectively. Lifestyle appears to be potentially etiologically significant in that the Edinburgh, Framingham, and Tampere studies all detected an increased prevalence of varicose veins in indi-

Table 24.1 Prevalence of Varicose Veins by Sex in Studies from Different Countries

Year	Country	Number	Prevalence of Varicose Veins	
			Male (%)	Female (%)
1966	Bohemia	15,060	6.6	14.1
1969	Egypt	467	–	5.8
1969	England	504	–	32.1
1972	India (south)	323	25.1	–
1972	India (north)	354	6.8	–
1973	Switzerland	610	–	29.0
1975	Cook Island (Pukapukans)	377	2.1	4.0
1975	Cook Island (Rarontongans)	417	15.6	14.9
1975	New Zealand (Maori)	721	33.4	43.7
1975	New Zealand (Europeans)	356	19.6	37.8
1975	Tokelau Island	786	2.9	0.8
1975	New Guinea	1,457	5.1	0.1
1977	Tanzania	1,000	6.1	5.0
1978	Switzerland	4,529	56.0	55.0
1981	France	7,425	26.2	–
1986	Brazil	1,755	37.9	50.9
1988	Sicily	1,122	19.3	46.2
1989	Germany	2,821	14.5	29.0
1990	Japan	541	–	45.0
1991	Czechoslovakia	696	–	60.5
1994	Turkey	850	34.5	38.3

Source: Adapted from Fowkes FR, Evans CJ, Lee AJ. Prevalence and risk factors of chronic venous insufficiency. Angiology 2001;52(S1): S5–S15. Adapted with permission.

viduals employed in occupations requiring prolonged periods of standing as compared with individuals employed in occupations that did not.[4–11]

Female gender and increasing parity have both been implicated as risk factors for varicose veins. In the Tampere study,[1] the risk of women developing varicose veins after 0, 1, 2, 3, or 4 or more pregnancies was 32, 38, 43, 48, and 59%, respectively. Varicose veins are hormonally sensitive to estrogen and progesterone, and increased estradiol levels have been shown to correlate with increased venous distensibility and varicose veins.[12,13] Hydrostatic effects of pelvic venous compression by the gravid uterus may compound the hormonal effects upon the veins, resulting in increased risk for lower extremity varicose vein formation. Overall lifetime exposure to these female reproductive hormones may contribute to the higher prevalence of varicose veins in women in general.

■ Lower Extremity Venous Anatomy

Nomenclature

Due to a lack of official guidelines, the nomenclature of the venous system of the lower extremity was historically inconsistent, resulting in widespread application of variable terminology and confusing abbreviations in the discussion of venous structures in the medical literature. In response to this problem, in 2002, an international interdisciplinary committee convened to standardize the venous nomenclature, resulting in publication of a consensus document that currently defines the accepted formal nomenclature of lower extremity venous anatomy. An additional update with refinements of terminology was published in 2005, and together these two documents define the currently accepted nomenclature of the lower extremity venous structures. Highlights of this consensus opinion are presented below.[14–16]

1. In the deep venous system, the term superficial femoral vein has been replaced by femoral vein to avoid mistaking the femoral vein in the thigh to be part of the superficial venous system. The profunda femoral vein has been redesignated the deep femoral vein.
2. In the superficial venous system, extensive nomenclature revisions were established. The saphenous veins have been formally labeled the great saphenous vein (GSV) and small saphenous vein (SSV), replacing numerous other terms including greater saphenous vein, long saphenous vein, short saphenous vein, and lesser saphenous vein. The anterior and posterior tributary veins have been renamed the anterior and posterior accessories of the GSV, and the Giacomini vein has been renamed the intersaphenous vein (**Fig. 24.1**).

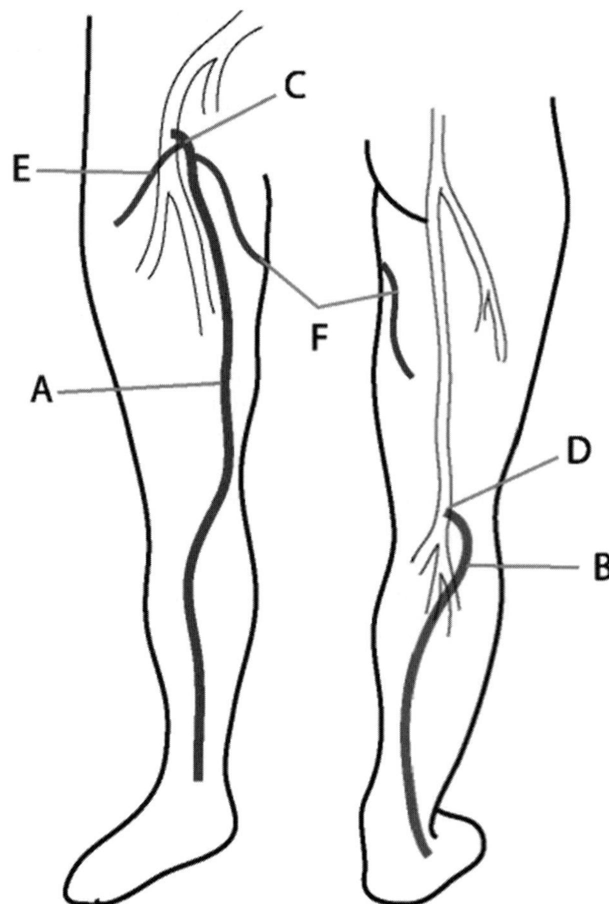

Fig. 24.1 Schematic representation of the superficial venous system of the lower extremity. **(A)** Great saphenous vein (GSV). **(B)** Small saphenous vein. **(C)** Saphenofemoral junction. **(D)** Saphenopopliteal junction. **(E)** Anterior accessory of the GSV. **(F)** Posterior accessory of the GSV.

Anatomy

The venous anatomy of the lower extremity consists of large capacitance deep venous system in the core of the leg, and a smaller capacitance superficial venous network near the surface. Technically, the superficial venous system also includes the epigastric veins and veins of the external genitalia. The two venous systems work together to carry the venous blood return from the extremity back to the central circulation. The deep and superficial systems connected at several consistent points: the saphenopopliteal junction (SPJ), the saphenofemoral junction (SFJ), and through an extensive system of horizontal bridging perforator veins. Anatomic studies estimate the presence of ~60 to 100 perforator veins in the lower extremity, which were historically grouped and named after eminent vascular surgeons, Hunter, Dodd, Boyd, and Cockett. These eponyms have been replaced by more anatomically descriptive terminology.[14–16]

The SFJ and SPJ are commonly implicated as primary sites of origin for venous reflux in the formation of varicose veins and also represent the central extension limits of endovenous saphenous thermal ablation. As such, these major deep-to-superficial connections merit additional discussion. The SFJ is bounded superiorly by the suprasaphenous valve and inferiorly by the infrasaphenous valve of the femoral veins. The SFJ also includes the GSV segment defined by the preterminal valve and terminal valves between which the tributary branches enter and drain (**Fig. 24.2**).[15] The SPJ represents the junction of the SSV to the popliteal vein, and has several common variants. The SSV may terminate directly in the popliteal vein, or commonly more superiorly at the suprapopliteal level. The SSV can also continue superiorly as the superior extension of the SSV and intersaphenous vein (formerly the Giacomini

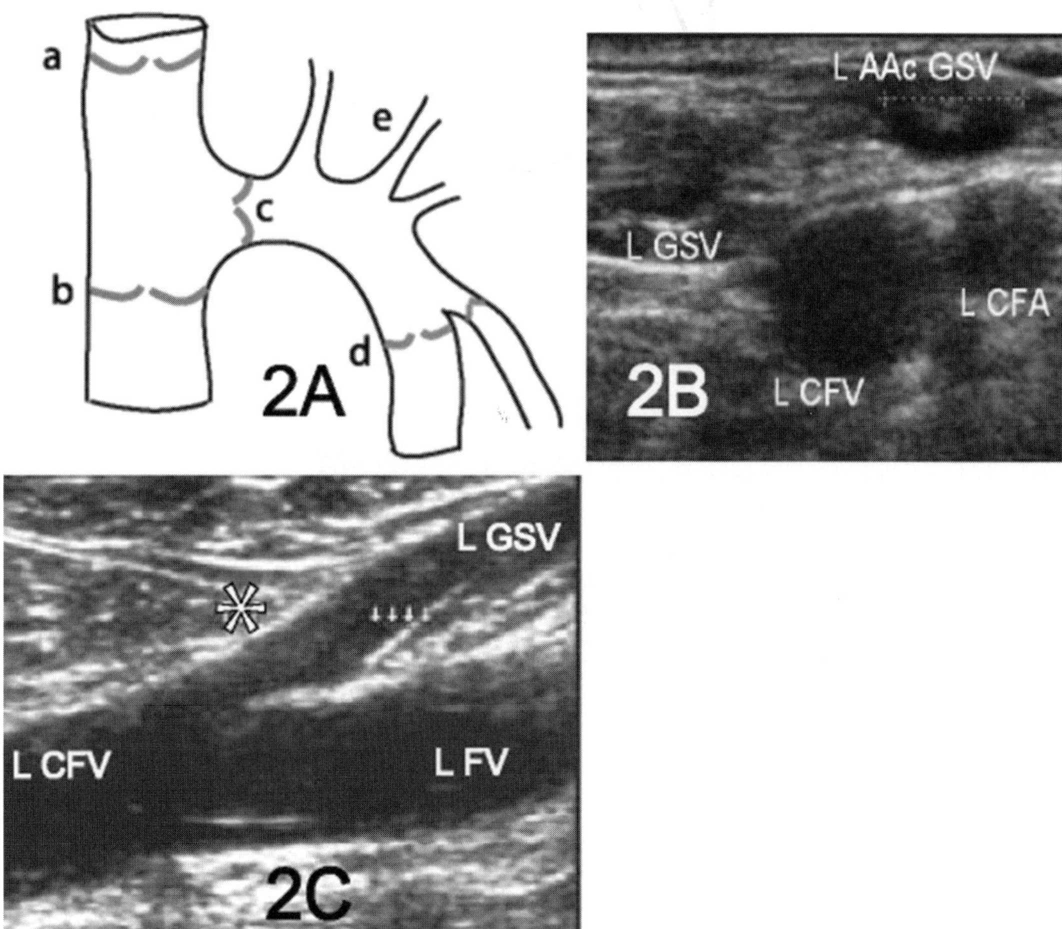

Fig. 24.2 Anatomy of the saphenofemoral junction (SFJ). **(A)** Schematic representation of the SFJ which is bounded superior by the suprasaphenous valve **(a)**, inferiorly by the infrasaphenous valve **(b)**, and within the great saphenous vein (GSV) by the preterminal valve **(d)** and terminal valve **(c)**.[15] **(B)** Axial ultrasound image of the left (L) saphenofemoral junction demonstrating the relationship of the L GSV to the L anterior accessory GSV (L AAc GSV), common femoral vein (L CFV), and common femoral artery (LCFA). **(C)** Longitudinal ultrasound image of the left SFJ (asterisk) showing the relationship of the L GSV to the femoral vein (L FV) and common femoral vein (L CFV).

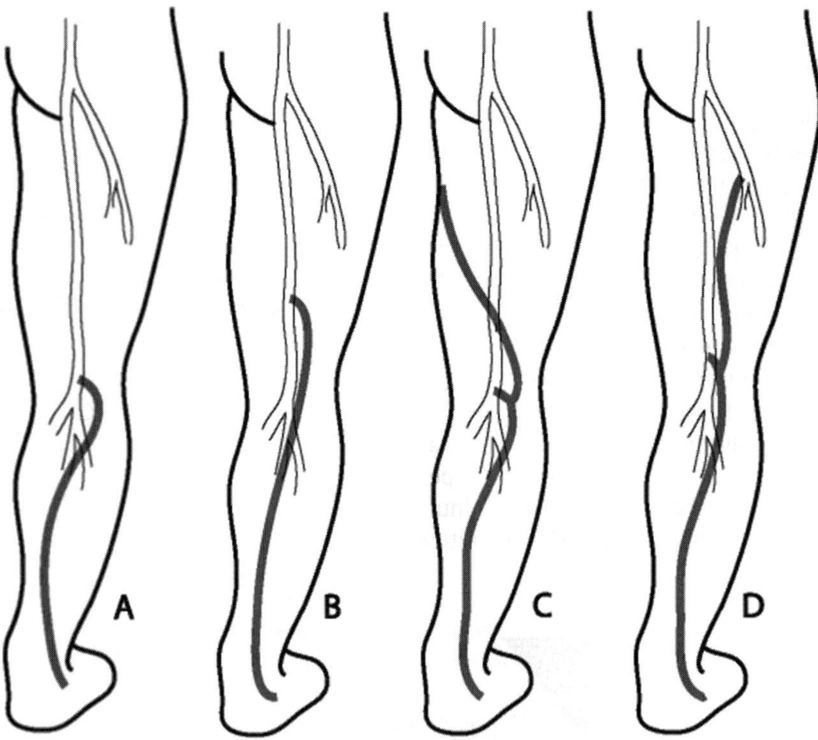

Fig. 24.3 Anatomic variants of the saphenopopliteal junction. **(A)** Most common pattern with short saphenous vein (SSV) insertion into the midpopliteal segment. **(B)** Superior extension of the SSV with high insertion into the upper popliteal/lower femoral vein. **(C)** Continuation of the superior extension of the SSV as the intersaphenous vein (formerly Giacomini vein) to anastomosis with posterior accessory of the great saphenous vein. **(D)** Uncommon variant in which the superior extension of the SSV enters into the deep femoral vein.

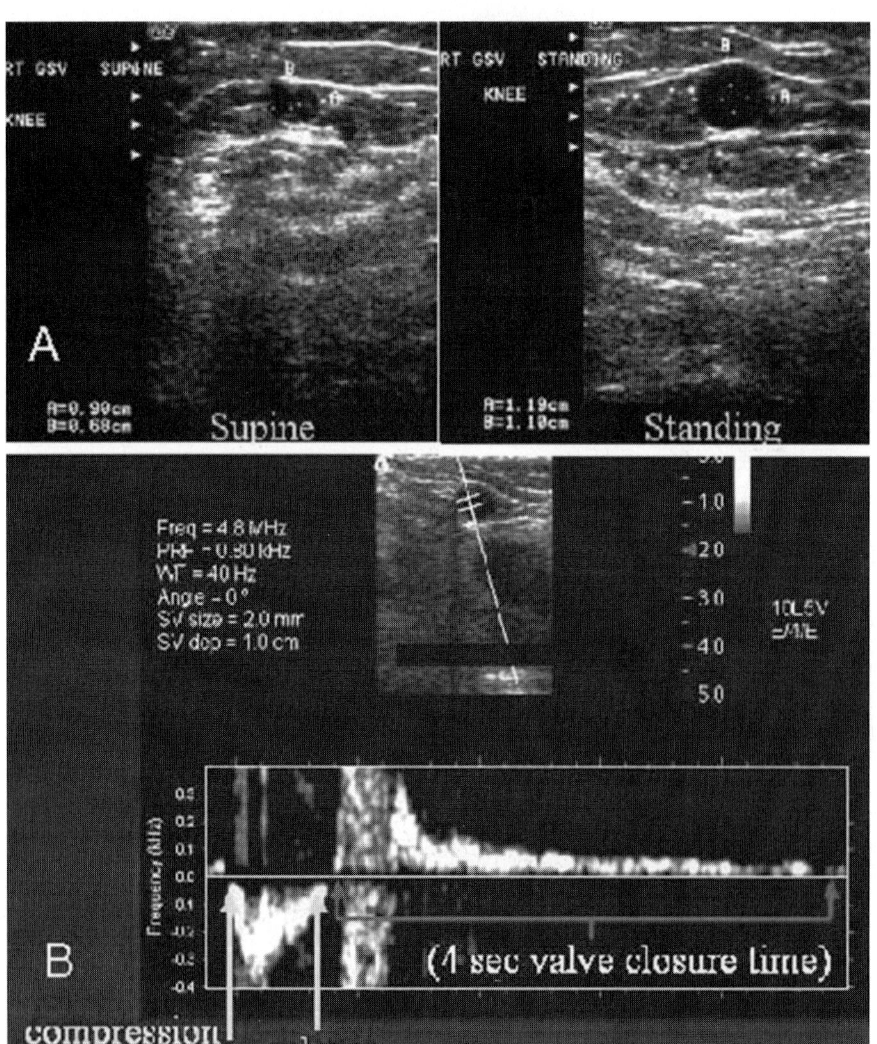

Fig. 24.4 Ultrasound evaluation of saphenous vein reflux. **(A)** Axial ultrasound images of the proximal great saphenous vein (GSV) in a patient with saphenous reflux. Note the marked dilatation of the GSV in the standing position. Also note characteristic “Egyptian eye” appearance of the GSV as it travels between the superficial and deep layers of fascia. **(B)** Spectral Doppler analysis of GSV reflux using calf compression. Compression is applied and then released (*arrows*), resulting in reversal of flow (reflux). The duration of the reflux is 4 seconds (passive valve closure time).

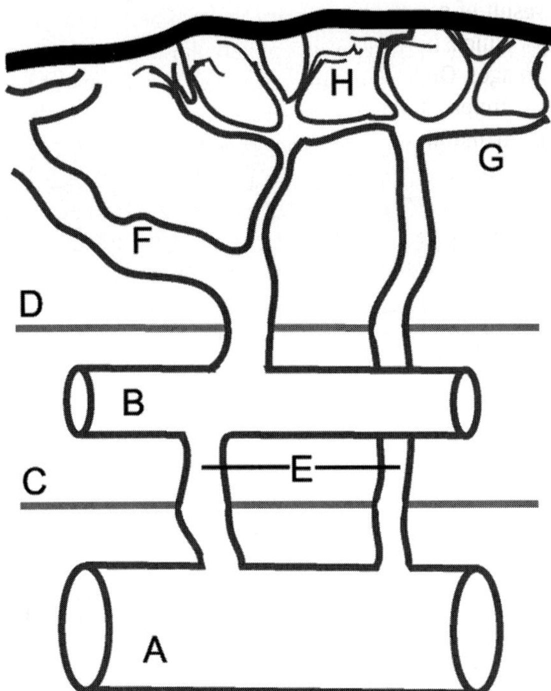

Fig. 24.5 Schematic representation of the cross-sectional distribution of venous structures from subdeep fascia to dermis. **(A)** Deep vein. **(B)** Saphenous vein running between the deep fascia **(C)** and superficial fascia **(D)**. Perforator veins **(E)** cross the fascial layers to directly connect saphenous and more superficial venous branches to the deep venous system. The saphenous vein joins tributary **(F)** and reticular branches **(G)**. Local venous incompetence in the reticular network can result in telangiectasia and venulectasia at the skin surface.

vein) which forms a direct connection to the posterior accessory of the GSV. Infrequently, the SSV may terminate directly into the deep femoral vein (**Fig. 24.3**).[17]

By definition, both the great and small saphenous veins are contained between superficial and deep fascial layers, and in cross-section have a characteristic "Egyptian eye" configuration (**Fig. 24.4**). If the saphenous vein crosses the superficial fascia into the subdermal tissues, it technically becomes a tributary vein.[18] Tributary veins are the largest nonsaphenous lower extremity branches, and share the suprafascial/subdermal space with a reticular vein network. Perforator veins connect both the saphenous veins and more superficial tributary and reticular venous branches to the deep venous system. Venous reflux in the reticular veins may give rise to venulectatic and telangiectatic patches on the skin surface. **Figure 24.5** presents a schematic diagram of the subfascial and subdermal venous structures.

■ Normal Venous Physiology

Both superficial and deep venous systems work together to carry the venous return from the leg to the central circulation. The venous load is normally distributed asymmetrically, with the deep system carrying ~90% of the volume load versus 10% in the superficial system. Flow direction in the venous system is normally unidirectional toward the heart in the superficial and deep veins, and from superficial to deep through the perforators. Normal venous flow direction is maintained through a system of one-way valves that prevent retrograde venous flow back into the leg(s), and from deep veins to the surface.

Intrinsic factors that assist in maintaining venous flow include venous contractions, arterial pressure, muscular contractions, respiratory movements, intrathoracic and intraabdominal pressure, and valve competency. Extrinsic factors include gravity, extrinsic compressive forces, and atmospheric pressure. Of the various factors that contribute to forward venous flow, the primary driving mechanism is contraction of the musculovenous pump of the calf and thigh.[19,20] During a normal contraction cycle, contraction of the muscles results in antegrade propulsion of the blood column, resulting in decreased calf venous volume and pressure. Muscular contraction around the perforators also provides a functional dynamic valve effect that helps prevent retrograde flow out the perforator. During the relaxation phase, the depressurized empty veins passively refill from below and from a superficial-to-deep flow of blood via perforator veins (**Fig. 24.6**). Neuromuscular disease,

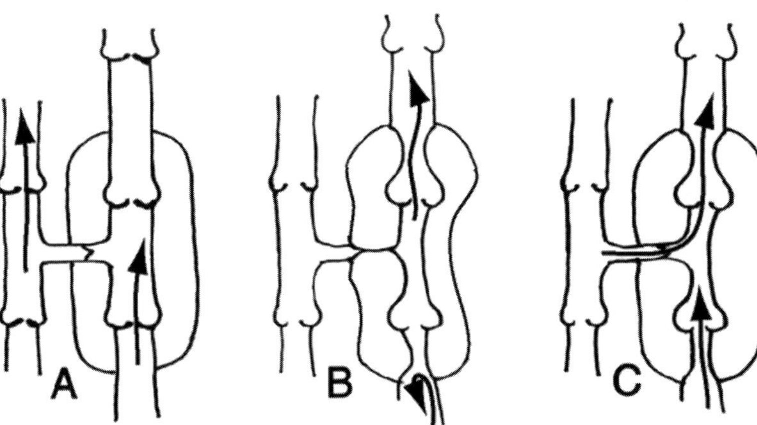

Fig. 24.6 Schematic representation of the calf musculovenous pump. **(A)** Neutral state during which there is passive unidirectional filling of the deep veins. When the deep venous volume increases and venous pressure increases, passive filling and contribution from the perforators slows and stops. **(B)** Contraction phase during which muscular contractions compress the deep veins and empty them in the antegrade direction. Intravenous pressure is high, impeding passive filling. Perforators also experience a functional compression that acts as an additional mechanism to prevent retrograde perforator reflux. **(C)** Relaxation phase during which muscles relax and the deep veins passively dilate. This decreases venous pressure and promotes passive refilling of the deep venous structures in preparation for the next pump cycle.

muscle wasting illness, or compartment disruption by fasciotomies can compromise pump function and exacerbate venous hypertension and insufficiency. Conversely, volume overload from severe venous reflux can compromise calf musculovenous pump contractility and impair calf ejection fraction, a detrimental effect that can reverse with correction of the venous insufficiency.[21]

■ Pathophysiology of Primary Venous Insufficiency

Currently two theories of primary varicose vein formation predominate. The first is the primary valvular incompetence theory, which postulates that venous reflux develops as a result of congenital paucity or weakness of the venous valves, which, in turn, results in valvular malfunction as the person ages. Once reflux develops, the vein segment below the incompetent valve is subject to hypertensive stress that results in dilatation, stretching of the valve, and propagation of the venous reflux in a central to peripheral direction.[22] This concept, first introduced by Sir William Harvey in 1628, is appealing in its simplicity, but does not explain why venous reflux frequently occurs below competent valves.

The second theory of varicose vein formation is the primary vein wall weakness theory, which proposes that the initial defect is one of vein wall composition, likely genetic in origin, which with time becomes compounded by extrinsic factors. The normal structure of the vein wall consists of a supporting collagen connective tissue matrix, elastic

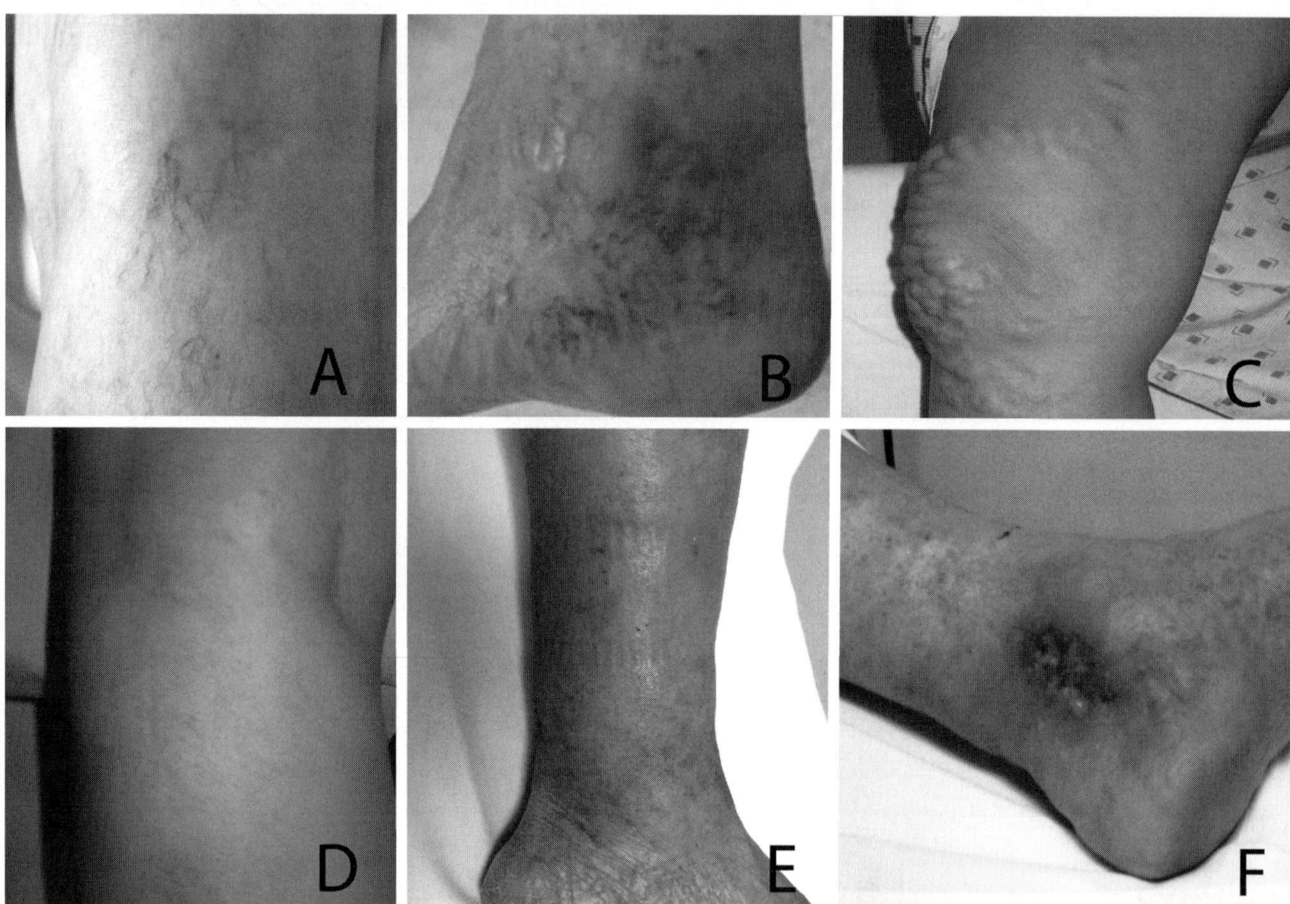

Fig. 24.7 Images representing the spectrum of skin changes seen with lower extremity venous insufficiency. **(A)** Telangiectasia (spider veins): the smallest form of varicose disease, usually manifesting as a cosmetic concern, rarely symptomatic. **(B)** Venulectasia: dilatation of veins slightly larger than spider telangiectasia. In this location at the medial malleolus, the pattern is termed corona phlebectatica, and has been implicated as an indicator of significant venous insufficiency more proximally in the leg. **(C)** Tributary varicose veins in the thigh showing the classic appearance of varicose veins originating from saphenous venous insufficiency. Treatment involves correction of the saphenous component followed by removal of the tributary varicose veins. **(D)** Reticular varicose veins: small subdermal varicose veins that may be isolated, or may be associated with saphenous vein reflux. Sclerotherapy is mainstay of treatment. **(E)**, Lipodermatosclerosis: a diffuse reactive inflammatory process to longstanding severe venous hypertension. Note the hyperpigmentation, induration, and skin retraction reflective of ongoing tissue degeneration and remodeling, often a precursor to ulceration. **(F)** Venous stasis ulcer: full thickness skin necrosis due to leukocyte infiltration with upregulation of oxygen free radical production and proteinase expression at the microcirculatory level. The resultant tissue destruction will not reverse until the venous hypertension is controlled or corrected.

fibers, and an organized vein wall muscular grid composed of smooth muscle cells arranged in longitudinal adventitial and intimal layers and a circumferentially oriented media layer. Histological studies of varicose veins reveal abnormal accumulation of collagen between the smooth muscle components, disrupting and distorting the muscular grid and compromising vein wall elasticity and strength. This results in vein dilatation, including expansion of the valve annulus causing separation of the leaflets and valvular reflux. The process affects the vein in a regional fashion interspersed between segments of normal vein, which results in the serpiginous appearance of the typical varicose vein.

Whether resulting from primary wall expansion, congenital valve weakness, or secondarily from postthrombotic valve damage, the presence of venous hypertension will incite activation of a complex cascade of inflammatory events that can ultimately lead to tissue destruction and ulceration. This process is the topic of intense ongoing debate and investigation, but it appears that high venous pressure alters vein wall stress mechanics and fluid shear stress mechanics. These hydrodynamic changes incite endothelial cell activation, red cell extravasation, and leukocyte trapping within the microcirculatory environment of the skin. Leukocyte entrapment may diminish capillary perfusion directly by luminal obstruction and promotion of thrombosis, or secondarily by associated upregulation of inflammatory processes including production of oxygen free radicals and elevated expression and activity of matrix metalloproteinases and other humoral factors. The increased inflammatory activity may lead to tissue remodeling and fibrosis seen in lipodermatosclerosis, as well as tissue degradation resulting in ulceration.[23–25]

■ Clinical Classification of Venous Insufficiency

The clinical and physical manifestations of CVI run the spectrum from asymptomatic cosmetic concerns to severe disability associated with advanced skin manifestations including frank ulceration. A spectrum of the physical manifestations of CVI is presented in **Fig. 24.7**. Several classification systems for CVI have been proposed,[26] of which the most widely used is the CEAP classification[27] that was first introduced in 1994. The CEAP classification system encompasses four dimensions: clinical, etiology, anatomy, and pathophysiology. The clinical dimension includes seven classes of clinical symptoms ranging from asymptomatic (C_0) to active ulceration (C_6). The etiology dimension defines the venous dysfunction as primary, secondary, or congenital; the anatomic classification includes deep, superficial, or perforating categories. The pathophysiological dimension classifies the venous problem as reflux, obstruction, or both (**Table 24.2**).

Table 24.2 The Four Dimensions of the CEAP Classification of Chronic Venous Disease of the Lower Extremities

A. CEAP Classification: Clinical	
Class	**Description**
0	No visible or palpable signs of venous disease
1	Telangiectasia or reticular veins
2	Varicose veins
3	Edema
4	Skin changes ascribed to venous disease: pigmentation, venous eczema, lipodermatosclerosis
5	Skin changes as defined above with healed ulceration
6	Skin changes as described above with active ulceration
B. CEAP Classification: Etiologic	
Category	**Notation and Definition**
Congenital	E_C – apparent at or recognized later
Primary	E_P – undetermined cause
Secondary	E_S – Known cause: postthrombotic, posttraumatic, other
C. CEAP Classification: Anatomic	
Segment #	**Area of Anatomic Involvement**
	Superficial veins (A_S)
1	Telangiectases or reticular veins
2	GSV: above knee
3	GSV: below knee
4	SSV
5	Nonsaphenous vein
	Deep veins (A_D)
6	Inferior vena cava
7	Common iliac vein
8	Internal iliac vein
9	External iliac vein
10	Pelvic vein: gonadal, broad ligament, other
11	Common femoral vein
12	Deep femoral vein
13	Femoral vein
14	Popliteal vein
15	Crural vein: anterior tibial, posterior tibial, peroneal
16	Muscular vein: gastrocnemius, soleus, other
	Perforating veins (A_P)
17	Thigh
18	Calf

(Continued on page 206)

Table 24.2 (*Continued*) The Four Dimensions of the CEAP Classification of Chronic Venous Disease of the Lower Extremities

D. CEAP Classification: Pathophysiologic	
Condition	**Notation**
Reflux	P_R
Obstruction	P_O
Reflux and obstruction	$P_{R,O}$

Source: From Kistner RL, Eklof B, Masuda EM. Diagnosis of chronic venous disease of the lower extremities: the "CEAP" classification. Mayo Clin Proc 1996;71:338–345. Reprinted with permission.

Although clearly useful for pretreatment stratification of patient status, the CEAP classification did not adequately quantify treatment outcomes, thus prompting the American Venous Forum to introduce a new venous classification system in 2000 (i.e., the Venous Severity Score [VSS] system).[28] The VSS has three elements: the venous clinical severity score (VCSS), the venous segmental disease score (VSDS), and the venous disability score (VDS), which are combined together to yield the VSS. The scoring criteria of the VCSS, VSDS, and VDS are presented in **Table 24.3.** Vali-

Table 24.3 Venous Severity Score (VSS) System of Venous Outcomes Assessment

A. Venous Clinical Severity Score (VCSS)				
Attribute	**Absent = 0**	**Mild = 1**	**Moderate = 2**	**Severe = 3**
Pain	None	Occasional, not restricting activity or requiring analgesics	Daily, moderate activity limitation, occasional analgesics	Daily, severe limiting activities or requiring regular use of analgesics
Varicose veins	None	Few, scattered; branch VVs	Multiple, GSV varicose veins confined to calf or thigh	Extensive: thigh and calf or GSV and SSV distribution
Venous edema	None	Evening ankle edema only	Afternoon edema, above ankle	Morning edema above ankle and requiring activity change, elevation
Skin pigmentation	None or focal, low intensity (tan)	Diffuse but limited in area and old (brown)	Diffuse over most of gaiter distribution (lower 1/3) or recent pigmentation (purple)	Wider distribution (above lower 1/3) and recent pigmentation
Inflammation	None	Mild cellulitis, limited to marginal area around ulcer	Moderate cellulites, involves most of gaiter area (lower 1/3)	Severe cellulitis (lower 1/3 and above) or significant venous eczema
Induration	None	Focal circum-malleolar (<5 cm)	Medial or lateral, less than lower third of leg	Entire lower third of leg or more
# Active ulcers	0	1	2	>2
Active ulceration, duration	None	<3 months	>3 months, <1 year	Not healed >1 year
Active ulceration, size	None	<2 cm diameter	2–6 cm diameter	>6 cm diameter
Compressive therapy	Not used or not compliant	Intermittent use of stockings	Wears elastic stockings most days	Full compliance: stockings and elevation

B. Venous Segmental Disease Score (VSDS)			
Reflux		**Obstruction**	
Score	**Segment**	**Score**	**Segment**
1/2	SSV	1	GSV (only if thrombosed from groin to below knee)
1	GSV	1	Calf veins, multiple
1/2	Perforators, thigh	2	Popliteal vein
1	Perforators, calf	1	Femoral vein
2	Calf veins, multiple (PT alone = 1)	1	Deep femoral vein
2	Popliteal vein	2	Common femoral vein
1	Femoral vein	1	Iliac vein
1	Deep femoral vein	1	IVC
1	Common femoral vein and above		
10	Maximum reflux score	10	Maximum obstruction score

Table 24.3 (*Continued*) **Venous Severity Score (VSS) System of Venous Outcomes Assessment**

C. Venous Disability Score (VDS)	
Score	**Criteria**
0	Asymptomatic
1	Symptomatic but able to carry out usual activities without compression therapy
2	Can carry out usual activities only with compression and/or limb elevation
3	Unable to carry out usual activities even with compression and/or limb elevation

Abbreviations: GSV, great saphenous vein; IVC, inferior vena cava; PT, posterior tibial; SSV, small saphenous vein; VVs, varicose veins.

dation studies of the VSS classification confirm that the VCSS and CEAP clinical scores are more sensitive gauges of clinical outcomes than the basic CEAP clinical class designation.[29,30]

■ Evaluation of Patient with Suspected Venous Insufficiency

Evaluation of suspected venous insufficiency includes a detailed medical history that includes documentation of symptom type and duration, prior treatments for venous insufficiency, past history of thromboembolic events, manifestations of peripheral vascular disease, family history of venous insufficiency, and current medications. **Table 24.4** presents an outline of the key aspects of the clinical history. The physical examination ideally should be performed with the patient standing upright to bring out major sites and patterns of varicose veins, and should include a circumferential and longitudinal assessment of the extremity with particular note taken of dermatological manifestations of venous insufficiency including edema, lipodermatosclerosis changes, hemosiderin deposition, and impending or active ulceration (**Fig. 24.7**).

Duplex ultrasound (DUS) has emerged as the imaging modality of choice for anatomic assessment of venous insufficiency. Advantages of DUS include ease of use and reproducibility of the exam, widespread availability, the ability to directly visualize and trace venous structures, and qualitative and quantitative detection of venous reflux. Standard US equipment includes a US unit capable of scanning and recording in grayscale, color, and pulse wave Doppler modes, and a 7.5 to 13.5 Hz linear array transducer. For most clinical applications, manual calf compression suffices for eliciting reflux during the exam, but automated inflation-deflation cuff systems are available if more standardized compressions are desired.

DUS evaluation of the suspected venous insufficiency is a two-part exam. The initial component is a standard supine study of the deep system with compression imaging

Table 24.4 Summary of Pertinent Aspects of the Clinical History in Assessment of a Venous Insufficiency Patient

Past Vascular History
Varicose veins and chronic venous insufficiency:
Onset, duration, affected sites
Prior vein treatments
Stripping, laser, sclerotherapy, inferior vena cava filter
Use of compression therapy
Prior thromboembolic events
Deep vein thrombosis
Superficial thrombophlebitis
Pulmonary embolism
Thrombophilias
Peripheral arterial insufficiency
Family history of varicose veins
Medications
Oral contraceptives
Anticoagulants
Antihyperglycemic drugs/insulin
Steroids
Symptoms
Cosmetic concerns
Leg fatigue, heaviness, pain
Itching, aching, restless legs
Exercise intolerance
Bleeding events
Thrombosis (superficial or deep)
Hyperpigmentation
Edema
Ulceration
Other Medical Illnesses
Malignancy
Stroke
Patent foramen ovale

to exclude congenital absence or hypoplasia of the deep veins, and to exclude deep vein thrombosis. The deep venous study is followed by an upright venous reflux exam that interrogates both the deep and superficial veins for retrograde flow. Specific goals of the study include

1. Determining anatomy, position, and competence of saphenous junctions
2. Determining the diameter and competence of superficial venous components including GSV, accessory GSVs, SSV, perforators, and deep venous system
3. Mapping all major varicosities to their source of reflux
4. Confirming status of deep system including assessment of reflux and exclusion of congenital absence, hypoplasia, or thrombotic occlusion[31]

Sonographic evidence of venous insufficiency includes dilatation of the superficial veins, and retrograde flow documented as color flow or pulse wave direction reversal. Normal venous diameter (which is generally considered to be 4 mm for the GSV, 3 mm for the SSV, and 3 mm for perforator veins in the upright position) can be dramatically increased in the presence of venous insufficiency (**Fig. 24.4A**). The duration of reversed flow on pulse wave tracing represents the passive valve closure time and provides a semiquantitative assessment of reflux severity (**Fig. 24.4B**). It should be noted that valve closure time alone does not fully define the severity of reflux in a given vein segment because mild venous reflux can result in low-amplitude retrograde flow and a protracted valve closure time, whereas severe valvular incompetence may result in high amplitude retrograde flow of shorter duration. That point notwithstanding, **Table 24.5** presents the accepted reflux duration criteria for venous insufficiency in the various components of the lower extremity venous system.[31,32]

Table 24.5 Upper Limits of Normal Duration of Retrograde Flow in Venous Segments of the Lower Extremity*

Vein Segment	Duration (seconds)
Common femoral vein	1.0
Femoral vein	1.0
Popliteal vein	1.0
Deep femoral vein	0.5
Deep veins of the calf	0.5
Great saphenous vein	0.5
Small saphenous vein	0.5
Perforator vein	0.35

*A minor amount of reflux is a normal finding with calf compression challenge of the venous system.
Source: From Labropoulos N, Tiongson J, Kang SS, Mansour A, Baker WH. The definition of venous reflux in the lower extremity veins. J Vasc Surg 2003;38(4):793–798. Reprinted with permission.

■ Conclusions

In recent years, significant advances in the minimally invasive treatment of lower extremity venous insufficiency and varicose veins have resulted in growing interest and awareness about these common medical problems by both the medical community and the public. Due to the effects of child bearing and hormonal factors, women are especially at risk for developing the primary effects and late debilitating sequelae of CVI. Understanding the basics of venous anatomy, physiology, and the clinical management of venous disease is an essential component of a comprehensive general women's health initiative.

References

1. Callam MJ. Epidemiology of varicose veins. Br J Surg 1994;81:167–173
2. Fowkes FR, Evans CJ, Lee AJ. Prevalence and risk factors of chronic venous insufficiency. Angiology 2001;52(S1):S5–S15
3. Cornu-Thenard A, Boivin P, Baud JM, de Vincenzi I, Capentier PH. Importance of the familial factor in varicose disease. J Dermatol Surg Oncol 1994;20:318–326
4. Laurikka JO, Sisto T, Tarkka MR, Auvinen O, Hakama M. Risk indicators for varicose veins in forty to sixty-year-olds in the Tampere Varicose Vein Study. World J Surg 2002;26:648–651
5. Evans CJ, Fowkes FGR, Ruckley DV, Lee AJ. Prevalence of varicose veins and chronic venous insufficiency in men and women in the general population: Edinburgh Vein Study. J Epidemiol Community Health 1999;53:149–153
6. Brand FN, Dannnenberg AL, Abbott RD, Kannel WB. The epidemiology of varicose veins: The Framingham Study. Am J Prev Med 1988;4(2):96–101
7. Sisto T, Reunanen A, Laurikka J, et al. Prevalence and risk factores of varicose veins in the lower extremities: Mini-Finland Health Survey. Eur J Surg 1995;161:405–414
8. Cesarone MR, Belcaro G, Nicolaides AN, et al. 'Real' epidemiology of varicose veins and chronic venous diseases: The San Valentino Vascular Screening Project. Angiology 2002;52(2):119–130
9. Hirai M, Naiki K, Nakayama R. Prevalence and risk factors of varicose veins in Japanese women. Angiology 1990;41:228–232
10. Fowkes FGR, Lee AJ, Evans CJ, et al. Lifestyle risk factors for lower limb venous reflux in the general population: Edinburgh Vein Study. Int J Epidemiol 2001;30:846–852
11. Hobson J. Venous insufficiency at work. Angiology 1997;48(7):577–582
12. Stansby G. Women, pregnancy, and varicose veins. Lancet 2000;355: 1117–1118
13. Ciardullo AV, Panico S, Bellati C, et al. High endogenous estradiol is associated with increased venous distensibility and clinical evidence of varicose veins in menopausal women. J Vasc Surg 2000;32:544–549
14. Caggiati A, Bergan JJ, Gloviczki P, Janter G, Wendell-Smith CP, Partsch H. International Interdisciplinary Consensus Committee on Venous Anatomical Terminology. Nomenclature of the veins of the lower limb: an international interdisciplinary consensus statement. J Vasc Surg 2002;36:416–422
15. Caggiati A, Bergan JJ, Gloviczki P, Eklof B, Allegra C, Partsch H. Nomenclature of the veins of the lower limb: extensions, refinements, and clinical application. J Vasc Surg 2005;41:719–724

16. Mozes G, Gloviczki P. New discoveries in anatomy and new terminology of leg veins: clinical implications. Vasc Endovascular Surg 2004;38:367–374
17. Tibbs DJ. Treatment of superficial vein incompetence. Varicose Veins and Related Disorders. Oxford, UK: Butterworth-Heinemann Ltd.; 1992:423–456
18. Khilnani NM, Min RJ. Duplex US for superficial venous insufficiency. Tech Vasc Interv Radiol 2003;6(3):111–115
19. Ludbrook B. The musculovenous pump of the human lower limb. Am Heart J 1966;71:635–641
20. Araki CT, Back TL, Padberg FT, et al. The significance of calf muscle pump function in venous ulceration. J Vasc Surg 1994;20(6):872–879
21. Padberg FT, Pappas PJ, Araki CT, Back TL, Hobson RW. Hemodynamic and clinical improvement after superficial vein ablation in primary combined venous insufficiency with ulceration. J Vasc Surg 1996;24(5):711–718
22. Goldman MP, Wiess RA, Bergan JJ. Varicose Veins and Telangiectasias: Diagnosis and treatment. 2nd ed. St. Louis, MO: Quality Medical Publishing; 1999:12–17
23. Schmid-Schonbein GW, Takase S, Bergan JJ. New advances in the understanding of the pathophysiology of chronic venous insufficiency. Angiology 2001;52:S27–S34
24. Coleridge Smith PD. Update on chronic venous insufficiency induced inflammatory process. Angiology 2001;52:S35–S42
25. Wollina U, Abdel-Naser MB, Mani R. A review of the microcirculation in skin in patients with chronic venous insufficiency: the problem and the evidence available for therapeutic options. Int J Low Extrem Wounds 2006;5(3):169–180
26. Antignani PL. Classification of chronic venous insufficiency: a review. Angiology 2001;52:S17–S26
27. Kistner RL, Eklof B, Masuda EM. Diagnosis of chronic venous disease of the lower extremities: the "CEAP" classification. Mayo Clin Proc 1996;71:338–345
28. Rutherford RB, Padberg FT, Comerota AJ, Kistner RL, Meissner MH, Moneta GI. Venous Severity Score: an adjunct to venous outcome assessment. J Vasc Surg 2000;31(6):1307–1312
29. Meissner MH, Natiello C, Nicholls SC. Performance characteristics of the venous clinical severity score. J Vasc Surg 2002;36:889–895
30. Kakkos SK, Rivera MA, Matsagas MI, et al. Validation of the new venous severity scoring system in varicose vein surgery. J Vasc Surg 2003;38:224–228
31. Coleridge-Smith P, Labropoulos N, Partch H, Myers K, Nicolaides A, Cavezzi A. Duplex ultrasound investigation of the veins in chronic venousdisease of the lower limbs – UIP consensus document. Part 1. Basic principles. Eur J Vasc Endovasc Surg 2006;31:83–92
32. Labropoulos N, Tiongson J, Kang SS, Mansour A, Baker WH. The definition of venous reflux in the lower extremity veins. J Vasc Surg 2003;38(4):793–798

25 Saphenous Vein Ablation

Robert J. Min

Dr. Boné first reported on delivery of endoluminal laser energy in 1999.[1] Since then, a method for treating the entire incompetent GSV segment has been described by Min and Navarro.[2,3] Endovenous laser treatment, which received U.S. Food and Drug Administration (FDA) approval in January 2002, creates nonthrombotic vein occlusion by delivering laser energy directly into the vein walls. Lasers with wavelengths of 810 nm, 940 nm, 980 nm, 1064 nm, and 1320 nm have all been used with reported success. Contact between the laser fiber and vein wall is necessary to cause sufficient damage to the vein resulting in wall thickening with eventual contraction and fibrosis. Over the past 7 years, reports of impressive clinical success and low complication rates have made endovenous laser the treatment of choice for eliminating reflux in incompetent saphenous veins.

■ Patient Selection

Medical treatment of varicose veins may be contemplated when symptoms persist despite conservative methods such as gradient compression hose and exercise. Other indications may include treatment or prevention of complications arising from chronic venous hypertension such as bleeding, superficial thrombophlebitis, and damage to the skin. Relative contraindications for endovenous laser include nonpalpable pedal pulses, inability to ambulate, acute deep venous thrombosis (DVT), general poor health, or pregnancy. An additional relative contraindication to all catheter-based endovenous ablation techniques are nontraversable vein segments either due to thrombosis or extreme tortuosity. Fortunately, this is an uncommon finding and should be recognized on pretreatment venous duplex ultrasound (DUS) mapping.

■ Technique

Prior to treatment, the abnormal venous pathways are mapped using Doppler ultrasound guidance and the veins to be treated are marked on the overlying skin with the patient standing. Additional important landmarks such as junctions, aneurysmal vein segments, and areas of significant blood inflow from tributaries or perforators should be marked on the skin.

The patient is placed horizontal on the table, allowing full access to the areas that are going to be treated. In general, patients being treated for great saphenous vein (GSV), accessory saphenous vein (ASV), or thigh circumflex vein (TCV) reflux are placed supine or in the appropriate oblique position to expose the course of the target vein. When the small saphenous vein (SSV) is to be ablated, the patient is placed prone with his or her feet hanging off the end of the table to relax the calf muscle and popliteal fossa. Treating an incompetent Vein of Giacomini or multiple sources of venous reflux may require repositioning and reprepping multiple times.

In almost all cases, the target vein is entered directly or access is gained via one of its principle tributaries. Tributary veins are more prone to venospasm and may be more difficult to access. Entry via a tributary should only be attempted if the vein is relatively straight and remains markedly enlarged in the horizontal position. The vein is usually punctured at, or just peripheral to, the lowest level of underlying reflux as determined by DUS. At this point, the vein diameter dramatically decreases just after it gives off a "refluxing escape" tributary and regains its competence. In many cases, GSV incompetence can occur segmentally. The reflux can completely spill out into a tributary vein, which then reenters the GSV at a lower level. In such a case, one should first access the lowest incompetent vein segment and treat all refluxing vein segments via one puncture, although more than one puncture is often necessary.

The target vein is entered with a 19- or 21-gauge needle using real time US guidance and single wall technique. Utilizing reverse Trendelenburg positioning and keeping the procedure room warm until access is obtained helps minimize shrinkage of the target vein. Other ancillary procedures advocated by some practitioners to maximize vein size include a heating pad or a small amount of nitroglycerin paste at the access point. Non-GSV segments are particularly prone to venospasm and particular care must be taken when accessing a tributary vein or a non-GSV such as the ASV, SSV, or TCV.

A 5F marked vascular sheath is inserted over a guide wire into the vein and passed through the entire abnormal segment and into a more central vein. A bare tipped laser fiber is inserted into the sheath. The sheath is then pulled back exposing a known length of the laser fiber tip and the fiber is fixed in place. Using US guidance, the sheath and fiber are withdrawn out of the deep veins and positioned within the superficial venous system at the junction as seen in **Fig. 25.1**. The fiber is left in this position during tumescent anesthesia administration and will be repositioned just prior to delivery of laser energy. Confirmation of the position can be made by direct visualization of the red aiming beam through the skin.

Tumescent anesthesia is a form of local anesthesia delivery, which utilizes large volumes of dilute anesthetic solutions permitting anesthesia of large areas. Proper use of tumescent anesthesia should make endovenous laser painless without the need of intravenous sedation or general anesthesia. In fact, it can be argued that sedation adds risk to endovenous laser treatment by inhibiting patient feedback during the procedure as well as delaying immediate postablation ambulation.

In addition to making endovenous laser painless, tumescent anesthesia is used to maximize efficacy and safety of treatment. Although venospasm may occur in portions of some accessed veins, proper delivery of tumescent fluid into the perivenous space is necessary to empty blood and to ensure compression of the vein around the laser fiber. Trendelenburg positioning or cooling the room to induce venospasm immediately before tumescent anesthesia will facilitate vein emptying. Contact between the vein walls and laser fiber tip will allow adequate transfer of laser energy to the target vein walls resulting in vein wall damage and subsequent fibrosis. Inadequate vein emptying with too much blood remaining within the vein will lead to nontarget heating. In the latter case if occlusion occurs, it will be the result of thrombosis with inevitable vessel recanalization.

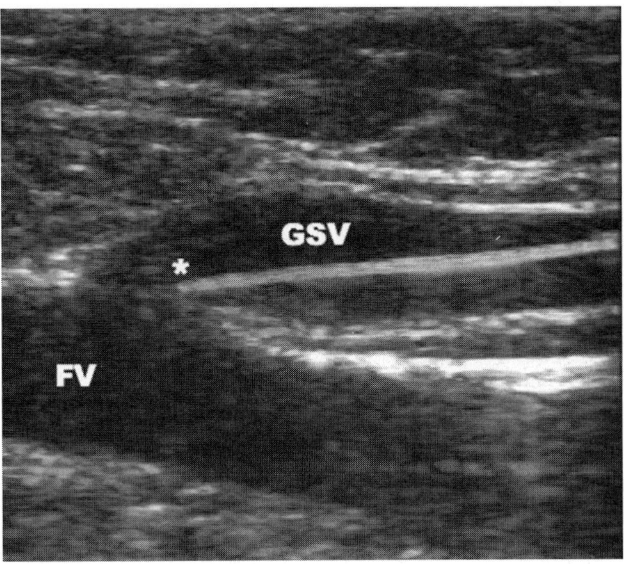

Fig. 25.1 Longitudinal ultrasound image at the saphenofemoral junction (patient's head is to the left) during laser fiber positioning. The fiber and sheath are pulled out of the femoral vein (FV) and positioned within the great saphenous vein (GSV). The fiber tip (*) will be repositioned after tumescent anesthesia delivery and prior to laser firing.

The surrounding cuff of tumescent fluid may also serve as a protective barrier and prevent heating of nontarget tissues, including skin, nerves, arteries, or the deep veins. Delivery of tumescent fluid in the proper plane can only be achieved with Doppler US guidance. This fluid is used to separate adjacent nontarget structures from the target vein. Some practitioners advocate injecting the fluid blindly or using highly pressurized devices to administer the tumescent fluid as is often done prior to liposuction. Although perhaps quicker, such systems offer less control compared with hand injection. For this reason, I prefer to deliver the tumescent anesthesia using hand pressure and a 1½ inch 25-gauge needle attached to a 20 mL syringe. For right-handed operators, the tumescent fluid is given from peripheral to central. Skin punctures are required every 3 to 5 cm until the proper perivenous tissue plane is located. Once this occurs, fluid will track more easily up and around the target vein and greater distances can be covered with each needle puncture.

To treat a 45 cm segment of vein, ~100 to 150 mL of 0.1% lidocaine neutralized with sodium bicarbonate may be required. This mixture can be made by diluting 50 mL of 1% lidocaine in 440 mL of normal saline and adding 5 to 10 mL of 8.4% sodium bicarbonate. If it is anticipated that larger volumes of tumescent anesthesia will be necessary, a concentration of 0.05% lidocaine can be used effectively. These amounts of lidocaine are well within the safe doses of 4.5 mg per kilogram of lidocaine without epinephrine and 7 mg per kilogram with epinephrine. Although many practitioners choose to use lidocaine with epinephrine to maximize venospasm and minimize bruising, we achieve adequate and complete vein emptying utilizing plain lidocaine and avoid the risk of toxicity related to epinephrine.

Following tumescent anesthesia delivery, ultrasound in the transverse plane is used to check for adequacy. A centimeter halo of fluid surrounding the target vein or separating the vein from the overlying skin is sufficient

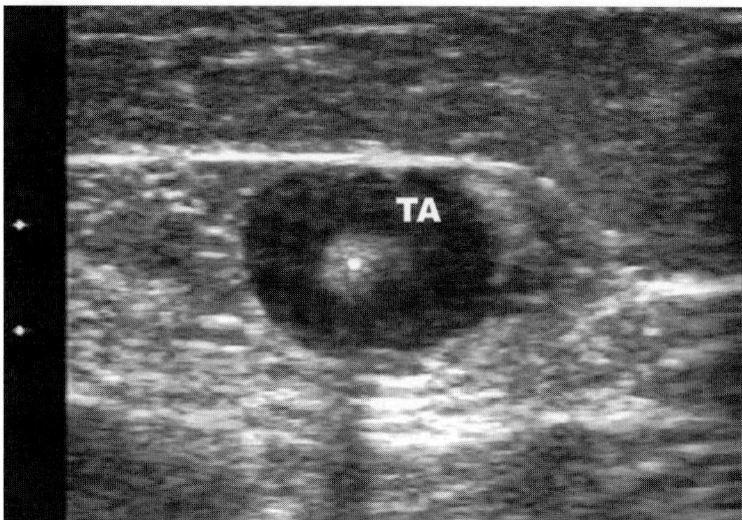

Fig. 25.2 Transverse ultrasound image of the vein walls compressed onto the laser fiber by a surrounding cuff of tumescent anesthesia (TA).

(Fig. 25.2). Proper delivery of tumescent anesthesia may be particularly important when performing endovenous laser of certain veins such as the SSV near the saphenopopliteal junction (SPJ) or the GSV below the knee due to their close proximity to nerves or arteries. Checking with color Doppler following tumescent anesthesia delivery can be useful when assessing adequacy of separation of arterial branches from the target vein.

Because the laser fiber can move during tumescent anesthesia administration, the laser fiber is repositioned prior to delivery of laser energy. For the GSV, the fiber tip is positioned 5 to 10 mm peripheral to the saphenofemoral (SFJ), usually at or just below a competent superficial epigastric vein. When treating the SSV, seeing the fiber tip can be difficult due to venospasm and the acute angle taken by the SSV as it dives to join the popliteal vein. Following delivery of tumescent anesthesia, the laser fiber tip may be more easily visualized with US **(Fig. 25.3)**. Accurate preprocedure marking of the SPJ is important, and when used with the red aiming beam will enable precise positioning of the laser fiber. Even in obese patients, this red light can be seen although dimming the room lights may be necessary. Optimally, the laser fiber tip is placed 10 to 15 mm peripheral to the SPJ where the SSV turns parallel to the skin just below the popliteal fossa.

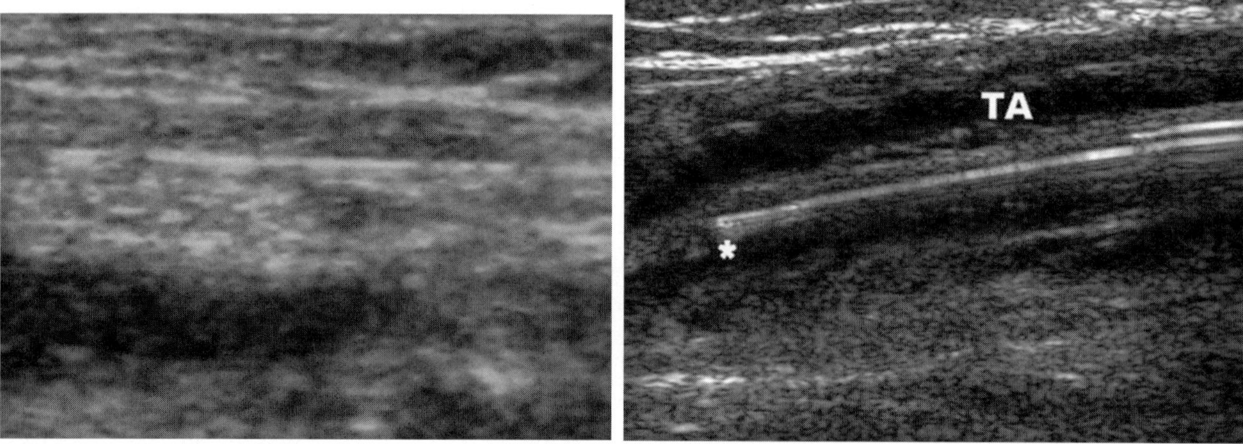

Fig. 25.3 **(A)** Longitudinal ultrasound image of the laser fiber within the small saphenous vein. Venospasm makes the fiber difficult to distinguish from the surrounding soft tissues. **(B)** Following delivery of tumescent anesthesia (TA), the laser fiber (*) is much easier to identify.

The vascular sheath and fiber are withdrawn together during laser activation (**Fig. 25.4**). In our practice, using the 810 nm diode laser (Diomed Holdings Inc, Andover, MA) laser energy is delivered using 14 W in "continuous mode." The amount of energy necessary to effect reliable vein ablation seems to be an average of 70 J per centimeter throughout the treated segment.[4] The average pullback rate to accomplish this is 2 mm per second. Although automatic catheter pullback devices are available, these are an unnecessary expense. Most manufacturers of endovenous laser ablation kits now provide marked vascular sheaths. Used in conjunction with the elapsed time display of the laser system, it is simple to regulate the pullback rate. This combination permits accurate and standardized delivery of laser energy.

Simple manual withdrawal also allows laser energy delivery to be customized to the particular vein segment being treated, which enhances treatment efficacy and safety. For example, when treating the GSV, higher laser energies are delivered to the most central portion of the vein with the first 10 to 15 cm of the vein treated with 140 J per centimeter. This is achieved by withdrawing the laser fiber at a rate of 1 mm per second. In general, the most central segment of the GSV is the most prone to treatment failure and is the least susceptible to venospasm. Thus, it is necessary to deliver proportionately larger amounts of tumescent anesthesia and greater laser energies to adequately treat this important portion of the vein. Higher laser energies may also be delivered in regions of blood inflow such as near junctions with incompetent tributaries or refluxing perforators. When treating vein segments close to the skin, the SSV near the SPJ, or the GSV below the knee, faster laser fiber withdrawal rates of ~3 mm per second are employed to minimize the risk of injury to nontarget tissues.

Class II (30 to 40 mm Hg) gradient compression hose are placed on the patient immediately following endovenous laser treatment and worn for a minimum of 2 weeks at all times, except to sleep or shower. The purpose of gradient compression hose is to lower the risk of superficial thrombophlebitis in tributary varices that will want to close once the underlying saphenous vein reflux is eliminated. Gradient compression, in addition to immediate ambulation following endovenous laser treatment, also increases the velocity of blood flow in the deep veins reducing the likelihood of DVT.

Most patients will have significant improvement or resolution of pretreatment leg symptoms within a month following endovenous laser treatment, but will require additional adjunctive procedures to completely eradicate the remaining varicosities and realize the full benefits of treatment. Sclerotherapy and ambulatory phlebectomy are the most commonly used techniques to accomplish this. The

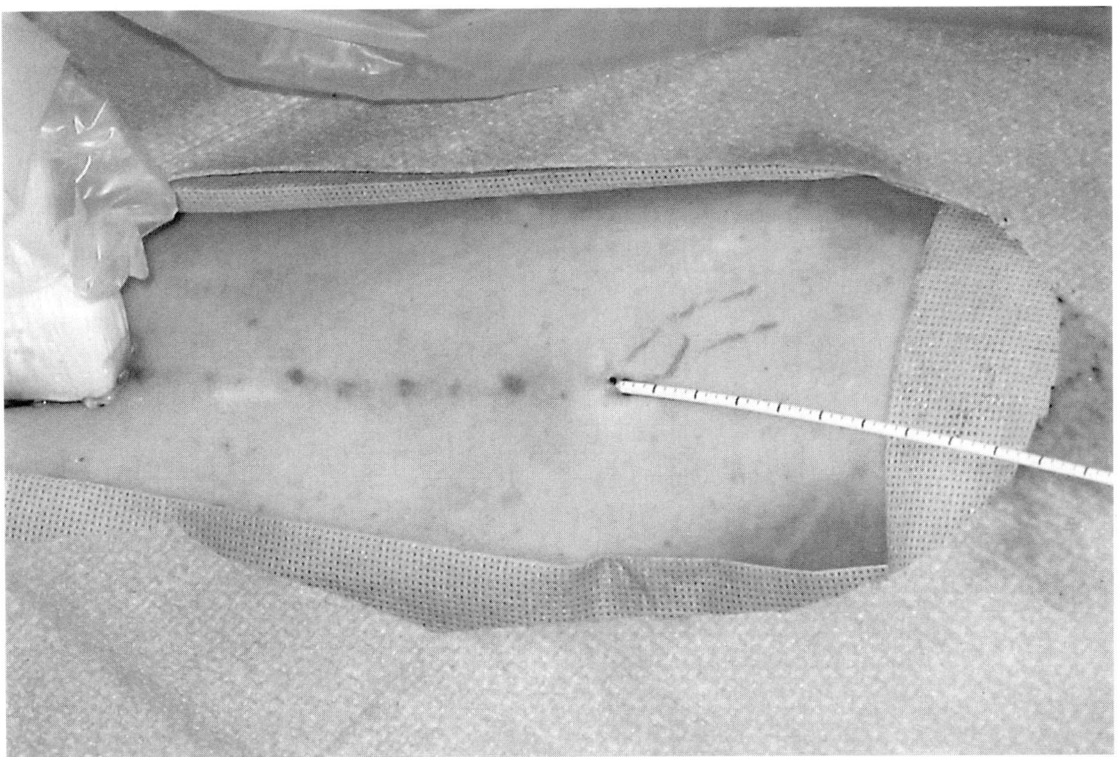

Fig. 25.4 Photograph demonstrating withdrawal of marked sheath at an average rate of 2 mm/s as laser energy is delivered from the junction to the vein entry point using 14 W in continuous mode.

ideal timing of adjunctive procedures has been debated. Those practitioners who advocate waiting note that most patients will experience reduction in the size and fullness of associated varices making ancillary treatments easier and more effective. Rarely, improvement is so dramatic and complete following endovenous laser ablation that additional procedures will not be necessary. Proponents of performing adjunctive procedures at the same sitting as endovenous ablation cite decreased treatment sessions and lower risks of superficial phlebitis, particularly in large thigh varicose tributaries following elimination of the underlying reflux. Occasionally, treatment of nonsurface tributary veins or persistence of clinically significant perforator reflux will require US-guided sclerotherapy with foam or strong liquid sclerosants.

■ Postendovenous Laser Follow-up

Many patients will develop ecchymosis over the treated site due to puncture of the vein during access and administration of tumescent anesthesia. This is of no medical consequence and will resolve within weeks following endovenous laser ablation. Some patients may experience mild discomfort over the treated vein beginning hours after the procedure and resolving within 24 to 48 hours. Many patients will also note delayed tightness and mild to moderate tenderness of the treated vein, particularly over the medial aspect of the lower thigh/knee. This sensation, described as a "pulling," will usually start at the end of the first week, reach a peak approximately 7 days following endovenous laser, and resolve by week two or three. This delayed pain does not correspond to presence or degree of bruising and is most likely caused by transverse and longitudinal retraction of the vein as the acute inflammation transitions to cicatrisation. Most patients feel better with gradient compression hose and ambulation with nonsteroidal antiinflammatories required in occasional cases.

■ Outcomes

The technical success of endovenous laser is defined as a procedure with successful access, crossing the segment to be treated, proper administration of tumescent anesthesia, emptying the vein adequately, and delivery of sufficient laser energy to the entire incompetent vein. Clinical success is defined as permanent occlusion of the treated vein segments with successful elimination of related varicose veins and improvement in the clinical classification of patients by a certain time interval after the procedure (**Fig. 25.5**).

In addition to clinical examination, DUS is essential for evaluating treatment success following endovenous laser. Most practitioners perform DUS within one week following endovenous laser, at completion of treatment, and yearly thereafter. DUS criteria for successful treatment are important to recognize. One week following endovenous laser, DUS imaging will reveal a noncompressible vein, minimally decreased in diameter, with echogenic, circumferentially thickened vein walls, and no flow seen within the entire treated vein lumen upon color Doppler interrogation. Adequate treatment should result in occlusion due to vein wall injury with resultant inflammation. If present, intraluminal thrombus should be minimal and a secondary phenomena, not the primary cause of occlusion, which would result in recanalization. At 3-month to 6-month follow-up, DUS should demonstrate continued target vein occlusion with marked reduction in vein diameter. The vein should be absent or only a minimal residual cord visible upon DUS imaging one year and beyond.[5,6]

Several investigators have reported outstanding success rates of endovenous laser ablation of the GSV.[7–15] These studies have consistently shown successful nonthrombotic occlusion of the saphenous vein in 90 to 100% of cases at 12- to 60-month follow-up with very rare recanalizations of previously occluded vein segments. Clinical improvement was noted in almost all cases following successful saphenous vein occlusion. Patient acceptance was high and adverse reactions were extremely rare with heat complications such as DVTs, paresthesias, or skin burns virtually nonexistent.

■ Discussion

Over the past 7 years, we have gained a better understanding of the usefulness of tumescent anesthesia in endovenous ablation. Emptying the vein with tumescent fluid is critical to ensuring treatment efficacy and safety. Because blood is a chromophore for all laser wavelengths used for endovenous ablation, too much blood will lead to inadequate vein wall damage. Occlusion by thrombosis will result in eventual vein recanalization and treatment failure. The goal is to maximize laser energy transfer to the vein walls by providing maximal contact of the vein walls and laser fiber tip. As mentioned earlier, another one of the goals of proper tumescent anesthesia is to separate nontarget structures from the target vein. US is critical in guiding delivery of dilute lidocaine into the proper location. The tumescent fluid should be delivered between the target vein and adjacent nontarget tissues. One can imagine that delivery of fluid in the wrong plane could compress adjacent structures against the vein exposing them to possible

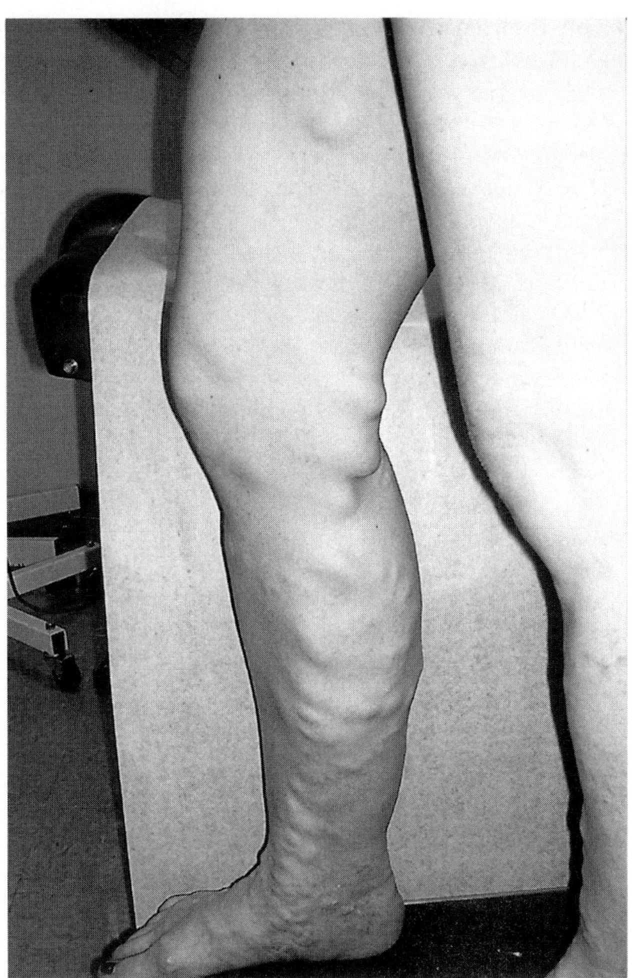

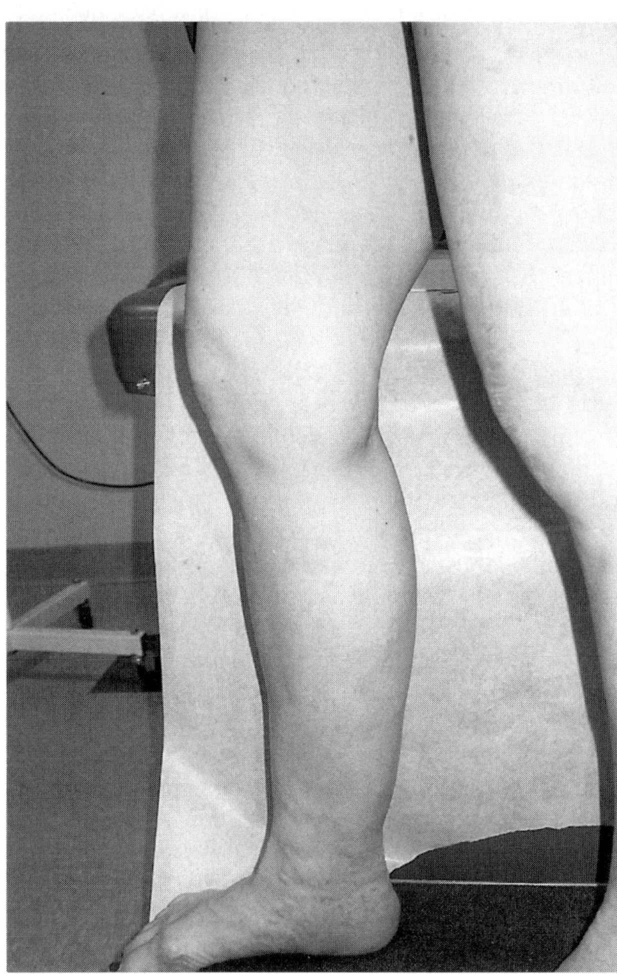

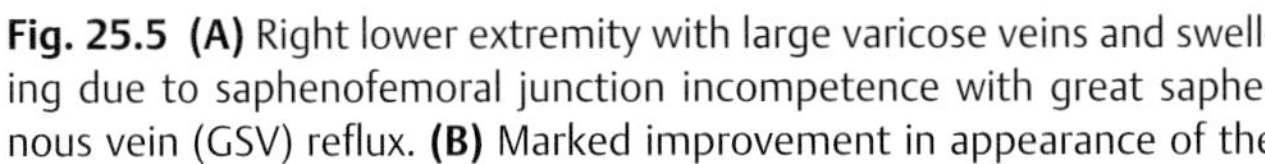

Fig. 25.5 (A) Right lower extremity with large varicose veins and swelling due to saphenofemoral junction incompetence with great saphenous vein (GSV) reflux. **(B)** Marked improvement in appearance of the leg 3 months following endovenous laser ablation of the GSV and sclerotherapy of associated varicosities.

injury during laser energy delivery rather than separating and protecting them. This is particularly important when treating veins known to travel in close proximity to nerves and arterial branches such as the GSV below the knee or the SSV.

The remarkably low rate of true adverse reactions following endovenous laser ablation compares favorably to other treatments of saphenous vein reflux such as surgery or other catheter-based procedures such as radiofrequency or chemical ablation. Complications related to endovenous techniques using radiofrequency have included skin paresthesias, skin burns, DVTs, and pulmonary emboli. Although liberal use of tumescent anesthesia has helped reduce the incidence of heat-related injury to adjacent nontarget tissues, there has been persistence of paresthesias (13 to 15%), clinical phlebitis (2 to 20%), thermal skin injury (4 to 7%), and DVT (1 to 16%) resulting from radiofrequency ablation.[16–19]

Although speculation exists regarding differences in success of endovenous laser versus radiofrequency ablation, there is limited published literature comparing these techniques. One recent study by Black et al demonstrated acceptable results with both procedures at 6 months with 100% (126/126) of veins closed with endovenous laser and 91.5% (118/129) closed with radiofrequency. Eight of the radiofrequency failures were retreated with radiofrequency. Interestingly, three veins failing repeat radiofrequency were successfully closed with endovenous laser treatment.[20] Despite these differences, it is important to emphasize that both of these minimally invasive techniques offers advances in safety and efficacy versus traditional surgical treatment of saphenous vein reflux.

The combined experience of multiple practitioners performing endovenous ablation over the past 7 years has led to greater understanding of this particular technique, but also of venous disease in general. Most failures seem to occur within the first year following treatment, with the majority of these becoming evident by 6 months and central vein segments being the most difficult to close.[21] Because these vein segments are exposed to the highest central venous pressures and are the least prone to venospasm, emptying the vein by using Trendelenburg positioning and tumescent anesthesia is especially important. Because transfer of laser energy to the vein walls via direct contact with the laser fiber tip is the predominant mechanism of action of endovenous laser ablation, maximizing this contact will result in the vein wall damage necessary for eventual fibrosis. It has been postulated by some investigators that absorption of laser energy by blood plays a role in homogeneous distribution of thermal damage to the inner vein wall.[22] It is apparent from more recent scientific studies and mathematical calculations that steam formation from blood absorption is grossly inadequate to result in significant vein wall damage.[23,24] Furthermore, because blood is a chromophore for all wavelengths used for endovenous laser, delivery of laser energy into a blood-filled vein will result in inadequate vein wall damage and nonocclusion or occlusion by thrombosis with eventual reopening.

Examination of treatment parameters has also led to optimization of endovenous laser technique. Studies by Timperman[4] and Proebstle[25,26] have shown that the success of endovenous laser is dependent upon amount of laser energy with treatment failures virtually nonexistent when at least 70 J are delivered per centimeter of treated vein. The vein reopenings seen within the first months following endovenous laser likely represent inadequate vein wall heating with thrombus recanalization. This is either because of excessively rapid pull back of the laser fiber or insufficient vein emptying resulting in poor transfer of thermal energy to the vein wall. True recanalizations of treated veins can occur, but appear to be uncommon. Initial vein wall diameter is unrelated to procedural success and there appears to be no size limit of vein that can be successfully treated with endovenous laser as long as adequate vein emptying and laser fiber to vein wall contact is achieved. Veins with initial diameters in excess of 30 mm have been successfully closed with endovenous laser by several practitioners.

Performing endovenous ablation of the GSV without division of each of the tributaries at the SFJ goes against a fundamental rule in saphenous vein surgery; however, endovenous ablation procedures seem to have lower recurrence rates compared with surgical ligation and stripping. Staying out of the groin, preserving venous drainage in normal competent tributaries, and removing only the abnormal refluxing segments may not incite neovascularization often seen following surgical treatment. Although true recanalization of ablated saphenous veins is uncommon, recurrence of varicose veins is not. Even successful endovenous ablation does not entirely eliminate someone's propensity to develop venous insufficiency. This can occur from untreated portions of the saphenous vein, incompetent tributaries, perforator reflux, or worsening of veins during pregnancy. Practitioners must counsel patients that venous insufficiency is a chronic condition.

Wavelengths of 810 nm, 940 nm, 980 nm, 1064 nm, and 1320 nm have all been used successfully for endovenous laser treatment. Despite attempts by industry or proponents of specific wavelengths to differentiate themselves, the techniques employing the various wavelengths are virtually identical. Because the primary mechanism of action for all of these wavelengths is the same – laser energy delivered to the vein wall via direct contact – classifying these lasers as hemoglobin-specific (810 nm, 940 nm, 980 nm) or water-specific (1320 nm) is inappropriate.[24] It is therefore not surprising that all wavelengths used for endovenous laser ablation have worked well; it is doubtful that one wavelength will excel above all others. Although perhaps scientifically disappointing, this is good news for patients because this is a consequence of the extremely high degree of success and extraordinarily low complication rate of the current technique.

References

1. Boné C. Tratamiento endoluminal de las varices con laser de Diodo. Estudio preliminary. Rev Patol Vasc 1999;5:35–46
2. Navarro L, Min R, Boné C. Endovenous laser: a new minimally invasive method of treatment for varicose veins-preliminary observations using an 810 nm diode laser. Dermatol Surg 2001;27:117–122
3. Min RJ, Zimmet S, Isaacs M, Forrestal M. Endovenous laser treatment of the incompetent greater saphenous vein. J Vasc Interv Radiol 2001;12:1167–1171
4. Timperman PE, Sichlau M, Ryu RK. Greater energy delivery improves treatment success of endovenous laser treatment of incompetent saphenous veins. J Vasc Interv Radiol 2004;15:1061–1063
5. Min RJ, Khilnani NM, Golia P. Duplex ultrasound of lower extremity venous insufficiency. J Vasc Interv Radiol 2003;14:1233–1241
6. Khilnani NM, Min RJ. Duplex ultrasound for superficial venous insufficiency. Tech Vasc Interv Radiol 2003;6:111–115
7. Min RJ, Khilnani N. Zimmet. Endovenous laser treatment of saphenous vein reflux: long-term results. J Vasc Interv Radiol 2003;14:991–996
8. Proebstle TM, Gul D, Lehr HA, Kargl A, Knop J. Infrequent early recanalization of great saphenous vein after endovenous laser treatment. J Vasc Surg 2003;38:511–516
9. Oh CK, Jung DS, Jang HS, Kwon KS. Endovenous laser surgery of the incompetent greater saphenous vein with a 980-nm diode laser. Dermatol Surg 2003;29(11):1135–1140
10. Sadick NS, Wasser S. Combined endovascular laser with ambulatory phlebectomy for the treatment of superficial venous incompetence: a 2-year perspective. J Cosmet Laser Ther 2004;6(1):44–49
11. Perkowski P, Ravi R, Gowda RC, et al. Endovenous laser ablation of the saphenous vein for treatment of venous insufficiency and varicose veins: early results from a large single-center experience. J Endovasc Ther 2004;11(2):132–138
12. Min RJ, Khilnani N. Endovenous laser ablation of varicose veins. J Cardiovasc Surg (Torino) 2005;46(4):395–405
13. Kabnick LS. Outcome of different endovenous laser wavelengths for great saphenous vein ablation. J Vasc Surg 2006;43:88–93

14. Ravi R, Rodriguez-Lopez JA, Trayler EA, Barrett DA, Ramaiah V, Diethrich EB. Endovenous ablation of incompetent saphenous veins: a large single-center experience. J Endovasc Ther 2006;13:244–248
15. Sadick NS, Wasser S. Combined endovascular laser plus ambulatory phlebectomy for the treatment of superficial venous incompetence: a 4-year perspective. J Cosmet Laser Ther 2007;9:9–13
16. Manfrini S, Gasbarro V, Danielsson G, et al. Endovenous management of saphenous vein reflux. J Vasc Surg 2000;32:330–342
17. Merchant RF, DePalma RG, Kabnick LS. Endovascular obliteration of saphenous reflux: a multi-center study. J Vasc Surg 2002;35:1190–1196
18. Rautio TT, Perala JM, Wiik HT, Juvonen TS, Haukipuro KA. Endovenous obliteration with radiofrequency-resistive heating for greater saphenous vein insufficiency: a feasibility study. J Vasc Interv Radiol 2002;13:569–575
19. Hingorani AP, Ascher E, Markevich N, et al. Deep venous thrombosis after radiofrequency ablation of greater saphenous vein: a word of caution. J Vasc Surg 2004;40:500–504
20. Black CM, Collins J, Hatch D, et al. Failure rates of endovenous radiofrequency compared to endovenous laser ablation. J Vasc Interv Radiol 2005; 16(2, Suppl 2)S52
21. Timperman PE. Prospective evaluation of higher energy great saphenous vein endovenous laser treatment. J Vasc Interv Radiol 2005;16:791–794
22. Proebstle TM, Sandhofer M, Kargl A, et al. Thermal damage of the inner vein wall during endovenous laser treatment: key role of energy absorption by intravascular blood. Dermatol Surg 2002;28:596–600
23. Mordon SR, Wassmer B, Zemmouri J. Mathematical modeling of endovenous laser treatment (ELT). Biomed Eng Online 2006;5:26
24. Mordon SR, Wassmer B, Zemmouri J. Mathematical modeling of 980 nm and 1,320 nm endovenous laser treatment. Lasers Surg Med 2007;39:256–265
25. Proebstle TM, Krummenauer F, Gul D, Knop J. Nonocclusion and early reopening of the great saphenous vein after endovenous laser treatment is fluence dependent. Dermatol Surg 2004;30:174–178
26. Proebstle TM, Moehler T, Herdemann S. Reduced recanalization rates of the great saphenous vein after endovenous laser treatment with increased energy dosing: definition of a threshold for the endovenous fluence equivalent. J Vasc Surg 2006;44:834–839

26 Sclerotherapy and Ambulatory Phlebectomy

Lowell S. Kabnick

Lower extremity venous insufficiency is a common condition that affects millions of people each year. Venous insufficiency frequently surfaces in the form of varicose veins or telangiectasia (spider veins); however, the disease can also result in hyperpigmentation, edema, and ulcers. Several risk factors are associated with the development of venous insufficiency, including family history, obesity, older age, pregnancy, and female gender.

Studies over the years have demonstrated that women are approximately twice as likely as men to develop the disease. In 2003, Criqui et al[1] studied 4422 limbs and found that 27.7% of women had varicose veins compared with 15% of men. In 2007, estimates showed that 19.4 million women and 8.9 million men in the United States over the age of 40 will present with varicose veins in 2007.[2]

Ambulatory phlebectomy (AP) and sclerotherapy (ST) are safe and economical procedures that have proven to be effective methods for treating incompetent veins. Patients are able to undergo these procedures in an outpatient setting, using local anesthesia with little or no recovery time. Sclerotherapy involves the intravascular injection of a sclerosing agent to produce endothelial damage and eventual fibrosis of the target vein. Ambulatory phlebectomy permanently removes undesirable veins through a small number of skin punctures, with minimal scarring or adverse effects. Treatment using sclerotherapy or ambulatory phlebectomy may be medically indicated if the veins are symptomatic, whereas asymptomatic veins are classified as a cosmetic procedure.

In this chapter several aspects of sclerotherapy and ambulatory phlebectomy are covered including treatment strategies, diagnostic methods, indications, contraindications, procedural techniques, and potential complications.

■ Treatment Strategies

When treating venous insufficiency, the goal is to first treat the highest point of reflux. Accepted treatment strategies to accomplish this include compression therapy, sclerotherapy, ambulatory phlebectomy, endovenous thermal ablation, and topical laser. Although each treatment modality has its specific advantages and indications, there is significant overlap.

Sclerotherapy and AP are similar treatment strategies; at present, there is a debate as to which is better. There is a lack of evidence-based literature to support the superiority of either procedure. Until conclusive evidence emerges, it is critical for the physician to be adept at both procedures.

Staged versus Unstaged Procedures

There is also substantial controversy over whether ST or AP should be performed at the same time that truncal reflux is being eradicated. The existing data suggest advantages to either ST or AP in conjunction with truncal reflux treatment and to performing the procedures independently. In a retrospective study by Welch,[3] the initial success of endovenous ablation to treat truncal reflux allowed most patients to defer subsequent stab phlebectomy. Conversely, in a controlled study by Mekako et al,[4] patients who underwent concomitant endovenous laser therapy and ambulatory phlebectomy did not need to return for ensuing phlebectomy procedures.

When considering the treatment algorithm, the physician must be selective and make decisions based on the needs of each individual patient. It is appropriate to combine procedures if the varicose veins involve the zone of influence regarding the truncal reflux. Staging is indicated if the varicose veins lie outside the zones of influence.

■ Diagnostic Methods

A complete history and physical examination should be performed for each patient. In most cases, a duplex ultrasound (DUS) is performed as part of the preoperative evaluation. Ultrasound examination allows for the identification of sources of reflux that may require treatment before moving forward with sclerotherapy or ambulatory phlebectomy of the target vein. Venous evaluation is also vital in diagnosing contraindications to ST or AP, thus avoiding serious complications. Photographs of the target veins should be taken to subsequently compare with the results of the procedure.

In addition, transillumination is beneficial for identifying reticular and feeding veins associated with telangiectasias. Common transilluminating devices include the Veinlite (TransLite, Sugar Land, TX) and VeinViewer (Luminetx Corp., Memphis, TN).

■ Sclerotherapy

Sclerotherapy is a method that has existed since the 1930s for the treatment of lower extremity varicosities. This technique involves the intravenous injection of a chemical agent into the lumen of a vessel. The agent produces endothelial damage to the vessel wall that causes initial thrombosis and subsequent fibrosis.

Indications

The intent of sclerotherapy is to effectively eliminate the target vein after the highest point of reflux is treated. The injection of an ideal sclerosing agent into a vessel induces an intense inflammatory response that results in endothelial damage. This leads to thrombus formation, fibrosis, and reabsorption of the vessel. ST is a versatile technique and is indicated to treat several levels of incompetent veins including varicose veins <8 mm, reticular veins (2 to 4 mm), telangiectasias (0.1 to 2 mm), recurrent varicosities, unsightly normal veins of the hands and feet, tributaries, perforators, and failed segments of endothermal ablation.

Indications vary according to the technique used and the skill set of the physician. Other areas appropriate for sclerotherapy treatment include small congenital malformations (such as hemangiomas), vascular malformations, and facial telangiectasia.

The primary limitation of sclerotherapy treatment is vein diameter; the sclerosing agent must make contact with the vein wall to cause endothelial damage. Blood flow within larger veins may dissipate the agent and prevent it from effectively interacting with the vein wall.

Types of Sclerotherapy Agents

Sclerosing agents can be grouped into categories based on their mechanism of action for producing endothelial damage. The currently available solutions are categorized as osmotic, alcohol, or detergent. Ideal characteristics of a sclerosing agent include ability to effectively damage the endothelium, low incidence of adverse events, and painless to inject. Each agent category and specific agent has its own advantages and disadvantages that should be considered when choosing an agent (**Table 26.1**).[5–8]

Table 26.1 Sclerosing Agent Comparison

Agent	Manufacturer	Category	FDA Approval	Advantages	Disadvantages
Hypertonic saline	Multiple	Osmotic	Off-label usage	Low risk of allergic reaction; wide availability; rapid response	Off label; painful to inject; hyperpigmentation; necrosis; rapid dilution; not recommended for facial veins
Sclerodex (hypertonic saline and dextrose)	Omega Laboratories, Canada	Osmotic	Not approved	Low risk of allergic reaction; low risk of necrosis; high viscosity	Not FDA-approved; stings when injected; hyperpigmentation
Chromex (72% chromated glycerin)	Omega Laboratories, Canada	Chemical irritant	Not approved	Low incidence of hyperpigmentation, necrosis, and allergic reaction	Not FDA-approved; weak sclerosing agent; highly viscous and painful to inject; may cause hematuria at high doses
Nonchromated Glycerin	Compounded at pharmacy	Chemical Irritant	Not approved	Low incidence of hyperpigmentation, necrosis and allergic reaction	Not FDA-approved; weak sclerosing agent; typically only used for telangiectasia
Scleromate (sodium morrhuate)	Glenwood, LLC, Englewood, NJ	Detergent	Approved	FDA-approved	High incidence of skin necrosis and anaphylaxis
Sotradecol (sodium tetradecyl sulfate)	Distributed by AngioDynamics, Inc., Queensbury, NY)	Detergent	Approved	FDA-approved; low risk of allergic reaction; potent sclerosant	Potential necrosis with extravasation; telangiectasia matting
Aethoxysklerol (polidocanol)	Kreussler Pharma, Ingelheim, Germany	Detergent	Not Approved	Very low risk of allergic reaction; painless to inject	Not FDA-approved; associated with telangiectasia matting

Abbreviations: FDA, U.S. Food and Drug Administration.
Sources: Data from Carlin MC, Ratz JL. Treatment of telangiectasia: comparison of sclerosing agents. J Dermatol Surg Oncol 1987;13:1181–1184. Goldman MP, Bergan JJ. Sclerotherapy Treatment of Varicose and Telangiectatic Veins. St. Louis: Mosby; 2001. Lewis KM. Anaphylaxis due to sodium morrhuate. JAMA 1936;107:1298–1299. Rabe E, Pannier-Fischer F, Gerlach H, et al. Abstract guidelines for sclerotherapy of varicose veins (ICD 10: I83.0, I83.1, I83.2, and I83.9). Dermatol Surg 2004;30:687–693.

Osmotic Agents

Osmotic agents are thought to cause dehydration of the endothelial cells through osmosis, which leads to endothelial destruction.[9] There are two primary agents used for lower extremity varicosities: hypertonic saline (23.4% sodium chloride) and a hypertonic saline and dextrose mixture, such as Sclerodex (Omega Laboratories, Montreal, Canada).

Alcohol Agents

Alcohol agents are weak sclerosants that cause irreversible destruction of endothelial cells upon contact. The main alcohol agent used for sclerotherapy is chromated glycerin 72% (Chromex, Omega Laboratories, Canada). Nonchromated glycerin is also utilized and is only available through compounding pharmacies. The typical mixture for this solution is two parts 72% nonchromated glycerin to one part 1% lidocaine with epinephrine.

Detergent Agents

Detergent agents are strong sclerosants that produce destruction of the target vein by aggregating on the endothelial wall to cause thrombosis. Currently, two agents are U.S. Food and Drug Administration (FDA-) approved for the treatment of lower extremity venous insufficiency: sodium morrhuate (Scleromate; Glenwood LLC, Englewood, NJ) and sodium tetradecyl sulfate (STS; Sotradecol, distributed exclusively in the United States by AngioDynamics Inc., Queensbury, NY). Although sodium morrhuate is FDA-approved, it is not a preferred detergent agent due to its high incidence of skin necrosis and anaphylaxis.[7]

Sotradecol was previously available in the United States through Elkins Sinn (then a division of Wyeth-Ayerst, Madison, NJ). In 2000 the company discontinued the production and marketing of STS because the integrity of the active pharmaceutical ingredient (API) could not be maintained to meet FDA standards. An industrial cleaning chemical was being used the make the API, which elevated the FDA concerns about the presence of contaminants. Sodium tetradecyl sulfate has a long history of safety and efficacy for use in sclerosing telangiectasia, reticular veins, and varicose veins. A major advantage of Sotradecol is that it is the only preferred, FDA-approved sclerosing agent currently available.

A third detergent agent is polidocanol (POL; Aethoxysklerol, Kreussler Pharma, Ingelheim, Germany). This agent is not FDA-approved; however, it is currently the only approved agent in Germany for sclerotherapy and has been utilized there for over 20 years. In previous studies comparing polidocanol to STS, fewer complications were reported with POL. It should be noted that these studies were conducted with the former industrial-grade STS manufactured by Elkins Sinn. The currently available Sotradecol is a more pure version of STS and there is a paucity of studies to evaluate this new agent.

Contraindications

Sclerotherapy has absolute and relative contraindications that are critical to review before commencing with patient treatment (**Table 26.2**).[8,10,11]

Technique

Preoperative Preparation

Before commencing with treatment, digital photographs of the target veins should be obtained to document the appearance before sclerotherapy is performed. Larger target veins, such as varicose veins should be traced with a surgical marker while the patient is standing as they may be difficult or impossible to identify during recumbency. Smaller veins such as telangiectasia and reticular veins typically do not require preoperative marking.

Surgical Plan

When sclerotherapy is combined with saphenectomy or endothermal ablation of the great or small saphenous veins, sclerotherapy below the knee should be performed second. If using a staging approach, the great or small saphenous veins should be treated first, and sclerotherapy

Table 26.2 Sclerotherapy Contraindications

Absolute Contraindications	Relative Contraindications
Known allergy to the sclerosant	Asthma
Acute cellulitis	Late complications in diabetes
Acute respiratory or skin diseases	Hypercoagulable state
Severe systemic disease	Leg edema
Phlebitis migrans	Advanced peripheral arterial occlusive disease
Acute superficial thrombophlebitis	Chronic renal insufficiency
Pregnancy	
Hyperthyroidism	
Bedridden patients	

Sources: Data from Rabe E, Pannier-Fischer F, Gerlach H, et al. Abstract guidelines for sclerotherapy of varicose veins (ICD 10: I83.0, I83.1, I83.2, and I83.9). Dermatol Surg 2004;30:687–693. Munavalli GS, Weiss RA. Complications of sclerotherapy. Semin Cutan Med Surg 2007;26:22–28. AngioDynamics, Inc. Sotradecol (sodium tetradecyl sulfate injection) prescribing information (PI). Queensbury: AngioDynamics, Inc; 2005.

should follow several weeks later. This method allows the existing truncal varicosities to decrease in size or disappear before further procedures.[12] Depending on the number and severity of diseased veins, several sclerotherapy treatments may be necessary to eliminate the veins. It is important to explain this process to patients and establish the expectation that several sessions could be required.

Equipment

Adequate lighting is essential to identify target veins and effectively perform sclerotherapy. A transilluminating device such as the Veinlite or VeinViewer may be used to enhance visualization of the target veins. A mayo stand is ideal for setting up the supplies for the procedure, which include normal saline, alcohol wipes, 2 × 2 gauze sponges, tape, syringes, butterfly needles, Kelly clamp, gloves, Q-tips, and hazardous waste containers (**Fig. 26.1**). In addition, the I use 30-gauge needles that are ½-inch in length for injection and Sotradecol is my sclerosing agent of choice. Although rare, anaphylaxis can occur and it is essential to have resuscitation equipment in the facility, as well as a facility protocol to handle an emergency.[13]

Procedure

After taking photographs and charting the location of the target veins, the sclerosing agent should be diluted with 0.9% saline according to the size of the vein. I recommend the following concentration dilutions for STS: 0.125 to 0.25% for telangiectasia; 0.25 to 0.5% for reticular veins; and 0.5 to 3.0% for varicose veins. Following dilution of the agent, multiple syringes are filled and assembled with the 30-gauge needles.

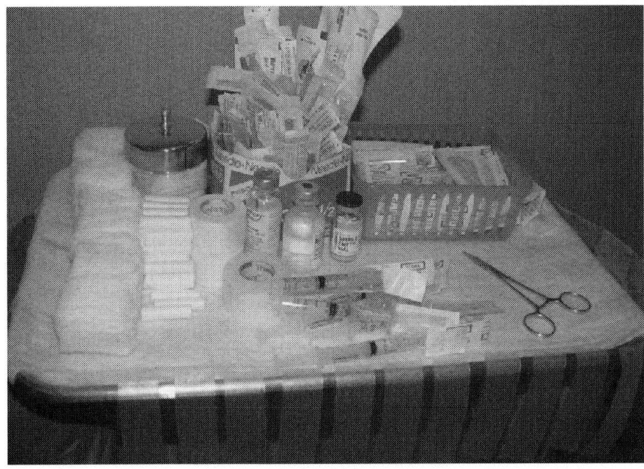

Fig. 26.1 Mayo stand set-up for a sclerotherapy procedure.

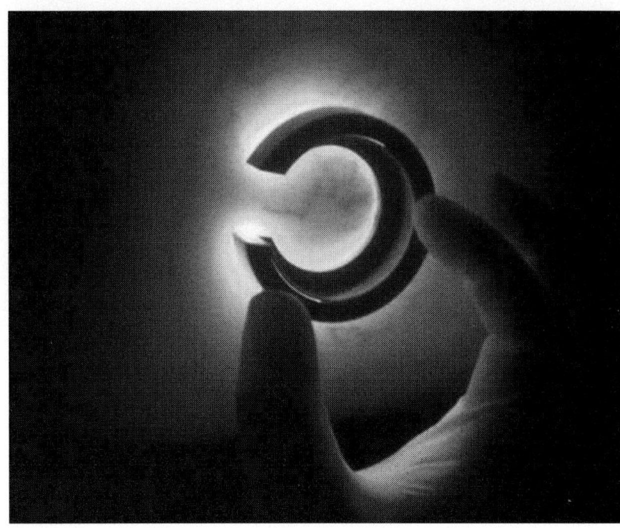

Fig. 26.2 Transillumination of veins using the Veinlite (TransLite, Sugar Land, TX).

Veins should be treated from largest diameter to smallest and from proximal to distal for best results. If treating small veins such as telangiectasia, transillumination can be advantageous in distinguishing veins (**Fig. 26.2**). The amount of STS injected per vein depends on the size of the vein; typically, telangiectasias require 0.1 to 0.2 mL. The operator should not inject more than a few centimeters from the puncture site and avoid forceful pressure during injection (**Fig. 26.3**). The application of pressure after each injection will aid in thrombus formation and increase procedural success. To help minimize bleeding, place 2 × 2 cotton gauze over each injection site and secure with tape. A typical initial sclerotherapy session consists of 10 to 20 injections, depending on the number and size of varicosities.

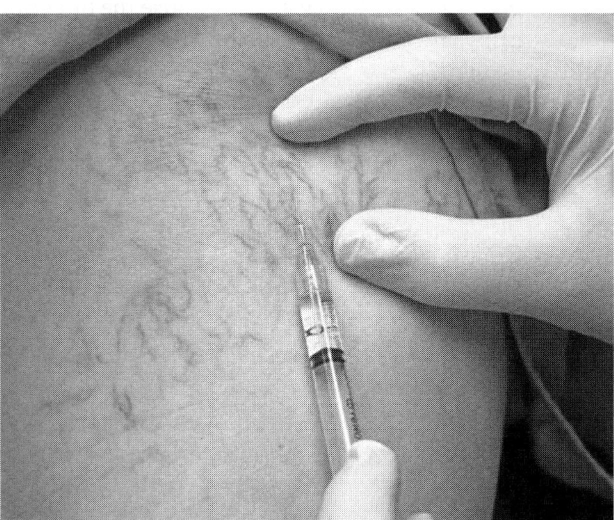

Fig. 26.3 Sclerotherapy injection of telangiectasia.

Discharge Recommendations

The patient should wear postprocedure a 30 to 40 mm Hg compression stocking for 24 hours for reticular veins and telangiectasia and 7 to 10 days for varicose veins and perforators. Although controversial, recent studies have demonstrated increased efficacy with postprocedure compression.[14] Subsequent to ambulation, patients can be discharged from the facility. Instruct the patient to return to activities of daily living, with no heavy aerobic exercise that would involve the lower extremities for 2 weeks. Advise the patient to avoid aspirin, ibuprofen, and other antiinflammatory medications for at least 48 hours. Tylenol may be used if needed. In addition, patients should refrain from sitting in a whirlpool, sauna, or hot bath for at least 48 hours postprocedure.

Complications

Complications vary according to the sclerosing agent utilized and the skill of the operator (**Table 26.3**).[11,13]

■ Ambulatory Phlebectomy

The term ambulatory phlebectomy refers to the technique in which varicose veins are extracted in an outpatient setting under local anesthesia using small punctures and hooks. This technique requires hemostatic compression and immediate ambulation. Synonymous terms used to describe this technique include ambulatory phlebectomy, stab avulsion, stab phlebectomy, microphlebectomy, and microextraction.

Table 26.3 Potential Complications Arising from Sclerotherapy

Potential Complications Arising from Sclerotherapy
Pigmentation changes
Telangiectatic matting
Allergic reactions and anaphylaxis
Ulceration
Cutaneous necrosis
Venous thrombosis
Inadvertent arterial injection (most common location is posterior or medial malleolar region)
Nerve damage (saphenous and sural nerves)
Superficial thrombophlebitis
Deep vein thrombosis
Pulmonary embolism

Sources: Data from AngioDynamics, Inc. Sotradecol (sodium tetradecyl sulfate injection) prescribing information (PI). Queensbury: AngioDynamics, Inc; 2005. Kabnick L. Sclerosants: spiders and superficial veins: results and techniques. Paper presented at: Society of Interventional Radiology Meeting; March 1–6, 2007; Seattle, WA.

Indications

As with sclerotherapy, the objective of ambulatory phlebectomy is to provide definitive treatment for removal of the target vein after the highest point of reflux is treated and/or eliminated. Varicose veins of any size, in any location excluding the cephalad end of the great or small saphenous vein, are candidates for ambulatory phlebectomy. Also appropriate for ambulatory phlebectomy are regional venous networks, reticular veins of the lateral subdermic plexus and popliteal fossa, as well as veins of the hands and feet.[15,16] Dilated veins in other parts of the body including the periorbital, abdominal, and chest areas, medial thigh perforators and small lateral perforators can also be removed by this technique with success.[17]

Contraindications

There are a limited number of contraindications to ambulatory phlebectomy (**Table 26.4**).

Technique

Preoperative Preparation

All target veins should be traced with a surgical marker while the patient is standing. Use of a permanent marker to trace the veins should be avoided because of risk of tattooing. After the patient has been placed in the recumbent position, the vein marks are adjusted using a transilluminator such as the VeinLite or VeinViewer. Because veins tend to shift, this subsequent adjustment adds to the efficacy and speed of extraction.[18,19]

Surgical Plan

The timing of ambulatory phlebectomy depends on the nature and type of other venous procedures being performed. When ambulatory phlebectomy is coupled with saphenectomy, endochemical, or endothermal ablation on the great or small saphenous veins, phlebectomy be-

Table 26.4 Ambulatory Phlebectomy Relative Contraindications

Ambulatory Phlebectomy Relative Contraindications
Infectious dermatitis or cellulitis in surrounding areas
Severe peripheral edema
Severe arterial insufficiency
Serious illness
Anticoagulated state (e.g., patient receiving warfarin)
Hypercoagulable state
Pregnancy

low the knee should be performed first. During saphenous treatment, a transient increase in endoluminal pressure in caudal veins can occur, which could result in bleeding if ambulatory phlebectomy is performed during the same stage. Staging of the procedures can help to eliminate this risk. Effective staging involves treatment of the great or small saphenous vein first, with ambulatory phlebectomy following several weeks after.

Anesthesia

Tumescent anesthesia exploits the principles of pharmacokinetics to achieve anesthesia of the epidermis, dermis, and subcutaneous tissues. The subcutaneous infiltration of a large volume of dilute buffered lidocaine and epinephrine causes the targeted tissue to become swollen and firm. When combined with 8.4% sodium bicarbonate solution, the lidocaine and epinephrine mixture takes on a more neutral pH, which allows for virtually painless injection into the patient.

Administration of Tumescent Anesthesia

The infiltration of dilute anesthesia in a perivascular position, epidermal and dermal, serves several purposes:

1. The anesthetic effect is long lasting, and sensation returns slowly.
2. With the use of longer needles and dilute solution, fewer needle punctures are required and there is less pain upon administration.
3. Tumescent technique causes more compression of surrounding tissues leading to less hematoma and ecchymosis.
4. Hydrodissection occurs around the vein, facilitating the removal.
5. Reduction of infection, usually limited to the incision site, is a result of the bacteriostatic and bacteriocidal properties of lidocaine concentration.[20]

The methods of delivering and mixing the ingredients of tumescent anesthesia vary among users. I use the following tumescent preparation for ambulatory phlebectomy:

- 445 mL of 0.9% saline
- 50 mL of 1% lidocaine with 1:100,000 epinephrine
- 5 mL of 8.4% sodium bicarbonate

Presently, most treatment providers use a regular syringe, a self-filling syringe, or a pump to deliver tumescent anesthesia. The latter two methods facilitate delivery of higher volumes of tumescent anesthesia. Microcannulas or 22-gauge (my preference) or 25-gauge needles are used for the delivery of the solution.

Equipment

Incisions or punctures can be made with various devices, including hypodermic needles and surgical blades. The most common instruments are 18-gauge needles, number 11 blades, and 15-degree ophthalmologic blades (my preference). The number 11 blade is designed to perform incision depths that are greater than what is needed for phlebectomy. From my experience, the number 11 blade causes greater scarring at the incision site. After phlebectomy is completed, ½-inch adhesive strips are placed to close the punctures.

Several different hooks are available for purchase, varying in size, shape, and sharpness. The most widely known are the Muller, Oesch, Tretbar, Ramelet, Verady, Dortu-Mortimbeau, and Kabnick-Goldman hooks.[21] When choosing phlebectomy instruments, it is important to try different hooks and to choose a set of hooks that are comfortable. The clamps used for the vein extraction should have a fine tip so that they can grip close to the skin. A serrated face is helpful in maintaining firm traction without slippage. The operator should have at least three fine mosquito clamps available, but five or more are preferable.

Procedure

After the tumescent anesthesia has been injected into the perivenous tissues, a microincision or puncture is made near the vein. Most incisions are oriented vertically, except around the knee, where they should be oriented along the tension lines (Langer lines). Once the hook has been inserted, the vein is grasped blindly and brought up and out of the opening. The vein is then grasped between clamps and transected by small scissors (**Fig. 26.4**). Using gentle

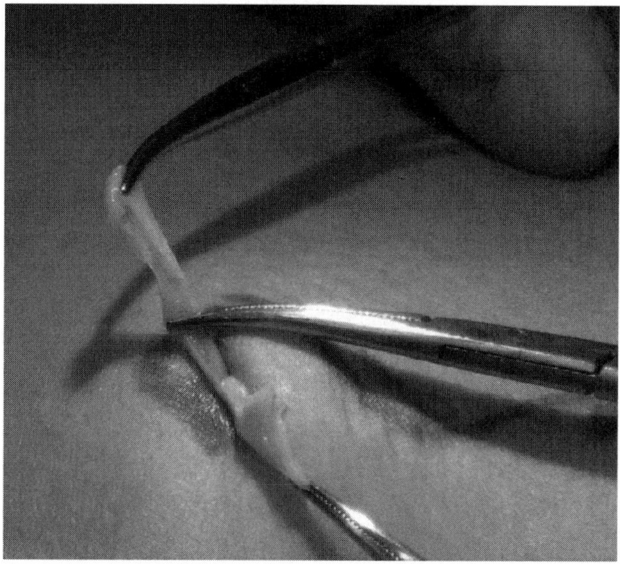

Fig. 26.4 Transection of vein during ambulatory phlebectomy procedure.

traction on the hemostat, one end of the varix is teased out of the puncture site. Successive mosquito clamps are applied to the varix as it is extracted from its position, keeping in mind that the vein will eventually tear. Very long segments can often be removed through a single puncture site. Once a segment has been extracted, the operator moves along the vein and makes another incision, and the process is repeated. The distance between incisions varies and depends on the treatment provider's experience and the size of the vein.

Removal of all parts of the varix, without leaving isolated segments behind, is ideal to reduce a possible inflammatory response from thrombosis of the retained segment. However, as long as most of the segment is removed, the patient should have an excellent result. Puncture sites should not require skin sutures if small incisions are made and postoperative compression is used.

The puncture sites should be covered with adhesive strips, sterile dressings, and wrapped with a soft gauze roll and stretch bandages. The stretch bandages should be started at the foot and wrapped up the leg, covering all the incisions. A 30 to 40 mm Hg compression stocking may also be used as an alternative to the stretch bandage. Postoperative compression plays a vital role in reducing complications, as well as reducing pain and bruising.

Discharge Recommendations

The patient can be safely discharged from the facility after ambulating. Discharge and follow-up recommendations are described in **Table 26.5**.

Complications

Complications arising from ambulatory phlebectomy are quite rare, but can occur (**Table 26.6**).[12,21–24]

Table 26.5 Discharge Recommendations Following Ambulatory Phlebectomy

1. Provide prescription for an oxycodone–acetaminophen combination tablet or capsule, with instructions to try acetaminophen initially
2. Schedule patient to return the following day for bandage removal and placement of a 30–40 mm Hg compression hose
3. Patient should wear compression hose 30–40 mm Hg for at least 2 weeks
4. Instruct the patient to return to activities of daily living, with no heavy aerobic exercise that would involve the lower extremities for 7–10 days
5. Leave adhesive strips in place for 2 weeks
6. Follow-up at 2 weeks, 8 weeks, 6 months, and 1 year

Table 26.6 Potential Complications Arising from Ambulatory Phlebectomy

- Anesthetic complications
  - Allergic reaction (e.g., to preservative, lidocaine)
  - Technique related (e.g., placement of injection)
  - Skin complications
    - Blister
    - Dimpling
    - Hypo- or hyperpigmentation (incision)
    - Induration
    - Infection
    - Pigmentation, transitory or permanent
- Complications of compression bandage
  - Blisters
  - Contact dermatitis
  - Ischemia
  - Skin necrosis
  - Swelling
- Vascular complications
  - Bleeding, seroma
  - Deep venous thrombosis
  - Matting
  - Pulmonary embolism
  - Superficial thrombosis
  - Telangiectasias
- Lymphatic complications
  - Lymphocele
  - Lymphorrhea
  - Persistent edema
- Neurologic complications
  - Dysesthesia (temporary or permanent)
  - Nerve damage – saphenous, sural, peroneal nerves
  - Temporary hypoesthesia
  - Traumatic neuroma

Sources: Data from Kabnick L. Should we consider a paradigm shift for the treatment of GSV and branch varicosities? Abstract presented at: UIP World Congress Phlebology Chapter Meeting; August 2003; San Diego, CA. Dortu J, Raymond-Martimbeau P, eds. Ambulatory Phlebectomy. Houston: PRM Editions; 1993. Ricci S. Ambulatory phlebectomy. Principles and evolution of the method. Dermatol Surg 1998;24:459–464. Olivencia JA. Complications of ambulatory phlebectomy. Review of 1000 consecutive cases. Dermatol Surg 1997;23:51–54. Kabnick LS, Ombrellino M. Ambulatory phlebectomy. Semin Intervent Radiol 2005;22:218–224.

■ Conclusions

To provide the most effective treatment of target veins, the treatment provider should be proficient at both sclerotherapy and ambulatory phlebectomy. These techniques should be applied according to the individual needs of each patient and based on which method will provide the best outcome. The size and type of target vein is a primary factor in technique selection; ambulatory phlebectomy is not appropriate for small telangiectasias, whereas large truncal veins should be avoided for sclerotherapy.

References

1. Criqui MH, Jamosmos M, Fronek A, et al. Chronic venous disease in an ethnically diverse population. Am J Epidemiol 2003;158:448–456
2. Millennium Research Group. US Markets for Varicose Vein Devices 2006. Toronto: Millennium Research Group, Inc; 2006
3. Welch HJ. Endovenous ablation of the great saphenous vein may avert phlebectomy for branch varicose veins. J Vasc Surg 2006;44:601–605
4. Mekako A, Hatfield J, Bryce M, et al. Combined endovenous laser therapy and ambulatory phlebectomy: refinement of a new technique. Eur J Vasc Endovasc Surg 2006;32:725–729
5. Carlin MC, Ratz JL. Treatment of telangiectasia: comparison of sclerosing agents. J Dermatol Surg Oncol 1987;13:1181–1184
6. Goldman MP, Bergan JJ. Sclerotherapy Treatment of Varicose and Telangiectatic Veins. St. Louis: Mosby; 2001
7. Lewis KM. Anaphylaxis due to sodium morrhuate. JAMA 1936;107: 1298–1299
8. Rabe E, Pannier-Fischer F, Gerlach H, et al. Abstract guidelines for sclerotherapy of varicose veins (ICD 10: I83.0, I83.1, I83.2, and I83.9). Dermatol Surg 2004;30:687–693
9. Weiss RA, Feied CF, Weiss MA. Vein Diagnosis and Treatment. New York: McGraw-Hill; 2001
10. Munavalli GS, Weiss RA. Complications of sclerotherapy. Semin Cutan Med Surg 2007;26:22–28
11. AngioDynamics, Inc. Sotradecol (sodium tetradecyl sulfate injection) prescribing information (PI). Queensbury: AngioDynamics, Inc; 2005
12. Kabnick L. Should we consider a paradigm shift for the treatment of GSV and branch varicosities? Abstract presented at: UIP World Congress Phlebology Chapter Meeting; August 27–31, 2003; San Diego, CA
13. Kabnick L. Sclerosants: spiders and superficial veins: results and techniques. Paper presented at: Society of Interventional Radiology Meeting; March 1–6, 2007; Seattle, WA
14. Kern P, Ramelet AA, Wutschert R, Hayoz D. Compression after sclerotherapy for telangiectasias and reticular leg veins: a randomized controlled study. J Vasc Surg 2007;45(6):1212–1216
15. Olivencia JA. Ambulatory phlebectomy of the foot. Review of 75 patients. Dermatol Surg 1997;23:279–280
16. Constancias-Dortu I. Indications for ambulatory phlebectomy. Phlebologie 1987;40:853–858
17. Weiss RA, Ramelet AA. Removal of blue periocular lower eyelid veins by ambulatory phlebectomy. Dermatol Surg 2002;28:43–45
18. Weiss R, Feied C, Weiss M. Vein Diagnosis and Treatment. New York: McGraw-Hill, 2001:198
19. Weiss RA, Goldman MP. Transillumination mapping prior to ambulatory phlebectomy. Dermatol Surg 1998;24:447–450
20. Schmidt RM, Rosenkranz HS. Antimicrobial activity of local anesthetics: lidocaine and procaine. J Infect Dis 1970;121:597–607
21. Dortu J, Raymond-Martimbeau P, eds. Ambulatory Phlebectomy. Houston: PRM Editions; 1993
22. Ricci S. Ambulatory phlebectomy. Principles and evolution of the method. Dermatol Surg 1998;24:459–464
23. Olivencia JA. Complications of ambulatory phlebectomy. Review of 1000 consecutive cases. Dermatol Surg 1997;23:51–54
24. Kabnick LS, Ombrellino M. Ambulatory phlebectomy. Semin Intervent Radiol 2005;22:218–224

27 Clinical Perspective: Venous Insufficiency and the Opportunity for Interventional Radiology

Gerald Niedzwiecki

The development of catheter-based endovascular techniques for the treatment of venous insufficiency has ushered in a new era in the treatment of venous disease. These catheter-based techniques have allowed multiple different specialties ranging from dermatology, gynecology, family practitioners, wound care physicians, and interventional radiologists to enter into the full treatment spectrum of venous disease. Previously, as high ligation and stripping were the gold standard therapy for saphenous insufficiency only a small group of vascular surgeons, general surgeons, and cardiothoracic surgeons would treat venous insufficiency of the saphenous vein. A body of literature as outlined in previous chapters now supports the superiority of endovascular techniques such as radiofrequency closure and endovenous laser therapy over high ligation and stripping. Not only are these techniques less painful, offer a shorter recovery time, and avoid the risks of general anesthesia, but they also avoid the late development of neovascularization in the groin. Combining these techniques with ambulatory phlebectomy and sclerotherapy allow any practitioner interested in these often challenging patients to treat all degrees of superficial venous insufficiency.

These technologic advances have afforded the interventional radiologist an "opportunity" to grow their practices into this area of medicine. At a time when many interventional radiologists are seeing parts of their practices migrate toward other practitioners, technology represents an opportunity for growth. However, treating the spectrum of venous disease is similar to treating women with symptomatic fibroids in that it requires a clinical practice for true success. In this setting, the interventional radiologist sees patients in an outpatient setting and provides consultation services in which the patient is clinically assessed, diagnostic testing is ordered and/or performed, and a treatment plan is formulated for the patient. These interactions with the patient allow the interventional radiologist to develop a traditional patient–physician relationship and to educate the patient regarding realistic outcome expectations. It is the latter that becomes easier for both the patient and physician when this relationship has been established.

Certainly, the treatment of venous diseases is not the only avenue to "break into" a clinical practice style. It is well recognized that interventional radiology over the past several years has been undergoing an evolution to a more clinically based practice style. Luminaries in the field of interventional radiology, the Society of Interventional Radiology, and just plain old hallway dialogues have focused on the need for interventional radiologists to develop offices and clinical practices and to accept direct referrals from primary care physicians to facilitate the management of specific disease states. A clinical practice style is extremely desirable in the treatment of peripheral arterial disease, for the assessment and treatment of patients with compression fractures or other causes of back pain, for patients with symptomatic fibroids, and for the treatment of patients with various forms of cancer. In fact, it would be easily defendable that a clinical practice is not only desirable, but should be the standard method of care for such patients. All of these patients require an initial evaluation, followed by treatment, and most importantly, postprocedure follow-up. These aspects of care all revolve around a clinical office in the outpatient setting.

Venous disease represents an opportunity for interventional radiology because all aspects of care for the patient with venous insufficiency, including the procedures themselves, can be performed in the office setting. In fact, patients often prefer this because an outpatient office is typically a much less complex experience for patients as compared with a day in any hospital. Of course, some patients may require sedation, which necessitates performing these procedures in a hospital setting because it may surpass what one is comfortable doing in the outpatient setting. However, these patients are few and far between and the need for that actually decreases as experience and confidence are gained with these procedures.

One obstacle experienced by interventional radiologists as they have attempted to establish an outpatient office-based practice has been the objections of their diagnostic radiology partners. These objections have typically revolved around the economics of such a venture. An outpatient office based on patient evaluation and management (E&M) often requires a great deal of time, but fails to generate the revenue that can be realized in the traditional radiology setting, despite the fact that assuming patient responsibility is arguably the most appropriate way to practice procedure-based medicine. Interventional radiologists do not usually see 20 to 30 patients per day; hence, the E&M coding associated with these visits will likely not even be enough to pay the overhead costs of the office and staff. This explains the hesitation on the part of many radiology practices to move in this direction. However, as appropriate practice expenses have been incorporated into saphenous vein ablation techniques in the office setting, a strong economic argument can be made to move in this direction. Incorporating the procedures to treat patients with varicose veins expands what can be offered to patients within an outpatient office setting and will often prompt the performance of other procedures as well. This allows the office setting in interventional radiology to be transformed from a “loss leader” that allows the right thing to be done for the patients, into at least a “break-even” proposition for the entire practice.

There are a myriad of reasons to embark into a clinical practice in interventional radiology, many of which have been alluded to earlier. It is certainly the right thing to do for patients and can potentially be a source of satisfaction for the practitioner. However, the “need” for a clinical practice can be crystallized when one looks to the future. Simply put, the arena of endovascular therapy is becoming increasingly crowded and no longer are interventional radiologists the only ones providing these services. Couple this with the fact that all other specialties involved in endovascular therapy already possess clinical practices, and one can quickly recognize that interventional radiology, as a vibrant, viable specialty, will become extinct if it does not evolve to at least match what our competition is providing. Luckily, the need for a clinically based practice to care for venous insufficiency patients and the treatments for venous insufficiency have fortuitously presented themselves as the vehicle for this evolution. This opportunity not only should be embraced, it must be embraced.

VII Breast Interventions

28 Forward Perspective: Interventional Radiology and the Breast

Kenneth R. Tomkovich

The field of interventional radiology is perhaps the most dynamic in all of medicine. Many of the procedures that are performed today were either nonexistent or heavily modified in the past 10 years. Uterine fibroid embolization, kyphoplasty, saphenous vein ablation, and many of the other procedures described in this text were not part of interventional radiology training programs in 1997. All of these as well as other procedures have been introduced, modified, or developed by interventional radiologists and incorporated into the practices and teaching programs during the past decade. The ability of interventional radiologists to adapt and apply new techniques and technology into their practices is probably the most important characteristic of this specialty.

With the recent development of clinical practices and specialization in areas such as interventional oncology, new opportunities for growth and practice development have been presented to interventional radiologists. Using imaging guidance, interventional radiologists have become an integral member of the oncology service line. Procedures including percutaneous biopsies, radiofrequency and cryoablations, arterial chemoembolizations, yttrium-90 microsphere embolotherapy, and vascular access are all part of the services offered by interventional radiologists practicing oncologic interventions. Yet there is one glaring omission in the practice of most interventional radiologists: the practice of breast interventions.

It is unclear the reason why the breast has been virtually omitted from the field of interventional radiology. As defined by the Society of Interventional Radiology, "Interventional Radiologists are board certified physicians who specialize in minimally invasive, targeted treatments performed using imaging for guidance. Their procedures have less risk, less pain and less recovery time compared to open surgery."[1] If this definition is accepted, then why omit care of the breast? In fact, the field of interventional radiology is well suited for breast care for many reasons. Interventional radiologists have training and expertise in performing biopsies safely and accurately in all areas of the body. Interventional radiologists have the most experience and expertise in percutaneous ablation procedures. Interventional radiologists may already care for some breast cancer patients through placement of vascular access for chemotherapy or through chemoembolization or radiofrequency ablation of metastatic disease. There are many procedures and applications of techniques unique to the breast, which can be learned and practiced by interventional radiologists.

■ Breast Biopsy

Once a lesion has been discovered, in any area of the body, a biopsy is required to direct treatment. Nowhere is this more important than in the breast. Patients with newly diagnosed breast lesions may have presented with a palpable growth or abnormality requiring imaging for further evaluation of the extent of disease or to look for disease in the contralateral breast.[2] Most often, women present for annual screening mammography and have a newly diagnosed lesion requiring further assessment with imaging and then biopsy. The standard of care in 2007 is to perform image-guided breast biopsy if possible rather than performing open surgical biopsies.[3] Patients will typically have a mammogram, which may or may not be combined with other imaging such as ultrasound or magnetic resonance imaging (MRI). Following the imaging workup, they will require a biopsy based on the interpretation of either a BI-RADS category 4 (suspicious) or 5 (highly suggestive of malignancy) abnormality. Some patients who have been given category 3 (probably benign) classifications are also presenting for biopsy in most cases because they are fearful of a growing lesion in their breast, may be planning pregnancy or breast augmentation procedures or have a breast cancer history or cancer in the opposite breast and need a more definitive diagnoses prior to therapy.[3] It is this last point that is most important in understanding why percutaneous breast biopsy is the standard of care today.

There are many options in treating breast cancer. The most obvious is surgical removal of the tumor. This can be accomplished through excisional biopsy, but more often than not this treatment is not definitive and patients would require a second open surgical procedure. The options presented to those with a percutaneous biopsy as the first diagnosis are many. Patients may have an additional, more detailed workup perhaps including a breast MRI prior to surgery. Patients may be given the options of neoadjuvant chemotherapy or hormone therapy prior to a surgical procedure in an attempt to shrink the size of the tumor and perhaps improve the surgical options for breast conservation. The tumor pathology can be accurately assessed including analysis of tumor markers such as estrogen and progesterone receptor sensitivity analysis. This can direct clinicians and patients with respect to the aggressiveness of the tumor and direct options for surgery and postsurgical care. Perhaps most importantly, percutaneous breast biopsy can be done safely and accurately in an outpatient setting avoiding the anxiety, extra time, and scarring, which are all associated with an open surgical procedure. Even with the improved accuracy of imaging and the use of digital mammography and MRI to help determine whether lesions of the breast are benign or malignant, nearly 80% of the biopsies recommended are still for benign lesions. It is important to be able to diagnose these benign breast lesions through percutaneous biopsy rather than open surgical procedures to avoid unnecessary surgery and scarring.

In general, when planning for a percutaneous image-guided breast biopsy it is important to review the imaging to choose the best approach for the patient. Even if one does not read mammography, breast MRI, or ultrasound on a regular basis there is no reason that the interventional radiologist cannot participate and effectively perform these biopsies. Certainly, the majority of biopsy procedures in other organs such as the liver or lungs were diagnosed by other imagers and presented for review by the interventionalist. Likewise, breast lesions, detected by other imagers, can be evaluated for biopsy by clinicians who did not make the initial interpretation. There is no reason the breast should be treated differently. In addition, the fact remains that as of today, all interventional radiologists are still first diagnostic radiologists who had to pass the board examination, including the sections on mammography and breast imaging. Therefore, interventional radiologists are better suited than other specialists to participate in percutaneous breast interventions because of their background and training.

As with any intervention, it is important to perform a brief history and physical examination prior to performing the procedure. Breast biopsies are no exception. It is very important to be aware of any medication or supplements such as aspirin, vitamin E, fish oils, or others that may predispose a patient to bleeding or hematoma, which is the most common complication from any percutaneous breast intervention.[4] I recommend that a patient stop all such medication or supplements for 5 days prior to any intervention or biopsy. Options for biopsy guidance include stereotactic, ultrasound, and MRI, and perhaps in the near future digital tomosynthesis. Fine-needle aspiration (FNA) biopsy is often performed with ultrasound guidance. Fine-needle aspirations obtain a suspension of cells with a small gauge needle through a back and forth motion while aspirating on a syringe or trapping a column of cells in the needle through motion. These cells can then be processed and analyzed for cytologic features.[5] This technique is not advisable except in situations where there is perhaps a mostly cystic lesion with or without a small solid or irregular component or in the case where there is a very large palpable lesion for confirmation of any already expected diagnosis. No tumor markers can be processed on FNA biopsies; often they are dependant on having a good histopathologist to process and interpret the findings. If performing FNA biopsies, it is most important to document concordance between the imaging findings and the pathology.[5]

Stereotactic breast biopsy is a mainstay of breast interventions. Lesions presenting as suspicious microcalcifications are most commonly approached with stereotactic guidance. Masses and areas of architectural distortion can also be biopsied with stereotactic technique. However, ultrasound guidance is the method of choice for these lesions if they can be identified sonographically. Lesions that are difficult to biopsy using stereotactic guidance are those which are very close to the chest wall, very superficial lesions, and those with very small or inconspicuous microcalcifications.[5] Stereotactic biopsy requires a dedicated table on which the patient lies in the prone position. The breast passes through a hole in the table and is positioned so as to best approach the lesion for biopsy. Through computer-generated coordinates based on position of the lesion relative to defined angles, the appropriate position and approach can be determined. Care should be taken to choose the shortest possible distance and to avoid any large or branching blood vessels, which may be near the biopsy site.[5] Once the calculations are made as to the depth and position of the target area, the breast is prepped in sterile fashion. After administration of 5 to 10 cc of 1% lidocaine solution, a 3 mm incision is made through which an 8- or 11-gauge biopsy needle is advanced up to the lesion under stereotactic guidance as per the manufacturer's instructions for depth. Confirmation imaging for needle placement is made and the needle is then deployed. Vacuum-assisted biopsy is then obtained from the site in a circumferential fashion. The number of cores obtained is dependent on what is being sampled and the gauge of the needle. I will typically obtain 12 cores using an 11-gauge needle and have most recently performed the majority of my stereotactic breast biopsies using an 8-gauge needle and only four cores. A specimen mammogram is suggested for all stereotactic biopsies particularly to document the removal of suspicious calcifications and to allow for separating the specimen into those with and without calcifications for pathologic analysis. After confirmation of the suspicious tissue in the biopsy specimen, a marker is placed at the biopsy site through the biopsy needle. I will typically close my incisions with ½ inch Steri-Strips (3M, St. Paul, MN) and apply a pressure dressing over the site. If there is bleeding at the biopsy site, it is important to main-

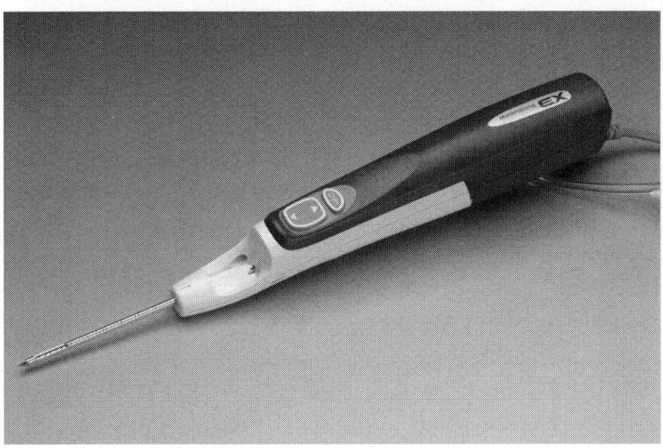

Fig. 28.1 Image of the Mammotome EX Vacuum-assisted hand-held biopsy needle. (Courtesy Ethicon Endo-Surgery, Inc., Cincinnati, OH.)

tain pressure to minimize the size of any breast hematoma and suture can be used to close the incision.

When a lesion is visible in the breast by ultrasound then percutaneous ultrasound-guided biopsy is the method of choice for obtaining a diagnostic sample of the tissue. The recent development of vacuum-assisted and stick freeze large-gauge hand-held biopsy devices have enabled clinicians to obtain larger samples under ultrasound guidance (**Fig. 28.1**). Although there may be a few circumstances in which FNA biopsy or spring-loaded core biopsy is performed in the breast, these are not the methods of choice for obtaining diagnostic samples and should not be utilized on a regular basis due to the availability, safety, and sample size of the vacuum-assisted or stick freeze large-gauge devices. Improper usage of FNA or small-gauge core needle biopsy can lead to a high percentage of false-negative biopsy results and unnecessary second biopsies due to discordance between imaging findings and pathology.[6–9] Whenever possible, an 11-gauge or larger biopsy device should be used to perform ultrasound-guided core breast biopsy.[10]

The Cassi needle (Sanarus Medical, Pleasanton, CA) uses stick freeze technology. To perform this procedure, a 19-gauge guiding needle is advanced through the lesion under ultrasound guidance (**Fig. 28.2A**). An automated freezing procedure using a carbon dioxide cartridge freezes the 19-gauge needle to the lesion and an outer 10-gauge cutting needle advances over the 19-gauge needle in a circumferential manner to obtain the core biopsy sample (**Fig. 28.2B**). In my experience, usually no more than three passes are required to sample the lesion in question adequately. One disadvantage to this device is the requirement of withdrawing the needle after each pass to retrieve the sample, which requires reinsertion to obtain additional cores. The Cassi device has a sharp leading 19-gauge needle, which can be very helpful in gaining access to lesions in dense breast tissue or to lesions located near the chest wall or deep within the upper outer quadrant.[10]

Several vendors have developed vacuum-assisted core needle biopsy systems. These typically are made in 8-, 11-, and 14-gauge sizes. The benefit of these devices is that they require only one needle insertion to obtain multiple core samples from the lesion and due to the large cores obtained under direct ultrasound observation the number of discordant results are quite few. In fact, ultrasound-guided large-gauge vacuum-assisted core breast biopsy done with the proper technique in experienced hands is as accurate, or better than open breast biopsy performed after needle localization. In addition, a marker can be placed through most devices at the biopsy site.[11] Vacuum-assisted biopsy has been shown to accurately diagnose atypical ductal

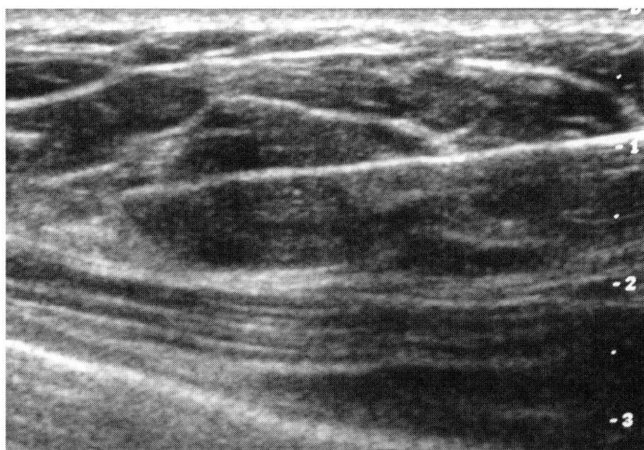

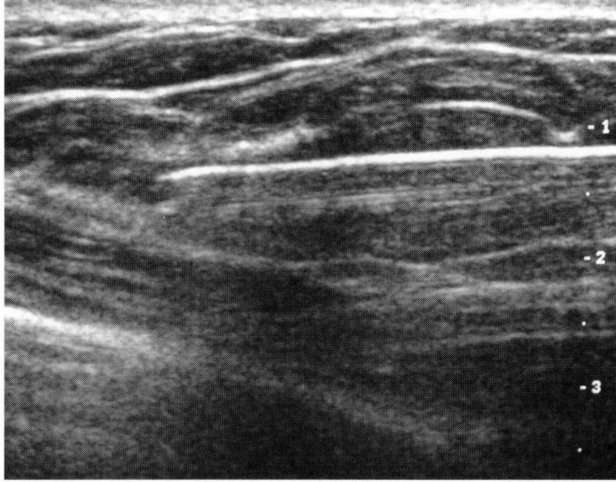

Fig. 28.2 Ultrasound images obtained during a percutaneous stick-freeze biopsy of a breast mass. **(A)** The 19-gauge guiding needle is seen advancing through the target lesion. **(B)** After a carbon dioxide cartridge freezes the 19-gauge needle to the lesion, an outer 10-gauge cutting needle is advanced over the 19-gauge needle to obtain the biopsy specimen.

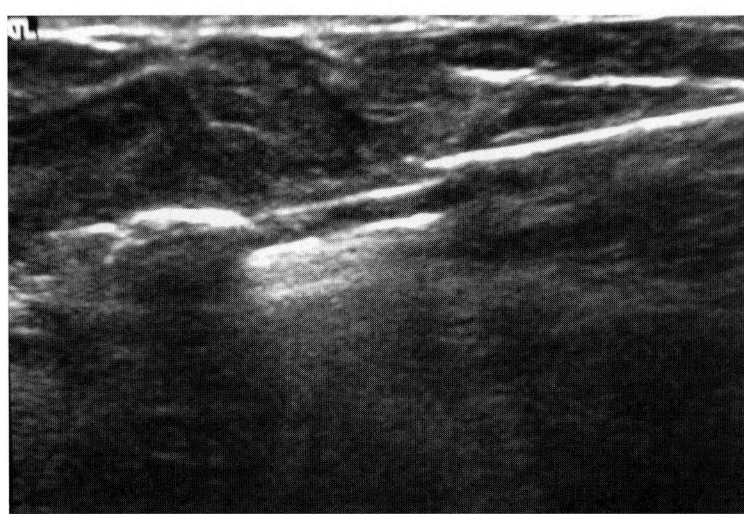

Fig. 28.3 Ultrasound image obtained during a vacuum-assisted biopsy of a breast mass. This demonstrates the position of the needle under the target mass, which enables the vacuum to draw tissue into the aperture for biopsy.

hyperplasia, ductal carcinoma in situ, and microcalcifications.[12–14] The breast is prepped and draped in sterile fashion. Local anesthetic is administered in the skin, along the biopsy tract, and distal to the biopsy site. A 3 mm incision is made through which the biopsy needle is advanced, under ultrasound guidance up to the lesion. The preferable approach is to have the needle under the mass so that the vacuum can draw the tissue into the aperture for biopsy, but this is not always possible (**Fig. 28.3**). The needle can be passed superior to or on the side of the lesion as long as the operator can document with certainty that the mass is being biopsied under direct visualization with ultrasound. After the vacuum is applied, the tissue is drawn into the aperture, and a rotating cutting device is then used to obtain a tissue sample.[15] After satisfactory sampling of the lesion, a localizing marker is placed, the device removed and good hemostasis is achieved with direct pressure. The incision is closed with ½ inch Steri-Strips and a pressure dressing is applied. The vacuum-assisted ultrasound-guided technique has also been used in the treatment of gynecomastia and for benign fibroadenomas.[16–18]

The increasing acceptance of breast MRI as a diagnostic tool has made it necessary for biopsies and localizations to be performed using MRI for guidance. This is particularly important in the case where a lesion is only seen on MRI. If a center is performing breast MRI then that center should also have the capability and expertise to perform MRI-guided breast localization and biopsy. Similar to ultrasound, many vendors have developed MRI-compatible biopsy needles and markers including vacuum-assisted mechanical rotating devices.[11] It is also important to think about future opportunities for growth and development in breast cancer diagnosis and intervention. Digital tomosynthesis is a technique in which thin-section tomographic images are obtained through the breast. The benefit is to eliminate artifact cast by adjacent normal breast tissue that may make a lesion or suspicious microcalcifications inconspicuous on conventional mammograms. Once the lesions are found, the challenge is then to accurately localize them for excisional biopsy or preferably to develop biopsy devices and techniques that can be used with digital tomosynthesis guidance. This challenge is also an opportunity for those of us in the field of interventional radiology to participate in the growth and development of these new techniques to improve the quality of care for women with breast disease.

■ Breast Ablation

Two decades ago, the majority of breast cancers were found when they became palpable masses and the treatment of choice was the radical mastectomy. Much has changed in the past 15 to 20 years with respect to the diagnosis and treatment of breast cancer. Today, breast conservation is the treatment of choice as cancers are detected at earlier stages and smaller sizes due to improvements in diagnostic imaging and better patient education about screening. Interventional radiologists have been at the forefront of developing thermal ablation techniques for the treatment of cancer. This was not the case 10 years ago when the possibility of using ablation therapy for treatment of liver, lung, kidney, and bone tumors was merely a hypothesis. The goal of any ablation therapy is to sufficiently heat or cool the abnormal tissue so as to cause cell death. The challenge is to now see if these techniques can be applied to the breast as they have been in other organs. Studies have been completed demonstrating the effectiveness of thermal ablation from a pathologic perspective and clinical trials are now ongoing to test the feasibility of percutaneous image-guided thermal ablation in patients with small focal breast cancer.[19]

The goal of conservative therapy is to treat tumors with as little tissue removal as possible. The next challenge is to effectively treat tumors with no surgery using image-guided ablation. To this end, more than 30 research articles have been published on the feasibility and success of the use of ablation for breast cancer.[20,21] The principles are quite similar to those for the treatment of lesions in other organs. The lesions must be localized with imaging guidance and the tip of the device, for cryoablation or radiofrequency ablation must be accurately placed within the lesion to be able to achieve an adequate margin of thermal injury so as to kill all viable tumor cells. Studies have been and are being performed testing radiofrequency ablation before surgical excision to assess for tumor viability. Early results have been mixed with some studies reporting complete necrosis and others viable tissue at surgical excision.[22,23,24] One recent promising study focused on treating patients with lesions 2 cm or less in size and reported no viable tumor at excisional biopsy performed 3 to 4 weeks following ablation.[25] Similar studies have utilized cryoablation and interstitial laser thermal ablation as a source of thermal injury in breast cancer.[26–30] The benefit to cryoablation is in the visualization of the ice ball as it forms under ultrasound guidance and the ability to protect the skin and chest wall through saline injection. Cryoablation has also been used to create a spherical guide to surgical excision in lesions 2 cm or less.[31] Perhaps the most promising form of ablation therapy for breast cancer is image-guided high-frequency ultrasound. Currently utilized for the treatment of uterine fibroids, there appears to be great potential for the treatment of breast cancer. Precise targeting of the tumor can be performed with MRI guidance and high-frequency ultrasound can be used to treat the tumors without the need for any incisions.[32–34]

The most common benign breast tumor is the fibroadenoma. Women may experience pain or discomfort from these lesions particularly in response to monthly hormone fluctuations.[35] Patients may also desire treatment for fibroadenomas when they are palpable for either cosmetic or psychological reasons.[10] Therefore, even though a benign histologic diagnosis is made, patients will often seek treatment due to symptoms or the presence of a palpable lump. Surgical excision has long been the treatment for the fibroadenoma but today, percutaneous image-guided cryoablation is a viable alternative. A device approved by the food and drug administration for ablation of fibroadenomas is the Visica system (Sanarus Medical Inc., Pleasanton, CA) (**Fig. 28.4**). Using ultrasound for guidance, a biopsy-proven fibroadenoma is first localized within the breast. The breast is then prepped and draped in sterile fashion and after administration of local anesthetic, the 13-gauge cryoprobe is

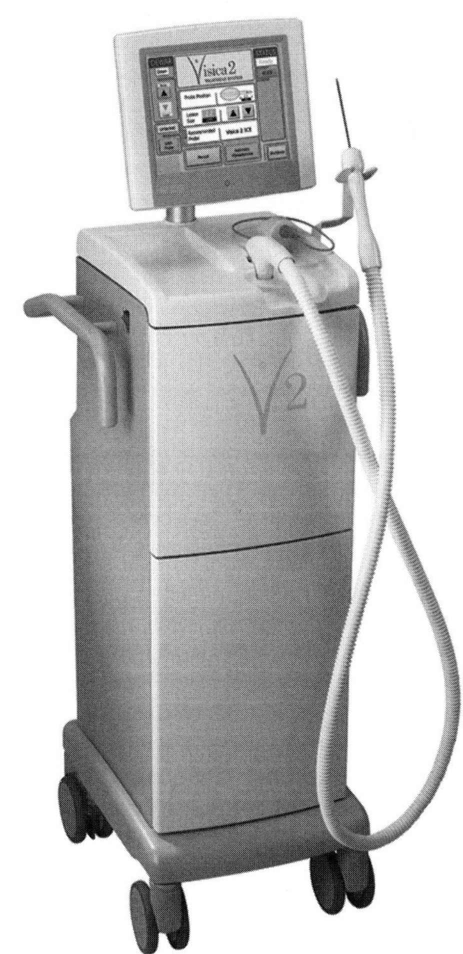

Fig. 28.4 Image of the Visica System, which can be used to ablate fibroadenomas within the breast. (Courtesy Sanarus Medical Inc., Pleasanton, CA.)

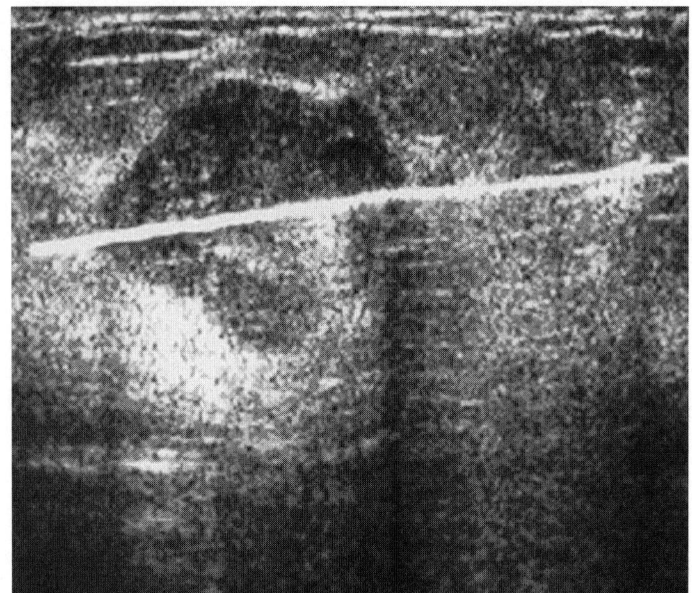

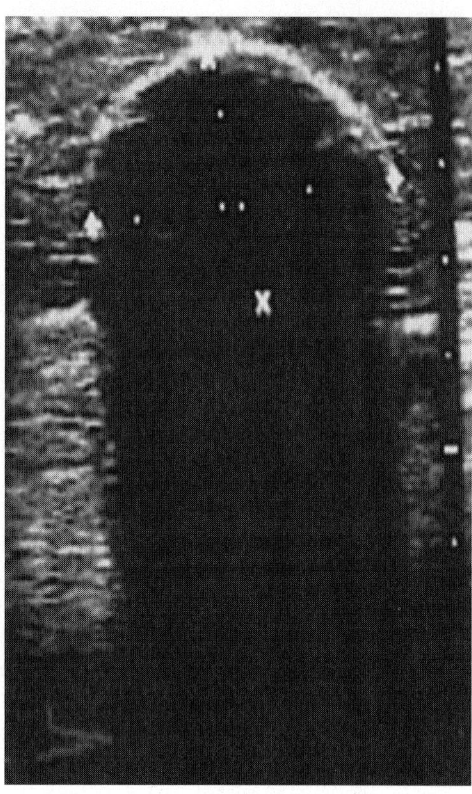

Fig. 28.5 Images obtained during a cryoablation procedure of a breast fibroadenoma. **(A)** Ultrasound image demonstrating the cryoprobe within the mass. **(B)** Ultrasound image demonstrating the appearance of the mass after the cryoablation procedure has been performed.

advanced into the mass (**Fig. 28.5A**). A freeze–thaw–freeze sequence is performed under ultrasound guidance for a time determined based on the size of the lesion (**Fig. 28.5B**). Following the procedure, the incision is closed with Steri-Strips and a pressure dressing is applied. A multicenter trial of 32 patients and 37 fibroadenomas reported a median volume reduction of 89% at one year and 99% at 2.6 years. The safety profile and satisfaction with outcomes were both reported as good.[36] The main advantage of percutaneous cryoablation is a smaller, if any, scar and no architectural distortion on mammography. In addition, the procedure can be performed in an outpatient office. Lesions that respond best to cryoablation are those that are 2 cm in diameter or smaller.[37] Percutaneous ultrasound-guided cryoablation of biopsy-proven benign fibroadenomas should be considered a primary treatment option for women desiring an alternative to surgery. This procedure is well within the scope of practice of interventional radiology.[10,11]

■ High-Dose Brachytherapy

Many women who require lumpectomy for breast cancer will undergo some form of radiation therapy. Whole breast radiation treatment was once the standard of care. Due to improvements in technique and through additional research, patients were then given the option of partial breast irradiation. Most recently, accelerated partial breast irradiation using interstitial brachytherapy has proven effective in a certain population of low-risk patients postlumpectomy.[11] The MammoSite balloon catheter system (Cytyc Surgical, Palo Alto, CA) has been introduced as a means of delivering partial breast brachytherapy (**Fig. 28.6**). The MammoSite catheter is a dual lumen device with one lumen for inflation of the balloon and the second lumen for administration of the high-dose iridium-192 source.[38] The MammoSite catheter can be placed at the time of lumpectomy surgery within the cavity or through a percutaneous ultrasound-guided technique as an outpatient, in-office procedure. The technique involves localizing the lumpectomy site with ultrasound guidance. After prepping the breast and administering local anesthesia, a small incision is made through which an introducer trocar is placed into the lumpectomy site. The trocar is removed and the MammoSite balloon catheter is placed into the lumpectomy cavity and inflated to profile (**Fig. 28.7**). The catheter is then secured in place and the patients receive high-dose brachytherapy for up to 7 days. The balloon catheter is removed percutaneously after completion of the therapy.[11] Reported possible complications with the device include infection, skin toxicity (erythema, hyperpigmentation, telangiectasias), seroma formation, and catheter failure.[39]

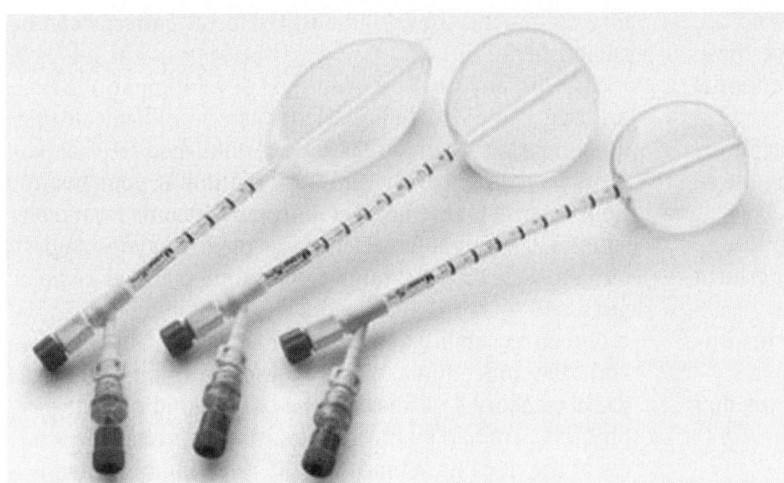

Fig. 28.6 Image of the MammoSite balloon catheter system (Cytyc Surgical, Palo Alto, CA), which is used for partial breast brachytherapy. (Courtesy of Hologic, Inc.)

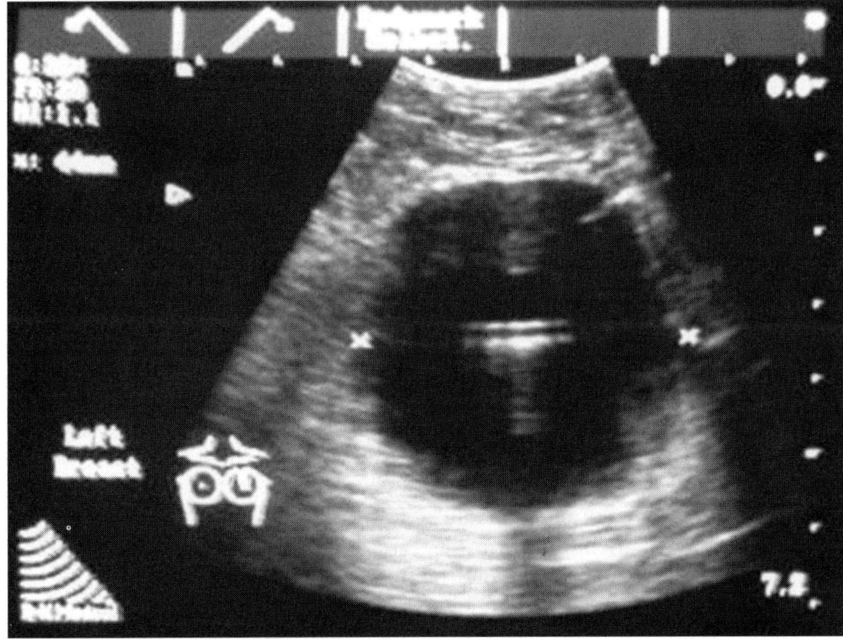

Fig. 28.7 Ultrasound image demonstrating the MammoSite catheter (Cytyc Surgical, Palo Alto, CA) placed within a lumpectomy cavity with the balloon inflated.

■ Practice Development

Imagine a scenario in which an interventional radiologist is presented with a computed tomography (CT) scan of the liver showing a lesion and instead of offering to biopsy it and treat it with an ablation procedure states, "I cannot treat this because I do not read CT scans. See the liver CT scan doctor." It is this very scenario that is being applied to diseases of the breast in many practices. Interventional radiologists in both office-based and hospital-based practices routinely evaluate images, which have already been interpreted by someone else for the purpose of performing image-guided interventions. Many patients who are then diagnosed with cancer through percutaneous biopsy techniques then return to the interventional radiologist for palliative and perhaps curative treatments of their cancers. Yet for some reason, when it comes to the breast, this is not frequently the case. Interventional radiologists are highly skilled when it comes to image-guided interventions, but infrequently participate in the care of women with breast disease. This should change. Many of the procedures described in this chapter were researched and developed by interventional radiologists. Interventional radiologists have the background to evaluate the images used for the diagnosis of breast disease and can then perform the image-guided interventions of the breast as they do in other areas of the body. Radiology groups should be made aware of the types of procedures available and the ability of an interventional radiologist to safely and accurately perform these procedures. It is then that these procedures will become a welcomed part of interventional radiology practice.

If the reader is interested in performing breast interventions, then you should answer the following three questions:

- Do I have the skills and time required to perform these procedures?
- Are these procedures being performed at my institution and if so by whom?
- What are the current referral patterns and how do I participate?

First, do you have the skills and time? In my practice, I am the only interventionalist in my group who performs these procedures. This is mainly due to my strong interest in the area of breast interventions and to my proficiency in ultrasound-guided procedures. If one is not skilled in ultrasound-guided biopsy or drainage or vascular access or does not feel capable of acquiring these skills then breast interventions are probably not for them. The techniques required for stereotactic biopsy are not as operator dependant, although they do require some practice to master. If a facility is certified by the American College of Radiology in stereotactic breast biopsy, then there are certain training requirements that must be met by physicians to maintain certification.[40] The skills for breast ablation and MammoSite placement are similar to those for ultrasound-guided biopsy. The techniques for all of these procedures can be learned through course study and hands-on training. There is also obviously a time requirement including patient consultation and image review. I must stress again that one does not have to read breast MRI, ultrasound, or mammography on a daily basis to be able to perform breast interventions. I devote ~50% of my time to breast interventions.

Second, who is performing these procedures now? If the answer is nobody, then this presents the ideal opportunity to build and enhance your existing practice. If surgeons or women's imagers are performing the breast interventions, then are they doing them because they want to or because they have to because there is nobody else who wants to do them? Does everyone in the women's imaging section want to perform large-gauge biopsies? Some certainly do and are very good at it, but others may welcome the opportunity to focus on imaging and give up some or all of the interventions. Some surgeons may want to perform percutaneous image-guided biopsies or ablation procedures, but many of the surgeons whom I have spoken to would rather devote their time to operating. This presents the interventional radiologist with a wonderful opportunity for practice development if referral patterns can be established.

As with any new procedure or development of a new practice, recruiting new patients can be difficult at first. It is important to understand the established referral patterns for breast biopsy and intervention at your institution. Referral for breast interventions can come from many sources. I get my referrals from oncologists, gynecologists, radiation oncologists, family practitioners, other radiologists, and surgeons. I have educated the radiologists in my group on my ability and desire to perform breast biopsies and other procedures. When a patient presents with a BI-RADS category 4 or 5 lesion, the patient and her referring physician are told by the radiologist interpreting the studies of the need for a biopsy. If the referring physician is a surgeon, then the patient is referred back to that surgeon for biopsy evaluation. If the referring physician is not a surgeon, then the referrer is told that the patient will require a biopsy and that they should consult with the physician or facility of their choice for biopsy. They are also given the option of having me review the images for possible biopsy. More than half of my referrals come from surgeons. Some of my referring surgeons are so busy that they will not see a patient in their office until I have completed my biopsy workup and they have pathology results. Most of the surgeons whom I work with will schedule appointments with their patients after I perform the biopsies so that they can deliver the results to their patients in person and discuss any follow-up or surgical options. I also have become a source of referrals for the surgeons. If a patient has not yet seen a surgeon and has a positive biopsy result requiring surgery I will deliver those results to the patient. I will consult their referring physician to see if they have a surgeon of choice. If they do not, I will then offer recommendations to the patient from a list of several surgeons whom I work with on a regular basis. Once the patient has made their choice, I will contact the surgeon to discuss the case. The surgeons often prefer this because the workup and biopsy are complete, the patients have a histologic diagnosis requiring surgery, and often tumor marker analysis is complete to guide postsurgical care.

Breast interventions can be performed safely in an office setting with the use of only local anesthesia. A model for cancer care is in place with increasing participation by the interventional radiologist. Working with surgeons, oncologists, radiation oncologists, and others who specialize in oncology, the interventional radiologist can provide services such as image-guided biopsy and drainage, vascular access, and embolization and ablation therapy to improve the care of the cancer patient. This comprehensive service should also be offered to breast cancer patients. Based on the extent of tumor and biopsy results, thermal ablation therapy may become the first option for patients with localized breast cancer. Following breast ablation, the patient may require placement of a balloon catheter for high-dose brachytherapy. The patient with breast cancer may require placement of long-term venous access for administration of chemotherapy. All of these services can be provided by interventional radiologists. Today, percutaneous cryoablation is a viable treatment option for patients with benign fibroadenomas who desire a nonsurgical option.

The future of the oncology service line for interventional radiology is bright. The opportunity to participate in the research and development of new procedures and devices aimed at treating diseases of the breast allows for validation of a specialty's ability to participate in the care of these patients. We as interventional radiologists should work with our colleagues in surgery, oncology, and diagnostic radiology in breast cancer care research. Caring for women with diseases of the breast should become part of the interventional radiology fellowship curriculum. Training programs should work with women's imaging departments at academic centers to incorporate breast interventions and breast intervention research into the core curriculum of interventional radiology.

In the United States, the lifetime risk of developing breast cancer for women is 13%. Breast cancer is the most common cancer among women; it is second only to lung cancer in deaths among women in the United States.[41] According to statistics provided by the American Cancer Society, in 2007 the estimated number of newly diagnosed breast cancers will be 182,460 not including an additional 67,770 cases of ductal carcinoma in situ.[42] It is very important that women be offered the best opportunity for the diagnosis and treatment of breast cancer. It is also very important that we in the field of medicine continue our efforts at improving the way we treat cancer. We must continue to educate our colleagues and ourselves regarding new and innovative ways to diagnose and treat diseases of the breast. We must also participate in research to advance the field of breast interventions. This specialty is rapidly growing and developing with each improvement in technology. The promise of breast digital tomosynthesis offers the opportunity to make new strides in the diagnosis and treatment of breast cancer. If we choose not to participate, we are doing a disservice to our specialty and our patients. The most important reason for our participation in the field of breast interventions is to improve the overall quality of care for women.

References

1. Society of Interventional Radiology. Interventional radiologists are.... Fairfax, VA: Society of Interventional Radiology; 2007. Available at: http://sirweb.org/index.shtml. Accessed June 26, 2007
2. Sickles EA. Periodic mammographic follow-up of probably benign lesions result of 3,184 consecutive cases. Radiology 1991;179:463–468
3. Silverstein MJ, Lagios MD, Recht A, et al. Image-detected breast cancer: state of the art diagnosis and treatment. International Breast Cancer Consensus Conference II. J Am Coll Surg 2005;201:586–597
4. Diebold T, Jacobi V, Krapfl EV, et al. The role of stereotactic 11g vacuum biopsy for clarification of BI-RADS trade mark IV findings in mammography. Fortschr Rontg 2003;175:489–494
5. Nurko J, Edwards MJ. Image-guided breast surgery. Am J Surg 2005;190:221–227
6. Uematsu T, Kasami M, Uchida Y, et al. Ultrasonographically guided 18-gauge automated core needle breast biopsy with post-fire needle position verification (PNPV). Breast Cancer 2007;14:219–228
7. Youk JH, Kim EK, Kim MJ, et al. Missed breast cancers at US-guided core needle biopsy: how to reduce them. Radiographics 2007;27:79–94
8. Margenthaler JA, Duke D, Monsees BS, et al. Correlation between core biopsy and excisional biopsy in breast high-risk lesions. Am J Surg 2006;192:534–537
9. Shulman SG, March DE. Ultrasound-guided breast interventions: accuracy of biopsy techniques and applications in patient management. Semin Ultrasound CT MR 2006;27:298–307
10. Tomkovich KR. Advanced breast interventions. Paper presented at: Western Angio and Interventional Society Annual Meeting; September 17–22, 2006; Kona, Hawaii
11. Tomkovich KR. Breast interventions: a primer for interventional radiologists. Tech Vasc Interv Radiol 2006;9:30–35
12. Joshi M, Duva-Frissora A, Padmanabhan R, et al. Atypical ductal hyperplasia in stereotactic breast biopsies: enhanced accuracy of diagnosis with the mammotome. Breast J 2001;7:207–213
13. Won B, Reynolds HE, Lazaridis CL, Jackson VP. Stereotactic biopsy of ductal carcinoma in-situ of the breast using an 11-gauge vacuum-assisted device: persistent underestimation of disease. AJR Am J Roentgenol 1999;173:227–229
14. Meloni GB, Dessole S, Becchere MP, et al. Ultrasound-guided mammotome vacuum biopsy for the diagnosis of impalpable breast lesions. Ultrasound Obstet Gynecol 2001;18:520–524
15. Iwuagwu O, Drew P. Vacuum-assisted biopsy device: diagnostic and therapeutic applications in breast surgery. Breast 2004;13:483–487
16. Iwuagwu OC, Calvey TA, Ilsley D, Drew P. Ultrasound guided minimally invasive breast surgery (UMIBS): a superior technique for gynecomastia. Ann Plast Surg 2004;52:131–133
17. Iwuagwu OC, Drew PJ. Ultrasound guided minimally invasive surgery for fibroadenomas. Arch Surg 2004;139:564
18. Fine RE, Boyd BA, Whitworth PW, et al. Percutaneous removal of benign breast masses using a vacuum-assisted hand-held device with ultrasound guidance. Am J Surg 2002;184:332–336
19. Fornage BD, Sneige N, Ross MI, et al. Small (≤ 2-cm) breast cancer treated with US-guided radiofrequency ablation: feasibility study. Radiology 2004;231:215–224
20. Huston TL, Simmons RM. Ablative therapies for the treatment of malignant diseases of the breast. Am J Surg 2005;189:694–701
21. Bland KL, Gass J, Klimberg VS. Radiofrequency, cryoablation and other modalities for breast cancer ablation. Surg Clin North Am 2007;87:539–550
22. Burak WE, Agnese DM, Povoski SP, et al. Radiofrequency ablation of invasive breast carcinoma followed by delayed surgical excision. Cancer 2003;98:1369–1376
23. Hayashi AH, Silver SF, van der Westhuizen NG, et al. Treatment of invasive breast carcinoma with ultrasound-guided radiofrequency ablation. Am J Surg 2003;185:429–435
24. Izzo F, Thomas R, Delrio P, et al. Radiofrequency ablation in patients with primary breast carcinoma: a pilot study in 2 patients. Cancer 2001;92:2036–2044
25. Oura S, Tamaki T, Hirai I, et al. Radiofrequency ablation therapy in patients with breast cancers two centimeters or less in size. Breast Cancer 2007;14:48–54
26. Stocks LH, Chang HR, Kaufman CS, et al. Pilot study of minimally invasive ultrasound-guided cryoablation in breast cancer. Paper presented at: the American Society of Breast Surgeons Meeting; April 24–28, 2002; Boston, MA

27. Pfleiderer SO, Freesmeyer MG, Marx C, et al. Cryotherapy of breast cancer under ultrasound-guidance: initial results and limitations. Eur Radiol 2002;12:3009–3014
28. Sabel MS, Kaufman CS, Whitworth PW, et al. Cryoablation of early stage breast cancer: work in progress report of a multi-institutional trial. Ann Surg Oncol 2004;11:542–549
29. Daniel BL. Intraprocedural magnetic resonance imaging-guided interventions in the breast. Top Magn Reson Imaging 2000;11:184–190
30. Mumtaz H, Hall-Craggs MA, Wotherspoon A, et al. Laser therapy for breast cancer: MR imaging and histopathologic correlation. Radiology 1996;200:651–658
31. Tafra L, Smith SJ, Woodward JE, et al. Pilot trial of cryoprobe-assisted breast-conserving surgery for small ultrasound-visible cancers. Ann Surg Oncol 2003;10:1018–1024
32. Gianfelice D, Khiat A, Amara M, et al. MR imaging-guided focused US ablation of breast cancer: histopathologic assessment of effectiveness – initial experience. Radiology 2003;227:849–855
33. Huber PE, Jenne JW, Rastert R, et al. A new noninvasive approach in breast cancer therapy using magnetic resonance imaging-guidance focused ultrasound surgery. Cancer Res 2001;61:8441–8447
34. Wu F, Wang ZB, Cao YD, et al. A randomized clinical trial of high-intensity focused ultrasound ablation for the treatment of patients with localized breast cancer. Br J Cancer 2003;89:2227–2233
35. Isaacs JH. Benign neoplasms. In: Marchant DJ, ed. Breast Disease. Philadelphia: WB Saunders; 1997:66–67
36. Kaufman CS, Littrup PJ, Freeman-Gibb LA, et al. Office-based cryoablation of breast fibroadenomas with long-term follow-up. Breast J 2005;11:344–350
37. Nurko J, Mabry CD, Whitworth P, et al. Interim results from the fibroadenoma cryoablation treatment registry. Am J Surg 2005;190:647–652
38. Niehoff P, Ballardini B, Polgar C, et al. Early European experience with the MammoSite radiation therapy system for partial breast brachytherapy following breast conservation operation in low-risk breast cancer. Breast 2006;15:319–325
39. Harper JL, Jenrette JM, Vanek KN, et al. Acute complications of MammoSite brachytherapy: a single institution's initial clinical experience. Int J Radiat Oncol Biol Phys 2005;61:169–174
40. American College of Radiology. Stereotactic breast biopsy. Reston, VA: American College of Radiology; 2007. Available at: http://acr.org/accreditation/stereotactic.aspx. Accessed July 7, 2007
41. Society of Interventional Radiology. Minimally invasive treatments for breast cancer. Reston, VA: American College of Radiology; 2007. Available at: http://sirweb.org/patPub/BreastCancerMain.shtml. Accessed
42. American Cancer Society, Inc. Cancer facts and figures 2008. Altanta, GA: American Cancer Society, Inc.; 2008. Available at: http://cancer.org. Accessed January 20, 2009

Index

Note: Page numbers followed by *f* and *t* indicate figures and tables, respectively.

A

B

C

D

E

F

G

H

I

J

K

L

M

N

O

P

R

U

V

W

Z